Advance Praise for *Bringing Psychotherapy to the Underserved*

"Too many societal groups suffer from a lack of access to adequate mental health services. Too often, practitioners and policy makers fail to recognize the nature and scope of service needs, or lack awareness of what they might do to help address the problem. This book provides an excellent guide to identifying and assisting in addressing and resolving such difficulties. A broad range of chapters by experts in systemic, discriminatory, geographical, migratory, and age-related barriers to quality mental health care offer details and guidance. I highly recommend this volume to those concerned about assisting underserved diverse populations."

—**Gerald P. Koocher**, PhD, ABPP, Former President, American Psychological Association (2006), Provost, Quincy College

"Louis Pasteur famously said that one should not ask those who suffer what is their country or what is their religion. Drs. Zimmerman, Barnett, and Campbell emphatically endorse this commitment to treating effectively all who suffer from mental disorders regardless of their socioeconomic status, ethnic/racial identity, sexual orientation, geographic location, religious affiliation, chronological age, national origin, and the like. A brilliant book that helps us see the 'invisible' and treat the 'underserved' among us. You will not read a more important mental health book than this!"

—**John C. Norcross**, PhD, ABPP, Distinguished Professor of Psychology, University of Scranton

"I have spent my professional life working for the betterment of marginalized, disenfranchised, and underserved people. This book speaks to the heart of my values and purpose. Veterans, sexual minorities, people living in poverty, rural, international, ethnic and racial minorities, and others are given voice. Readers become aware of barriers and challenges and importantly effective treatment plans tailored to these populations. I am thrilled that this book captures the spirit and resilience of these people and gives them visibility."

—**Rosie Phillips Davis,** PhD, ABPP, Professor, Counseling, Educational Psychology & Research, The University of Memphis

Bringing Psychotherapy to the Underserved

Challenges and Strategies

Edited by
JEFFREY ZIMMERMAN, JEFFREY E. BARNETT,
AND LINDA F. CAMPBELL

OXFORD
UNIVERSITY PRESS

OXFORD
UNIVERSITY PRESS

Oxford University Press is a department of the University of Oxford. It furthers the University's objective of excellence in research, scholarship, and education by publishing worldwide. Oxford is a registered trade mark of Oxford University Press in the UK and certain other countries.

Published in the United States of America by Oxford University Press
198 Madison Avenue, New York, NY 10016, United States of America.

Library of Congress Cataloging-in-Publication Data
Names: Zimmerman, Jeffrey, editor. | Barnett, Jeffrey E., editor. |
Campbell, Linda F., 1947– editor.
Title: Bringing psychotherapy to the underserved : challenges and strategies /
edited by Jeffrey Zimmerman, Jeffrey E. Barnett, Linda F. Campbell.
Description: New York : Oxford University Press, [2020] |
Includes bibliographical references and index.
Identifiers: LCCN 2019031788 (print) | LCCN 2019031789 (ebook) |
ISBN 9780190912727 (pbk) | ISBN 9780190912741 (epub) |
ISBN 9780190912734 (updf) | ISBN 9780190912758 (online)
Subjects: LCSH: Cultural psychiatry. | Psychotherapy—Cross-cultural studies. |
Mental illness—Social aspects—Cross-cultural studies. |
Minorities—Mental health services. | Medically underserved areas.
Classification: LCC RC455.4.E8 B76 2020 (print) | LCC RC455.4.E8 (ebook) |
DDC 616.89/14—dc23
LC record available at https://lccn.loc.gov/2019031788
LC ebook record available at https://lccn.loc.gov/2019031789

1 3 5 7 9 8 6 4 2

Printed by Marquis, Canada

This book is dedicated to all those who are underserved, and to those who dedicate themselves to providing desperately needed psychotherapeutic services with compassion and grace.

Contents

Acknowledgments

The concept for this book follows an initiative Jeff Zimmerman began during his 2017 presidential year for the Society for the Advancement of Psychotherapy, Division 29, American Psychological Association. One of the central initiatives was to increase the Society's awareness and participation in activities that address the needs of the underserved. The concept of addressing this in written form was formed in discussion with our editor, Sarah Harrington (Oxford University Press), who simply asked, "Have you thought about writing about this important initiative?" Thank you, Sarah, for providing us the opportunity to try to make a difference to the underserved.

We also want to thank our contributors, who have been dedicated and hard-working. Their diversity in experience and approach serves to make this book rich in ideas across so many different areas.

We have also learned, and continue to learn, from the underserved with whom we work. Thank you for teaching us how to be more responsive to your needs.

And, thank you to our spouses, Lauren Behrman, Stephanie Barnett, and Alan Campbell, who have supported us in so many ways through the years, giving us the encouragement to go beyond our self-imposed boundaries as we strive to make a difference.

Jeffrey Zimmerman, Ph.D., ABPP
Jeffrey E. Barnett, Psy.D., ABPP
Linda F. Campbell, Ph.D.

About the Editors

Jeffrey Zimmerman, Ph.D., ABPP, Jeff has worked with the underserved since the 1970s during his training in rural Mississippi and then later in West Virginia and Connecticut. More recently, he is doing more international work and seeing the need for psychotherapy to be made available in a culturally sensitive way throughout many parts of the world. At present, Jeff works in New York providing psychotherapy, training, and consultation. He strongly believes that other cultures have lots to teach us about how to provide psychotherapeutic services in general, and especially to the underserved, and looks forward to the evolution of this important process.

Jeffrey E. Barnett, Psy.D., ABPP, Jeff is a licensed psychologist as well as professor of psychology and associate dean for the social sciences and graduate programs at Loyola University Maryland. He is actively engaged in the education and training of graduate students and practicing mental health professionals to promote more ethical and effective practice with all populations in need. Consistent with the mission of Loyola University Maryland, he has focused his efforts on bringing quality mental health services to those who typically experience barriers to needed care. As a former Army psychologist, he has worked to ensure that all military service members, their families, and veterans have access to needed mental health services that are provided in a timely, sensitive, and effective manner.

Linda F. Campbell, Ph.D., Linda is a professor in the Counseling and Human Development Department at the University of Georgia and is director of the Center for Counseling, which is the training clinic for the counseling psychology doctoral program. Her area of expertise is ethics; however, more recently she has focused on training doctoral students to work with people living in poverty and marginalized populations. She is a native of West Virginia and has had a longstanding commitment to working with underserved populations through her clinic and through community sites where she has developed behavioral health training opportunities for students. Her work represents the belief that from those to whom much is given, much is expected.

Contributors

Jeffrey E. Barnett, PsyD, ABPP
Department of Psychology
Loyola College of Arts and Sciences
Loyola University Maryland

Marcella A. Beaumont, MA
Division of Counseling and Educational Psychology
University of Missouri-Kansas City

Jonathan M. Campbell, PhD
Department of Educational, School, and Counseling Psychology
University of Kentucky

Linda F. Campbell, PhD
Department of Counseling and Human Development Services
University of Georgia

Alec Cecil, EdD
Psychologist and Volunteer in Disaster Mental Health
American Red Cross

Tracy J. Cohn, PhD
Licensed Clinical Psychologist
Radford University
Associate Professor, Psychology
Radford University

Changming Duan, PhD, ABPP
Department of Educational Psychology
University of Kansas

Héctor Fernández-Álvarez, PhD
Fundación Aigle

Charles Gaba, BS
ACASignups.net

Rodney Goodyear, PhD
Center for Advanced Professional Education, School of Education
University of Redlands

Maria del Pilar Grazioso, PhD
Proyecto Aiglé Guatemala and Universidad del Valle de Guatemala

Douglas C. Haldeman, PhD
College of Psychology
John F. Kennedy University

Gordon I. Herz, PhD
Forward Psychology Group, LLC,
Independent Practice

Jessica Horine, BA
Division of Counseling and Educational Psychology
University of Missouri-Kansas City

K. C. Kalmbach, PhD
Texas A&M University—San Antonio,
College of Arts & Sciences,
Department of Science and Mathematics (Psychology)

Diana Kirszman, PhD
Fundación Aigle

Meri Lubina, MA
Proyecto Aiglé Guatemala
and Universidad
del Valle de Guatemala

Gina Magyar-Russell, PhD
Department of Pastoral Counseling
Loyola University Maryland

Bruna Martins, PhD
Department of Psychological and Brain Sciences
University of Massachusetts Amherst

Hamid Mirsalimi, PhD, ABPP
Department of Psychiatry and Behavioral Sciences
Emory University

Aurora Molitoris, MPH, MA
Department of Psychology
University of Missouri-Kansas City

Bret A. Moore, PsyD, ABPP
Warrior Resiliency Program-San Antonio

Johanna E. Nilsson, PhD
Department of Psychology
University of Missouri-Kansas City

Angela Scarpa, PhD
Department of Psychology
Autism Clinic & Center for Autism Research
Virginia Tech

Emily M. Selby-Nelson, PsyD
Cabin Creek Health Systems

Ric G. Steele, PhD, ABPP
Clinical Child Psychology Program
University of Kansas

Sally Stratmann, BA
Department of Psychology
University of Missouri-Kansas City

Pei-Chun Tsai, PhD
Department of Psychology
Radford University

Susan Krauss Whitbourne, PhD, ABPP
Department of Psychological and Brain Sciences
University of Massachusetts Amherst

Elizabeth Nutt Williams, PhD
Professor of Psychology
St. Mary's College of Maryland

Introduction

Underserved communities exist throughout the United States and the rest of the world. The Health Resources and Services Administration (2017) identifies geographic areas across the nation as having a "shortage designation" based on too few health and mental health professionals to meet the needs of the population. At present, over 4,000 areas across the United States have received this designation, affecting over 106 million people (Kaiser Family Foundation, 2017). While only 9% of counties (284 counties) in the United States have no behavioral health providers (psychologists, counselors, social workers, psychiatrists, and psychiatric nurse practitioners), 17% of rural counties (221 counties) have no behavioral health providers (Larson, Patterson, Garberson, & Andrilla, 2016). Further, Thomas, Ellis, Konrad, Holzer, and Morrissey (2009) found that over 77% of all counties had a severe shortage of mental health providers. Thus, significant shortages of mental health providers exist throughout the nation, resulting in numerous underserved communities where residents do not have access to needed mental health treatment services.

In addition to the absence of mental health professionals in many geographic areas, a range of additional factors exist that result in a lack of access to needed mental health care for many individuals. In addition to shortages of mental health professionals, Mental Health America (2017) identifies a number of barriers many individuals face that limit their ability to access needed care. These include lack of insurance or inadequate insurance and insufficient finances to cover costs such as co-pays and uncovered treatments, and when mental health professionals do not participate in their insurance. These factors contribute to the fact that 20.3% of adults in the United States are unable to obtain needed mental health treatment services (Mental Health America, 2017).

There is also a wide range of groups of individuals whose mental health needs often go unmet. Such groups include LGBTQ individuals, members of racial and ethnic minorities, religious individuals, the elderly, individuals with developmental and intellectual disabilities, Native Americans, trauma survivors, and refugees and members of immigrant communities. There may be a number of barriers to access to needed mental health services for these individuals, such as a paucity of mental health professionals with the clinical competence needed to work with these populations (e.g., lack of knowledge about these groups, lack of experience or interest in working with them). Language and cultural differences may also create barriers to access to needed mental health services.

The World Health Organization World Mental Health Survey Consortium (2004) has estimated that between 35.5% and 50.3% of individuals in developed countries and between 76.3% and 85.4% of individuals in less developed countries with mental health difficulties that meet diagnostic criteria as set forth in the American Psychiatric Association's *Diagnostic and Statistical Manual of Mental Disorders* do not have access to needed treatment. This equates to over 450 million people worldwide with unmet mental health treatment needs (Leung et al., 2009). Additionally, there may be many areas around the world where natural and other disasters occur that are in remote locales and/or the disaster makes it difficult for mental health professionals to access these areas, leaving urgent mental health needs unmet (Marsella & Pedersen, 2004).

This book is designed to help mental health professionals who provide psychotherapy increase their awareness of the key issues related to many different cohorts of underserved peoples. We focus on many underserved communities, in their many different forms, both within and outside the United States. We have attempted to provide in one volume a wide-ranging discussion of the issues of many underserved peoples and are so pleased to bring you chapters written by experts in their respective fields, offering their thoughts and very practical advice.

We have divided the book into five sections. Section 1 addresses systemic factors and the underserved. These include issues related to the health system, care of military members and veterans, and natural and manmade disasters. Section 2 addresses issues related to discrimination against people due to their ethnic status, economic disadvantages, sexual orientation, and religion. Section 3 focuses on people who are in transition and due to where they are located. This includes civilians and refugees of war, immigrants, those in rural locations, and people in underserved countries. For example, we highlight a program in Latin America. Section 4 addresses people who are often overlooked as being underserved, including children, older adults, and those with intellectual and developmental disabilities.

Each of these chapters follows the same format to bring you a more consistent reading experience. The authors begin by discussing the scope and offer a description of the area they are addressing. They then discuss barriers to service delivery, how to create or improve cultural competence, and effective strategies and empirically supported treatments. They conclude by discussing future steps.

The last section addresses other challenges and focuses on the more general areas of ethics and research. The ethics chapter addresses overarching considerations when a mental health professional provides services (e.g., scope of practice, competence, multicultural competence, tele-mental health, compassion fatigue). The final chapter explores current research strategies, looks at less often employed methodologies in the area of mental health disparities, and speaks to what is still needed in order to develop new and effective treatment models that are accessible from geographic, language, and cultural perspectives.

Overall, whether you read this book cover to cover or pick particular chapters that are of interest, we hope it is a valuable resource for you as you strive to approach underserved communities in socially responsible, culturally sensitive, ethical, and effective ways.

Jeffrey Zimmerman
Jeffrey E. Barnett
Linda F. Campbell

References

Health Resources & Services Administration. (2017). Mental health in America—Access to care data. Retrieved from http://www.mentalhealthamerica.net/issues/mental-health-america-access-care-data

Kaiser Family Foundation. (2017). Mental health care health professional shortage area (HPSAs). Retrieved from http://www.kff.org/state-category/providers-service-use/health- professional-shortage-areas/

Larson, E. H., Patterson, D. G., Garberson, L. A., & Andrilla, C. H. A. (2016). Supply and distribution of the behavioral health workforce in rural America. Data Brief #160. Seattle, WA: WWAMI Rural Health Research Center, University of Washington. Retrieved from http://depts.washington.edu/fammed/rhrc/wp-content/uploads/sites/4/2016/09/RHRC_DB160_Larson.pdf

Leung, S.-M. A., Clawson, T., Norsworthy, K. L., Tena, A., Szilagyi, A., & Rogers, J. (2009). Internationalization of the counseling profession. In L. H. Gerstein, P. P. Heppner, S. Aegisdottir, S.-M. A. Leung, & K. L. Norsworthy (Eds.), *International handbook of cross-cultural counseling* (pp. 111–127). Los Angeles, CA: Sage.

Marsella, A. J., & Pedersen, P. B. (2004). Internationalizing the counseling psychology curriculum: Toward new values, competencies, and directions. *Counselling Psychology Quarterly, 17*(4), 413–423.

Mental Health America. (2017). Mental health in America—Access to care data. Retrieved from http://www.mentalhealthamerica.net/issues/mental-health-america-access-care-data

Thomas, K. C., Ellis, A. R., Konrad, T. R., Holzer, C. E., & Morrissey, J. P. (2009). County-level estimates of mental health professional shortage in the United States. *Psychiatric Services, 60*(10), 1323–1328.

World Health Organization World Mental Health Survey Consortium. (2004). Prevalence, severity, and unmet need for treatment of mental disorders in the World Health Organization World Mental Health Surveys. *Journal of the American Medical Association, 291*(21), 2581–2590.

SECTION 1

UNDERSERVED BY SYSTEMIC FACTORS

1

Health Systems Issues and the Underserved

Gordon I. Herz and Charles Gaba

A number of factors endemic to the U.S. health system contribute to barriers to meeting the mental health needs of the underserved. Important variables include the economic barrier of continued gaps in affordable third-party coverage for care, perceived and actual costs of care, insufficient numbers of clinicians relative to the number of individuals in need of mental health services, and training and workforce gaps to meet specific needs (e.g., culture, disability, geographic) of the population. Approaches being developed to counter the limited-access problem include increasing economic support for coverage of services, expanding the workforce, incorporating ethics and cultural competence in clinical training, educating consumers about real costs of care, and developing volunteer and charitable models of service provision. Future developments to decrease health system barriers are likely to include technological advances.

The Scope and Description of the Problem

Mental health needs continue to rise in the face of limited options for services. Ironically, the awareness and destigmatization of mental health needs, primary and specialty care referral, self-initiated pursuit of services, and integration of mind–body, whole-person care reflect increased demand for mental health services. The National Institute of Mental Health (NIMH, 2017a) reports that nearly 20% of adults in the United States are living with a mental illness but only half of them receive needed treatment. The NIMH (2017a) further reports that an estimated 4.2% of U.S. adults (~10.4 million people) are living with a serious mental illness that results in functional impairment serious enough to interfere with major life activities. Variability in these findings is reported, with mental illness being found more frequently in women, younger adults, American Indians/Alaska Natives, and those reporting two or more races. These variations in the prevalence of serious mental illness throughout the population likely has implications for those who are underserved relative to those with potentially adequate access, particularly if there is an intersection with economic resources (NIMH, 2017a).

Although underserved groups are often also marginalized, socioeconomic, geographic, workplace, and other factors contribute to the status of underserved. One example of the underserved illustrated here is the college student population, and an example of both marginalized and underserved is the older adult population. These two groups exemplify the impact of inadequate health care provision in our current system.

The College Student Population

Broad concerns about the availability of mental health services for students are becoming apparent, if not reaching "crisis" proportions. Anxiety and depression are the most common clinician-assessed presenting problems in large samples of college counseling centers, according to the Center for Collegiate Mental Health (CCMH)'s 2017 report (CCMH, 2018). Suicidal ideation and threat of harm to self increased for the seventh consecutive year among students requesting treatment, commensurate with a 28% increase in "rapid access" services and an 8% decrease in routine treatment at college and university health services (CCMH, 2018). College and university health services utilization increased by five to six times the rate of institutional enrollment during the preceding five years, primarily associated with "threat to self" characteristics (CCMH, 2018).

In 2016, the prevalence of major depression was highest among 18- to 25-year-olds, at 10.9% (NIMH, 2017b). Average undergraduate enrollment among 1,275 institutions was 6,265 in 2016, with the 10 highest undergraduate enrollments averaging nearly 45,000 (Powell, 2017). If 10% of undergraduates on a campus of 45,000 experience an episode of major depression during an academic year, 4,500 students could be in need of treatment for this condition alone. With students receiving an average of 4.5 sessions each, there could be a potential need in excess of 20,000 visits on a large campus setting for students, just for major depression. The crisis in mental health needs on campuses is well recognized (Novotney, 2014; Taylor, 2006).

Exacerbating the college student need for mental health services is the third-party payor factor. Many students are retained on their parents' insurance policies until age 26 under the current Affordable Care Act. Students often do not want their parents to know of their health service treatment at school. Further, university student insurance is designed to provide basic health care needs and may not be sufficient for the length of treatment needed and may not be applicable for given diagnoses. Given these increasing needs, college and university health services need to continually recalibrate their parameters for provision of care. That is, short-term psychotherapy for diagnoses that can be improved in limited sessions are prioritized, resulting in other cases being referred out—which reintroduces the cost factor for college students with limited means.

Older Adults

A second example of mental health care needs for a population that is both marginalized and underserved is older adults. This group is projected to reach 16% of the U.S. population by 2020 (Department of Economic and Social Affairs, United Nations, 2010), or nearly 54 million people (Statista, 2017). Fifteen percent of older adults in the United States are diagnosed with a personality disorder and approximately 11% experience an anxiety disorder. Approximately 7% experienced a mood disorder and 4% experienced substance use disorder in the year prior to this study (Reynolds, Pietrzak, El-Gabalawy, Mackenzie, & Sareen, 2015). About 15% of the U.S. population is covered under Medicare (not all enrollees qualify based on age alone), with the most recent figures showing an enrollment of 59.7 million individuals as of August 2018 (Centers for Medicare and Medicaid Services [CMS]/Office of Enterprise Data & Analytics, 2018a) and a projected enrollment of 64 million in 2020 (AARP Public Policy Institute, 2012). Most of the psychotherapy provided to Medicare beneficiaries is provided by clinical psychologists (~48% of the almost 10 million sessions provided in 2016) and licensed clinical social workers (~45%), with psychiatrists providing slightly less than 6% and other health specialties about 2% (Herz, 2018). In 2016, there were 98,559 of these clinicians participating in Medicare (41,347 licensed clinical social workers, 29,062 psychologists, and 28,150 psychiatrists). With just under 57 million enrollees in Medicare in 2016, these data project a ratio of about 578 enrollees in Medicare to one mental health specialist available. This ratio does not suggest mental health needs for all enrollees but rather indicates the parameters of potential provision given the number of enrollees. Consider these data in the context of the mental health needs of older adults, the number of visits typically needed for effective treatment, and the fact that the older adult population will only be increasing, and one begins to grasp the extent to which older adults currently are and will in the future be underserved, and the scope of this challenge. The older population and mental health services are discussed in greater depth in Chapter 13.

These two groups illustrate a greater systemic need for mental health services across the general population. Factors inherent in the growing scope of mental health needs include the following:

- Individuals "fall through the cracks" of our health system in that health care systems formulate parameters based on income, health status, age, disabilities, and other metrics that determine who is included in the service plan. An often-heard example is one of making just too much money or not making enough to qualify for a specific plan.
- The problem of health disparities cuts across many individual classifications, with education, socioeconomic class, and income contributing to individuals being left out of health systems. Advocacy for equal treatment, understanding inclusion and exclusion in one's plan, knowledge of plans and specific benefits, access to information about costs and payment plans, and seeking consultation when options are unclear might now be familiar to those accustomed to being left out of health systems.
- Mental health treatment is still stigmatized among cultures, within families, and resulting from personal beliefs. Ironically, mental health is portrayed more frequently in the media, is featured in health programming, and in some areas carries positive attributes. The fact remains that mental health treatment is still not as concretely understood as treatment for diabetes, high blood pressure, or other physical health treatments; therefore, clients may be uncertain about what will occur in treatment and what it will mean to them.
- Literacy disparities are often overlooked, even though reading levels, comprehension, and the ability to ask pertinent questions are significant factors in access to mental health care. Prospective clients may be embarrassed about being in a situation in which they don't know what to say, don't understand what is being said, or may end up looking foolish, and this prevents them from coming forward for help. They may fear they will be declared "crazy" or that the mental health professional will declare them unfit or unstable and will interfere with their lives. Even though most individuals who have knowledge about health systems would know these fears are unfounded, a segment of the population does not.

For-profit health care systems face rising costs and the pressure to increase profit margins. And because our health care system is predominantly for profit, the factors involved in mental health care are always in a state of tension between care and cost. Even though insurance companies develop algorithms and standards of treatment for mental disorder diagnoses, treatment plans are still a long way from consensual clinical practice guidelines, with some exceptions (e.g., post-traumatic stress disorder, depression). Predominantly, physical medicine has developed guidelines and standards of practice that are questioned by very few. Allowance for mental health treatment can reside in the hands of sometimes-capricious administrators. The wide variety of plans, with varying premiums, co-pays, lifetime and annual caps, and other parameters, can challenge the health literacy of even those who are highly educated. The cost of health care is prohibitive for many individuals. Even if the premiums are affordable (or paid by one's employer), a high deductible could exclude payment for all costs except life-threatening events. The precarious state of health care and costs in the United States positions reasonable levels of coverage out of reach for many individuals.

Barriers to Service Delivery

Throughout the history of health care delivery in the United States, challenges to access have been variable but always present. The high cost of health care, notwithstanding periodic attempts to resolve the situation, has persisted. Technology and new market products signal significant increases in cost for insurance companies, resulting in rising costs for the consumer. Changing policy positions at the state and federal level continue to be catalysts in fluctuating criteria for benefits. The health care workforce, particularly in the mental health field, continues to be variable, with changing scope of practice, level of skills, and particularly cultural competence to serve the diverse patient population in need.

Economic Barriers

When the Patient Protection and Affordable Care Act (ACA) was signed into law in 2010, nearly 18% of the nonelderly population in the United States was uninsured, or about 46.5 million individuals (Kaiser Family Foundation [KFF], 2018). Their choices were either to pay full price for all medical treatment if they could afford it, to obtain care in the emergency department, or to forgo care. The ACA was an effort to resolve, or at least mitigate, overall coverage and other issues. Goals included (a) expanding health care coverage to as many people as possible; (b) helping to make that coverage as comprehensive as possible; (c) making health care as affordable as possible in the process; and (d) eliminating the worst abuses being carried out by insurance carriers. Some of these goals have been achieved, some have not; some have failed due to poor design and/or implementation, some due to subsequent alterations in the law; and some are still in "too soon to tell" status. One potentially telling measure is that, by early 2018, about

12.5% of nonelderly adults were uninsured (Keith, 2018), down from 18% before the ACA's implementation.

Even though these goals are certainly meritorious and have resulted in more individuals having some coverage for health care, significant problems remain, some of which were not resolved by the ACA and some of which were created by the ACA. Some state legislatures have chosen not to accept the Medicaid expansion, thereby resulting in higher costs for low-income individuals than if they lived in Medicaid expansion states. Part of the sustainability formula for the ACA was the requirement that all individuals buy insurance. In some states the cost of simply paying the premiums was unaffordable, resulting in fines that also were unaffordable. Subsequently, the requirement to buy insurance was struck down by the courts, thereby returning to a larger segment of the population being without health insurance.

Political and Policy Barriers

Approximately 27.4 million nonelderly Americans remain uninsured (KFF, 2018). While 37 states (including Washington, DC) have expanded Medicaid under the ACA, 14 states have not done so, including two of the largest in the country: Texas and Florida (KFF, 2019b). Low-income Americans in these states may have few affordable health care options. In 2017, nearly 40% of the 22 million non-citizens residing in the United States were undocumented immigrants (KFF, 2019a). These 8.8 million persons would be ineligible for either Medicaid via ACA expansion or for private ACA exchange policies, even if they were willing and able to pay full price.

Another serious problem is network breadth, an issue that could be related to a systemic obstacle that will be further addressed—workforce limitations. More and more insurance carriers have been dropping preferred provider organization (PPO) plans in favor of increasingly narrow health maintenance organizations (HMOs; Henry, 2016). While the ACA does have minimum network size requirements (National Association of Insurance Commissioners, 2019), networks appear to be becoming more limited (Livingston, 2018).

As noted earlier, some of the ACA's problems to date have been inherent in its design or initial management; others may be due to efforts to alter the law at the federal or state level. Examples include the following:

- Curtailment in funding for ACA "navigators," individuals or organizations "trained to help consumers, small businesses and their employees find health care through the ACA marketplace" (Wisconsin Public Radio, 2018)

- Changes in ACA planned budgeting for insurance market "stabilization" programs such as the "risk corridors" that, after implementation of the ACA, were anticipated to increase premiums (Center on Budget and Policy Priorities, 2014) and increase efforts by health insurance companies to limit enrollment (Kaiser Health News, 2016)
- Executive branch orders implementing "policy . . . to seek the prompt repeal of the Patient Protection and Affordable Care Act" (Executive Office of the President, 2017)
- Discontinuance of cost sharing reduction (CSR) reimbursement payments to insurance carriers who were contractually owed the money, resulting in average premium increases in 2018 of about 14% (Gaba, 2018)
- Legislation enacted that "repeals the penalty for individuals who fail to maintain minimum essential health coverage as required by the Patient Protection and Affordable Care Act" (commonly referred to as the "individual mandate") (U.S. Congress, 2017). This legislation became effective January 1, 2019, and was estimated to potentially result in reduced enrollment by 2.8 to 13 million Americans, to potentially increase premiums for some insurance plans by 3% to 13% (Commonwealth Fund, 2018), and to potentially cause a significant number of healthier people enrolled in ACA-compliant policies to drop their coverage, further contributing to higher premiums for unsubsidized enrollees in 2019 and beyond (Congressional Budget Office, 2018).

Direct Costs to the Individual

The American Psychological Association (APA, 2018c) found the most frequently cited reason for not receiving services among those with a self-perceived unmet need was the inability to afford treatment, with 38% reporting this reason. Given the perceived cost barrier, how much does mental health treatment actually cost?

This is of course difficult to answer in that there are many variables that may influence cost, such as the reason for seeking treatment, whether medication or inpatient treatment is necessary, geographic variation, the type of provider, and others. But some information is available to the public (indeed, it is increasingly available), improving the transparency of potential costs and possibly dispelling myths. Online "lookup" resources are becoming available for consumers, though they tend to show considerable variability in estimates, possibly because these databases are still "stabilizing" in terms of the number and sources of charges submitted and paid that they incorporate.

For example, Healthcare Blue Book (https://www.healthcarebluebook.com/) estimates the "fair price"—defined as "the price that you should reasonably expect a medical service to cost if you shop for care" based on "actual amounts health plans have paid on claims"—for a 45-minute therapy visit to be $107 (range $79 to $207+) in a Midwest metropolitan area with a population of about 200,000. The "fair price" for the same therapy session length in Los Angeles is estimated to be $94. FairHealth Consumer (https://www.fairhealthconsumer.org/) estimates the price of a 45-minute therapy session to be $236 for an uninsured person in the same Midwest metropolitan area, and $225 in Los Angeles. In the large Medicare sample (Data.CMS.gov), the average charge actually submitted for more than 48,000 individuals for 45- to 50-minute sessions in 2016 by all providers billing Medicare was about $162. The Agency for Health Care Research and Quality (2018) reported the average out-of-pocket expense for a visit to a psychiatrist in 2016 was $88, more expensive than a typical visit to a pediatrician (average of $40) but less expensive than visits to other medical specialists, such as an obstetrician/gynecologist (average of $92) or a cardiologist (average of $108). Such information could quite reasonably be used to educate consumers to address the perceived inability to afford psychotherapy. This might also help clinicians and social service agencies to establish benchmarks to form a basis for possible fee reductions for those who are less able to afford treatment.

Costs of Mental Health Care Across the U.S. Health Care System

Another way to potentially grasp the cost challenges could be to understand the total burden of costs in the United States. In 2016, the Agency for Healthcare Research and Quality (AHRQ)/Medical Expenditure Panel Survey (MEPS) reported mental disorders to be the third most commonly cited reason for obtaining medical care (after hypertension and hyperlipidemia), with 39.2 million adults 18 and over—16.2% of the population—being treated for mental health conditions among conditions with at least 10% prevalence (Soni & Mitchell, 2016). It may be surprising, but the number and relative percentage of people treated for mental health conditions exceeded those treated for trauma-related conditions, diabetes, and heart conditions. However, the average expense per person for mental health conditions was $1,779, well below the per-person costs of treatment for heart conditions ($3,794), trauma-related disorders ($3,070), and diabetes ($2,565). Furthermore, about 27% of the per-person mental health expenses were for office-based/outpatient treatment, with the bulk of expenses (~45%) for prescriptions. About 16% of the costs were paid on an out-of-pocket basis, with the rest almost evenly divided among private insurance (26%), Medicare (27%), and Medicaid (23%) (about 7% "other"). Medicaid's highest proportion of expenditures is, in fact, treatment of mental disorders (23.3%), followed by hypertension (16.6%) and diabetes (16.3%) (Soni & Mitchell, 2016, p. 3). This of course suggests that some of those who may be underserved on the basis of financial need (i.e., receiving Medicaid) do have some potential for funded access to care.

Finally, at local, national, and global health levels, another way to ask the question and identify meaningful ways to limit cost obstacles to mental health care is to ask: What are the costs of *not* making care accessible? What are the cost savings generated by providing care?

Workforce Limitations

In the context of the sheer volume of people potentially seeking mental health services, and cost burdens at the national and individual level, the availability of mental health clinicians must be considered. Studies have estimated a shortage of approximately 45,000 psychiatrists for a U.S. population of 300 million (Carlat, 2010). A recent report to the Council on Social Work Education and National Workforce Initiative Steering Committee estimated that there were 352,000 state licensed social workers in the United States; the number of social workers for a population of 100,000 ranged from 80 to 572, a significant disparity across the country (George Washington University Health Workforce Institute, 2017). The APA reported that there were an estimated 106,000 licensed psychologists in the United States in 2016, also with considerable variability in geographic distribution, ranging from zero to 3,600 per county (APA, 2016). In this "first independent workforce analysis commissioned by the American Psychological Association," recent estimates were that supply is expected to be sufficient for the demand under "baseline . . . Affordable Care Act and . . . geographic equivalence" scenarios," but that supply fell short by 20,000 to 25,000 psychologists in 2015 in the context of racial/ethnic equivalence ratios. This metric is intended to project demand should the entire U.S. population have service utilization patterns similar to the insured non-Hispanic White population in metropolitan areas (APA, 2018a). The report also found that increasing the number of graduates by 10% and delaying retirement by two years would narrow but not eliminate the gap between supply and unmet need (APA, 2018a). The report estimated a national demand of about 101,000 additional full-time-equivalent psychologists by 2030, an increase of 6% above 2015 levels (APA, 2018b).

Gaps in Availability of Culturally and Diversity-Sensitive and Competent Clinicians

Gaps in mental health care have been noted for specific groups, such as immigrant children and families of diverse backgrounds who live in households in which English may not be the primary spoken language. For these individuals, the cultural context for mental illness is not based in Western perspectives and therefore is not aligned with the diagnoses and treatment practices of their clinicians (Alegria, Atkins, Farmer, Slaton, & Stelk, 2010). The Substance Abuse and Mental Health Services Administration (SAMHSA, 2018) reported that almost 40% of lesbian, gay, and bisexual (LGB) adults had a mental illness in the year preceding their 2015–2016 survey, but only about 27% received mental health treatment in that same period. Children and adults with physical or mental disabilities were historically institutionalized and continue to be marginalized. Individuals with disabilities continue to be victims of health disparities and evidence higher unmet health care needs, chronic diseases, and lower general health outcomes than other populations (Krahn, Walker, & Correa-De-Araujo, 2015). Other underserved populations include children, veterans, and rural populations (APA, 2018c).

Creating Cultural Competency

SAMHSA's description of cultural competence suggests that both individuals and organizations can be culturally competent (SAMHSA, 2016). Such an understanding implies that individual clinicians, organizational and agency settings, and our society more broadly can work toward cultural sensitivity in the process of providing mental health care. All levels of change toward competency should be enacted, from internalized clinician attitudes and behaviors, to agency structures, to societal levels of access and availability. In a sense, this provides something of a framework for considering how to proceed.

At the individual clinician level, this concept could include inculcating "lifelong learning" as a professional value and expectation, particularly in expanding one's knowledge in relation to particular groups. This may be promoted in professional ethics codes as well as in particular treatment guidelines, and especially in the interaction among these. For example, Principle E of the APA's Ethics Code (APA, 2017) urges psychologists to respect the rights, dignity, and welfare of all people, to protect those whose vulnerabilities may impair their decision making, and to eliminate their own biases and prejudices. One marginalized group that is particularly vulnerable to exploitation and maltreatment is older adults. Guideline 2 of the APA's "Guidelines for Psychological Practice with

Older Adults" encourages psychologists to be aware of their attitudes and beliefs about aging and to assess the potential impact of their biases on their diagnoses and treatment of older adults. Psychologists are urged to seek consultation or further education about these issues when indicated (APA, 2014). Such expectations are increasingly embedded in a range of professional educational standards and clinical practice guidelines.

Training in cultural competency has increasingly become a part of requirements promoted in health service psychology for licensing and in other legislative and regulatory contexts. Cultural competence in health care services has been elevated in importance by local, state, and federal governmental entities. The visibility and the negative impact of disparities in health and health care on the population have resulted in a growing call for mandatory cultural competence training (Graves, Like, Kelly, & Hohensee, 2007).

At agency and organizational levels, some aspects of promoting access to care for diverse populations have been mandated at federal and/or state levels, for example in language access in health care settings (Chen, Youdelman, & Brooks, 2007) or for persons who are hard of hearing (National Association of the Deaf, 2018).

Effective Strategies and Empirically-Supported Treatments

The ACA was instrumental in expanding available coverage for those potentially seeking mental health care. Furthermore, the ACA mandated coverage inclusion of mental health and substance use disorder services in policies sold in the United States. Before considering specific solutions to the barriers, a review of the impact of the ACA on systems and individuals is helpful.

Since the ACA went into effect, much of the gain in coverage has come via the ACA's "Medicaid expansion" provision, which raises the Medicaid eligibility income threshold from prior levels, which varied by state, up to 138% of the federal poverty level (around $16,600/year for a childless adult, or roughly $34,000/year for a family of four). As of this writing, 37 states (including Washington, DC) have expanded Medicaid under the ACA (KFF, 2019b), increasing the number of Americans for whom coverage could potentially become affordable.

Beyond the increased number of people who have gained health care coverage under the ACA, the scope of coverage has also improved dramatically. Since January 1, 2014, all major medical health care policies sold in the United States are required to cover 10 "essential health benefits," which include mental health and substance use disorder services and behavioral health treatment. The ACA also removed the maximum caps on annual and/or lifetime coverage in health care policies sold in both the individual and group markets, while adding maximum caps on out-of-pocket enrollee expenses, beyond which the insurance carrier is required to cover the balance. Other provisions of the ACA potentially fostered consumer access to coverage and care, such as elimination of the practice of "rescission," by which an insurer could eliminate coverage when an enrollee might have a new diagnosis. This might particularly affect access to mental health care, as many consumers purchasing insurance policies may well not consider the possibility that they or a family member might have a new onset of a mental health condition, or purchase a policy with this benefit in mind.

Other important components of the ACA particularly relevant to potential access to coverage and care are "guaranteed issue" and "community rating." Guaranteed issue means that insurance carriers cannot refuse to enroll a person based on the person's health status or medical history. Community rating means enrollees may no longer be charged more based on their health status, medical history, or gender. Potential biases against those with prior or current mental health conditions (or other conditions against which insurers may want to discriminate) may thus be minimized. Indeed, under the ACA, insurance carriers may no longer ask potential enrollees for their medical history. Policies must be offered to anyone who is willing to pay the premiums, with pricing taking into account only the rating area where the enrollee lives, with some variability (up to three times as much) due to age; the only health factor that can be taken into account is whether the enrollee is a tobacco user (Tobacco Control Legal Consortium, 2014).

Potential solutions to health care barriers seem to fall into several categories: addressing economic barriers, workforce barriers, and specific clinical population/consumer needs. Each of these areas might be approached locally (e.g., at a community or state level), at the national level, or with global initiatives. A model allowing categorization of potential solutions might look like the one in Table 1.1, which could help identify unmet/under-addressed areas for potential intervention.

Table 1.1 Categorizing Obstacles and Potential Needs

	Focus of intervention	
Potential level of intervention	**Workforce/clinicians**	**Economic**
Local (community, state)	Volunteer organizations Cultural competency	Charities Religious organizations
National	Volunteer organizations Cultural competency	Health care policy and funding Insurance industry
Global	Cultural competency	International aid

Tested examples or initiatives may not exist in some of these areas, but this may be a useful way to think about meaningful interventions, how efforts toward decreasing barriers have been implemented, and how initiatives may interact in different domains. Strategies and empirically supported efforts have included fostering cultural competence, expanding the workforce, and pursuing initiatives directed toward specific populations, public education, and global initiatives.

Expanding the Workforce

Enlarging the available pool of health care professionals will require long-term planning and likely revamping of training models. Other ways to expand available mental health care are to engage already licensed professionals in volunteering additional services in ways that are sustainable for the professional as well as the consumer. Two highly successful models may serve as examples. Volunteers in Psychotherapy (VIP, see http://www.ctvip.org/) operates at the community level, with treatment hours donated by licensed clinicians. Consumers "pay" for therapy received on a completely private basis by doing volunteer work at other nonprofit organizations, charities, or other community agencies. VIP has been in operation for nearly 20 years and has received multiple grants as well as awards and recognition. The organization has provided more than 7,500 therapy sessions to 650+ individuals or families in the local community. Consider a "multiplier" effect if such a model were to be implemented in other communities; indeed, VIP makes consultation available to recreate or adapt the model in other locales and settings.

A similar example is the "Give an Hour" organization (see https://giveanhour.org/), whose mission is to be "to develop national networks of volunteer professionals capable of responding to both acute and chronic conditions that arise within our society." The group provides free and confidential mental health care and initially served veterans and their families, since expanding to other populations. Care is provided by volunteer mental health professionals who agree to donate one hour per week for at least a year. Operating on a nonprofit basis, Give An Hour's funding is through donations and grants, and the group has a national reach in terms of mental health professionals who donate their services. Clearly, such models provide "win–win–win" approaches in terms of harnessing already available mental health professional resources, with funding streams that have proven sustainability, and have the potential to provide services to those who may not have the individual resources. In the case of VIP, consumers of services are able to directly give back to their local community with volunteer activities.

Efforts are underway to address health care needs through a number of avenues, though the question remains whether growth will catch up with demand. For example, at the federal level, the Health Resources and Services Administration (HRSA) is an agency within the U.S. Department of Health and Human Services that provides educational programs, holds conferences, disseminates information, and is the grantor for Graduate Psychology Education grants and many other behavioral health grants. HRSA is the primary federal agency focused on marginalized populations, particularly rural residents, those from lower socioeconomic groups, the geographically isolated, and the medically vulnerable. The agency operates through a number of mechanisms, such as providing training grants as well as loans, scholarships, and scholarship repayment programs that enable practitioners to work in rural and other underserved areas. HRSA has specific initiatives in the prevention and treatment area of substance abuse through training for behavioral health professions. HRSA also supports training and treatment in combined primary and behavioral health services (https://bhw.hrsa.gov/grants/mentalbehavioralhealth). HRSA grants include funding for training programs in psychology and social work, for example, "to train psychologists to work with underserved populations." Strategies to expand the psychiatry workforce that have been identified include updating training models, addressing financial burdens for psychiatrists in training, and maximizing patient/clinician ratios by use of newer technologies such as telemedicine, and integration of psychiatry including co-location with primary care (https://www.thenationalcouncil.org/wp-content/uploads/2017/03/Psychiatric-Shortage_National-Council-.pdf). While these strategies do not necessarily increase the number of psychiatrists available, the initiatives might increase the efficiency of mental health care delivery and increase ease of access for underserved groups. Similar approaches have been taken in psychology training, for example to increase exposure early in training to geriatric populations, address training funding needs, expand mentoring opportunities, as well as internship and training site opportunities, for example with the U.S. Department of Veterans Affairs (VA) system (Hoge, Karel, Zeiss, Alegria, & Moye, 2015).

Addressing Health System Obstacles for Specific Populations

Innovative programs have been developed and evaluated for many groups who are underserved due to health system obstacles. For example, college and university systems are taking many approaches such as extending the number of sessions, hiring more clinicians, extending hours of operation, hiring case managers to assist students with the insurance process, and making appointments for referrals to off-site psychotherapists (Fairyington, 2018). Other approaches include moving toward "triage" and "urgent care" models, with clinicians and appointment availability dedicated to students with high-risk needs (Meek, 2018). Programming specific to the health needs of traditionally underserved groups even within student populations, such as transgender, gender nonconforming, and non-binary students, is being developed—for example, toward an "informed consent" model that would eliminate any required mental health screening prior to obtaining hormone treatment, as long as the student is able to provide informed consent (Williams, 2018). Ironically, such models may increase access to general health care rather than mental health care per se among these students (while potentially increasing access to mental health care by other students), bypassing mental health assessment and written consent when unnecessary.

Another example of innovative approaches to mental health care for older adults is tele-mental health. The effectiveness of tele-mental health interventions for older adults is becoming increasingly evident (Grady et al., 2011). Telehealth is proving to be of great potential for rural populations. Given that there were 60.4 million enrollees in Medicare at the end of 2018, 51 million of whom were enrolled based on age 65+ (CMS/Office of Enterprise Data & Analytics/Office of the Actuary, January, 2019), this traditionally underserved population has great potential to benefit from increased access to mental health care via this modality. Indeed, in a recent report to Congress, Centers for Medicare & Medicaid Services (CMS, 2018a) cited that in 2016, 85.4% of telehealth beneficiaries (74,547) were diagnosed with a mental health disorder and approximately 37% of those were diagnosed with major depressive, bipolar, and schizoaffective disorders, with psychotherapy being among the most frequent modalities of treatment.

Public Education

Obstacles to care such as perceived ability to handle concerns individually and without treatment or knowing where services may be found could be remedied through public education. Many such efforts exist, such as the National Alliance on Mental Illness's "Ending the Silence" presentations, https://www.nami.org/Find-Support/NAMI-Programs/NAMI-Ending-the-Silence). Nationwide initiatives that are carried out at the local community level may be particularly effective, such as "National Depression Screening Day," which serves to inform individuals across the nation of important mental health education and connect consumers of health information with support services (https://mentalhealthscreening.org/programs/initiatives). Finally, as noted in relation to individual costs of care, educating the public may dispel myths about perceived financial burdens and spread the news that mental health care may be increasingly affordable to individuals and families. Note that considering the cost of mental health treatment in this manner intersects individual clinician and practices, national and state economic policies, and consumer education.

What Might Be Done on a Global Health/International Basis?

The World Health Organization (WHO, 2018) reported that every dollar spent to treat depression, anxiety, and the more common mental illnesses results in a return of four dollars in terms of improved health and ability to work. Analyses indicate that health care costs projected from 2016 to 2030 for untreated depression and anxiety across low-, middle-, and high-income countries will result in a global economic loss of $1 trillion per year.

Economic losses alone of course do not measure the toll in terms of human suffering, foreshortened lives, and other humanitarian burdens. All of these considerations should serve as powerful incentives to improve access to mental health care, in the United States and internationally. We have previously discussed the ratio of consumers to mental health clinicians. The same WHO study reported that there may be as few as two mental health workers per 100,000 people in some low-income countries, in contrast to 70+ workers per 100,000 in high-income countries (WHO, 2018).

In its companion "Mental Health Action Plan 2013–2020" (WHO, 2013), WHO identifies four major objectives:

- Strengthen effective leadership and governance for mental health
- Provide comprehensive, integrated, and responsive mental health and social care services in community-based settings
- Implement strategies for promotion and prevention in mental health
- Strengthen information systems, evidence, and research for mental health.

Each of these has specific targets that provide the foundation for measurable action and success by member states toward global goals and associated measures that are periodically collected and reported through the Mental Health Atlas project. Given the emphases that include integrated and community-setting–based care, and preventive services, could these not be scaled down to more local community efforts? And what of individual clinicians and small or larger practice groups, as well as training models and settings and research programs, incorporating these as principles to drive future work? Such approaches would truly have the potential to act locally from a global perspective, expanding access to mental health care for those who remain underserved.

Future Steps

Keeping in mind the model previously described to categorize obstacles and potential needs, clinicians could begin by considering levels of systems at which they have interest and skills (or skills gaps) for intervention. In terms of practice building or developing advocacy interests, clinicians might well consider identifying unmet needs at local or broader levels. At the most "local" level, clinicians could self-evaluate and consult with peers about gaps in training and make efforts to decrease gaps with further education and training. Identified needs could fulfill continuing education (CE) for licensure requirements. CE credit could be available for evaluating community-based outpatient mental health programs (Wisconsin Department of Regulation & Licensing, 2011), or issues related to cultural/ethnic diversity (e.g., New Mexico Regulation & Licensing Department, 2019).

At a community level, interventions might be offered to underserved groups within communities or those more particular to a local setting. For example, a survey of the number of skilled nursing facilities in an identifiable region, including a review of psychologically relevant variables such as the prevalence of anxiety or depressive symptoms or pain among residents, with resources such as https://www.medicare.gov/NursingHomeCompare/compare.html might, would readily yield a substantial number of agencies and individuals that may lack adequate services at both organizational consultation and individual treatment levels. Allying with statewide organizations (e.g., American Health Care Association, https://www.ahcancal.org/about_ahca/pages/default.aspx could readily broaden the potential level of intervention. Similarly, populations underserved and more unique to a particular locale, such as immigrants/refugees, might be identified (e.g., https://www.dhs.wisconsin.gov/minority-health/population/asian-pophistory.htm). Knowledge, skills, and needs gaps identified by the clinician/practice introduce the potential for services. Given the potentially unmet needs among college students, and the relative ease of identifying relevant settings in the community, there could be great potential to offer services on an individual practitioner or practice group consortium basis.

At a more complex level of intervention, clinicians likely would need specialized training and guided experience in participating in activities geared toward influencing policy. Advocacy at this level is not necessarily a part of graduate-level training, but fortunately many such opportunities are available (e.g., https://www.apa.org/advocacy, https://www.socialworkers.org/Advocacy/Policy-Issues, and https://www.psychiatry.org/psychiatrists/advocacy). As with underserved individuals and groups, advocacy needs for the mental health professions and the individuals and communities served are greater than available resources.

But the rewards of joining with others to serve those greater goals are undoubtedly worth efforts to rise to the challenges.

Most recently, CMS has announced payment policies by which clinicians could be paid for brief communication technology-based service for the purpose of patient check-in with the practitioner to determine need for an in-person appointment or for remote evaluation of patients' video recordings, which would enable practitioners to be separately paid for reviewing patient-transmitted photo or video information or internet interprofessional consultation (CMS, 2018a). CMS was an "early adopter" of reimbursed psychotherapy via "telehealth" under specified conditions (Ballie, 2001) and continues to expand technologies and services available.

The VA serves as a model for leading-edge application of telehealth services. The VA utilizes telehealth in providing services to veterans in remote or rural areas, to those who have limited mobility, and to those who for various reasons cannot engage in in-person services. The Seattle VA maintains mobile units in remote areas of Washington state through which veterans can receive synchronous services from mental health professionals who are located at the VA in Seattle. These adaptations increase access to treatment and promote a healthier population.

While reimbursement for use of such technologies for service delivery may not be available for all mental health clinicians early during implementation, and consistency in coverage may be elusive at this time (Wicklund, 2018), opportunities nevertheless are potentially great (Bryant, 2018). Forward-looking clinicians undoubtedly would do well to remain alert to possibilities and develop skills and knowledge for this likely expanding domain, with its potential to bring reimbursed services to those who may otherwise be underserved.

References

AARP Public Policy Institute. (2012). Who relies on Medicare? Profile of the Medicare population. Retrieved from https://www.aarp.org/content/dam/aarp/research/public_policy_institute/health/who-relies-on-medicare-factsheet-AARP-ppi-health.pdf

Agency For Healthcare Research and Quality. (2018). Expenses for office-based physician visit by specialty and insurance type, 2016. Retrieved from https://meps.ahrq.gov/data_files/publications/st517/stat517.pdf

Alegria, M., Atkins, M., Farmer, E., Slaton, E., & Stelk, W. (2010). One size does not fit all: Taking diversity, culture and context seriously. *Administration and Policy in Mental Health, 37*(1–2), 48–60.

American Psychological Association. (2014). Guidelines for psychological practice with older adults. *American Psychologist, 69*(1), 34–65.

American Psychological Association. (2016, March). Datapoint: Where are the highest concentrations of licensed psychologists? *Monitor on Psychology, 47*(3), 13.

American Psychological Association. (2017). *Ethical principles of psychologists and code of conduct* (2002, amended June 1, 2010, and January 1, 2017). Retrieved from http://www.apa.org/ethics/code/index.aspx

American Psychological Association. (2018a). *A summary of psychologist workforce projections: Addressing supply and demand from 2015–2030*. Washington, DC: Author.

American Psychological Association. (2018b). APA fact sheet series on psychologist supply and demand projections 2015–2030: Unmet need. Retrieved from https://www.apa.org/workforce/publications/supply-demand/unmet-need.pdf

American Psychological Association. (2018c). Addressing the mental and behavioral health needs of underserved populations. Retrieved from https://www.apa.org/advocacy/workforce-development/gpe/populations.aspx

Ballie, R. (2001). Medicare will now cover some telehealth psychotherapy services. *Monitor on Psychology, 32*(10), 84.

Bryant, M. (2018). Telebehavioral health finding its niche. Retrieved from https://www.healthcaredive.com/news/telebehavioral-health-finding-its-niche/525740/

Carlat, D. (2010). 45,000 more psychiatrists anyone? *Psychiatric Times, 27*(8). Retrieved from https://www.psychiatrictimes.com/adhd/45000-more-psychiatrists-anyone

Center on Budget and Policy Priorities. (2014). Repealing health reform's risk corridors would boost deficits and premiums. Retrieved from https://www.cbpp.org/blog/repealing-health-reforms-risk-corridors-would-boost-deficits-and-premiums

Center for Collegiate Mental Health. (2018, January). 2017 annual report (Publication No. STA 18-166). Retrieved from https://ccmh.psu.edu/publications/

Centers for Medicare & Medicaid Services. (2018a). Information on Medicare telehealth. Retrieved from https://www.cms.gov/About-CMS/Agency-Information/OMH/Downloads/Information-on-Medicare-Telehealth-Report.pdf

Centers for Medicare & Medicaid Services. (2018b). Final policy, payment, and quality provisions changes to the Medicare physician fee schedule for calendar year 2019. Retrieved from https://www.cms.gov/newsroom/fact-sheets/final-policy-payment-and-quality-provisions-changes-medicare-physician-fee-schedule-calendar-year

Centers for Medicare & Medicaid Services/Office of Enterprise Data and Analytics. (2018c, September). Hospital/medical enrollment, August 2018. Retrieved from https://www.cms.gov/Research-Statistics-Data-and-Systems/Statistics-Trends-and-Reports/CMSProgramStatistics/Dashboard.html

Centers for Medicare & Medicaid Services/Office of Enterprise Data & Analytics/Office of the Actuary. (2019, January). CMS fast facts. Retrieved from https://www.cms.gov/research-statistics-data-and-systems/statistics-trends-and-reports/cms-fast-facts/index.html

Chen, A., Youdelman, M., & Brooks, J. (2007). The legal framework for language access in healthcare settings: Title VI and beyond. *Journal of General Internal Medicine, 22*(Suppl 2), 362–367.

Commonwealth Fund. (2018). The effect of eliminating the individual mandate penalty and the role of behavioral factors. Retrieved from https://www.commonwealthfund.org/publications/fund-reports/2018/jul/eliminating-individual-mandate-penalty-behavioral-factors

Congressional Budget Office. (2018). Federal subsidies for health insurance coverage for people under age 65: 2018 to 2028. Retrieved from https://www.cbo.gov/system/files?file=2018-06/53826-healthinsurancecoverage.pdf

Department of Economic and Social Affairs, United Nations. (2010). *World population aging 2009*. New York, NY: United Nations.

Executive Office of the President. (2017). E.O. 13765, 82 FR 8351, pp. 8351–8352.

Fairyington, S. (2018). What campus mental health centers are doing to keep up with student need. Retrieved from https://thriveglobal.com/stories/campus-mental-health-crisis-health-centers-student-needs/

Gaba, C. (2018). Rate hikes. Retrieved from http://acasignups.net/2018-rate-hikes

George Washington University Health Workforce Institute. (2017, October). Profile of the social work workforce. Retrieved from https://www.socialworkers.org/News/Research-Data/Workforce

Grady, B., Myers, K., Nelson, E., Belz, N., Bennett, L., Carnahan, L., . . . Voyles, D. (2011). Evidence-based practice for telemental health. *Telemedicine Journal and E-Health*, *17*(2), 131–148.

Graves, D., Like, R., Kelly, N., & Hohensee, A. (2007). Legislation as intervention: A survey of cultural competence policy in health care. *Journal of Health Care Law and Policy*, *10*(2), 339–361.

Henry, J. (2016). Are insurers ditching PPOs? Retrieved from https://www.healthcaredive.com/news/are-insurers-ditching-ppos/423291/

Henry J. Kaiser Family Foundation. (2018). Key facts about the uninsured population. Retrieved from https://www.kff.org/uninsured/fact-sheet/key-facts- about-the-uninsured-population/

Henry J. Kaiser Family Foundation. (2019a). Health coverage of immigrants: Fact sheet. Retrieved from https://www.kff.org/disparities-policy/fact-sheet/health-coverage-of-immigrants/

Henry J. Kaiser Family Foundation. (2019b). Status of the state Medicaid expansion decisions: An interactive map. Retrieved from https://www.kff.org/medicaid/issue-brief/status-of-state-medicaid-expansion-decisions-interactive-map/

Herz, G. (2018). Psychotherapy in Medicare update—10 million+ sessions likely provided for the first time in 2017. Retrieved from http://drherz.us/psychotherapy-in-medicare-update-10-million-sessions-likely-provided-for-the-first-time-in-2017/

Hoge, M., Karel, M., Zeiss, A., Alegria, M., & Moye, J. (2015). Strengthening psychology's workforce for older adults: Implications of the Institute of Medicine's report to Congress. *American Psychologist*, *70*(3), 265–278.

Kaiser Health News. (2016). Licking wounds, insurers accelerate moves to limit health-law enrollment. Retrieved from https://khn.org/news/licking-wounds-insurers-accelerate-moves-to-limit-health-law-enrollment/

Keith, K. (2018). Two new federal surveys show stable uninsured rate. *Health Affairs Blog*. Retrieved from https://www.healthaffairs.org/do/10.1377/hblog20180913.896261/full/

Krahn, G., Walker, D., & Correa-De-Araujo, R. (2015). Persons with disabilities as an unrecognized health disparity population. *American Journal of Public Health*, *105*(Suppl 2), S198–S206.

Livingston, S. (2018). Most ACA exchange plans feature a narrow network. Retrieved from https://www.modernhealthcare.com/article/20181204/NEWS/181209976/most-aca-exchange-plans-feature-a-narrow-network

Meek, W. (2018). How Brown University radically transformed its approach to student mental health. Retrieved from https://thriveglobal.com/stories/brown-university-student-mental-health/

National Association of the Deaf. (2018). Questions and answers for health care providers. Retrieved from https://www.nad.org/resources/health-care-and-mental-health-services/health-care-providers/questions-and-answers-for-health-care-providers/

National Association of Insurance Commissioners. (2019). Network Adequacy. Retrieved from https://www.naic.org/cipr_topics/topic_network_adequacy.htm.

National Institute of Mental Health. (2017a). Mental illness. Retrieved from https://www.nimh.nih.gov/health/statistics/mental-illness.shtml

National Institute of Mental Health. (2017b). Major depression. Retrieved from https://www.nimh.nih.gov/health/statistics/major-depression.shtml

New Mexico Regulation & Licensing Department. (2019). Continuing education requirements. Retrieved from http://www.rld.state.nm.us/boards/Psychologist_Examiners_Requirements_and_Continuing_Education.aspx

Novotney, A. (2014). Students under pressure: College and university counseling centers are examining how best to serve the growing number of students seeking their services. Retrieved from http://www.apa.org/monitor/2014/09/cover-pressure.aspx

Powell, F. (2017). 10 universities with the most undergraduates. Retrieved from https://www.usnews.com/education/best-colleges/the-short-list-college/articles/2017-12-05/10-universities-with-the-most-undergraduate-students

Reynolds, K., Pietrzak, R., El-Gabalawy, R., Mackenzie, C., & Sareen, J. (2015). Prevalence of psychiatric disorders in U.S. older adults: Findings from a nationally representative survey. *World Psychiatry*, *14*(1), 74–81.

Soni, A., & Mitchell, E. (2016, May). Expenditures for commonly treated conditions among adults age 18 and older in the U.S. civilian noninstitutionalized population, 2013. Statistical Brief #487. Rockville, MD: Agency for Healthcare Research and Quality. Retrieved from http://www.meps.ahrq.gov/mepsweb/data_files/publications/st487/stat487.pdf

Statista. (2017). Population projections for the United States from 2015 to 2060 (in mil lions). Retrieved from https://www.statista.com/statistics/183481/united-states-population-projection/

Substance Abuse and Mental Health Services Administration. (2016). Cultural competence. Retrieved from https://www.samhsa.gov/capt/applying-strategic-prevention/cultural-competence

Substance Abuse and Mental Health Services Administration. (2018). The need to focus on individuals with serious mental illness includes the LGBT community. Retrieved from https://blog.samhsa.gov/2018/03/28/the-need-to-focus-on-individuals-with-serious-mental-illness-includes-the-lgbt-community/#.W80GbVVKipo

Taylor, Y. (2006). Review: "College of the overwhelmed: The campus mental health crisis and what to do about it." *Journal of College and Character*, *7*(8). Retrieved from https://www.tandfonline.com/doi/abs/10.2202/1940-1639.1223

Tobacco Control Legal Consortium. (2014). How the Affordable Care Act affects tobacco use and control. Retrieved from https://www.integration.samhsa.gov/health-wellness/How_the_Affordable_Care_Act_Affects_Tobacco_Use_and_Control.pdf

U.S. Congress. (2017). Public Law 115-97, 115th Congress. Retrieved from https://www.congress.gov/bill/115th-congress/house-bill/1

Wicklund, E. (2018). Reimbursement barriers still plague telemental health expansion. Retrieved from https://mhealthintelligence.com/news/reimbursement-barriers-still-plague-telemental-health-expansion

Williams, M. (2018). UW-Madison to make changes to transgender health care: University Health Services plan to move to informed consent model. Retrieved from https://www.wpr.org/uw-madison-make-changes-transgender-health-care

Wisconsin Department of Regulation & Licensing. (2011). Application to receive CE credit for voluntary, uncompensated evaluation assistance with the Wisconsin Department of Health Services. Retrieved from https://dsps.wi.gov/Documents/fm2945.pdf

Wisconsin Public Radio. (2018). Federal money for ACA sign up assistance declines again: Wisconsin down to 1 'navigator' agency; some states will have none. Retrieved from https://www.wpr.org/federal-money-aca-sign-assistance-declines-again

World Health Organization. (2013). Mental health action plan 2013-2020. Retrieved from https://www.who.int/mental_health/publications/action_plan/en/,

World Health Organization. (2018). Mental health atlas 2017. Retrieved from https://www.who.int/mental_health/evidence/atlas/mental_health_atlas_2017/en/

2

Delivering Psychological Services to Military Members

K. C. Kalmbach and Bret A. Moore

Currently, service members in the U.S. Armed Forces[1] make up 0.04% of the nation's adult population (U.S. Department of Defense [DoD], 2017)[2]. In voluntarily taking on this role, military members are immersed in an all-encompassing culture and are required to make countless personal sacrifices, often experiencing trauma or other stressors that most civilians will never face. Over the past two decades, a grateful nation has provided unprecedented levels of support for the many brave servicemen and women who choose this career path. It may therefore come as a surprise to some that, despite this support, many military members[3] remain underserved in the area of mental health. Challenges include system and access barriers; health providers' lack of familiarity with military injuries, needs, and culture; and military members' own stigma-related reluctance to seek treatment.

This chapter will provide mental health clinicians with suggestions for practice grounded in a review of the literature and integrated with the professional experience of the authors, both of whom have extensive experience working with this population. We will outline the challenges and detail the qualities necessary to work effectively with psychotherapy clients who are military members.

The Scope and Description of the Problem

In many ways, September 11, 2001, ushered in an era of unprecedented change for U.S. service members and those tasked with their care. Although veterans from

[1] The U.S. Armed Forces comprise five branches: Army, Marines, Navy, Air Force, and Coast Guard (in wartime). The National Guard and Reserve components are also included in total force demographics.

[2] The views expressed herein are those of the authors and do not reflect the official policy or position of Army Regional Health Command - Central, the U.S. Army Medical Department, the U.S. Army Office of the Surgeon General, the Department of the Army, the Department of the Air Force and Department of Defense or the U.S. Government.

[3] The term *military member* will be used when referring to active-duty service members and veterans as a group.

all eras face unusual challenges, a number of factors aggregate to create a unique risk profile for veterans of post-9/11 conflicts. For combat troops, the proliferation of devastating improvised explosive devices required a state of chronic hypervigilance for survival. Unlike any prior era, a significant portion of the military became battle-weary as a result of multiple deployments. In fact, since 2001, a quarter of all service members have been deployed three or more times; prior eras saw a smaller percentage of service members deployed to war zones, and typically only once. Health care providers adjusted rapidly to an evolving picture of complicated mental health conditions (MHCs),[4] including post-traumatic stress disorder (PTSD), traumatic brain injury (TBI), and related polytrauma. Although there is variability among the branches, one thing is clear: The prevalence of MHCs in the active-duty military rose over the past decade, peaking in 2012–2013, when it reached an average of 24% for all branches combined. Fortunately, however, the same data also appear to reflect a modest downward trend since that time (cf. 20% in 2016) (Deployment Health Clinical Center [DHCC], 2017).

A Complicated Clinical Profile

As military medicine rapidly upskilled to cope with new and complicated injuries, survival rates improved. More seriously injured and blast-exposed service members were surviving than in previous eras, but they were surviving with polytraumatic injuries requiring lifelong care. Known as the "signature wounds" of Iraq and Afghanistan, PTSD and TBI estimates increased steadily. Survival in war zones, especially for those who are repeatedly deployed, requires a mental "battle hardening"; this often means habituating to ever-present trauma, violence, and death. While perhaps adaptive in combat, these changes can increase the risk of MHCs and high-risk behaviors, including substance abuse and suicidal ideation (Brenner et al., 2008).

Mental Health Conditions

In 2008, RAND released *The Invisible Wounds of War*, a seminal research report that found that 31% of returning combat-deployed service members met criteria for a primary MHC: PTSD or depression, 11.2%; TBI, 12.2%; and TBI comorbid with PTSD and/or depression, 7.3%. Importantly, only slightly more than half of those

[4] We have intentionally chosen to use the term *mental health condition* (MHC) when discussing clinical categories that may span psychological/emotional (e.g., depression) as well as neurophysiological (e.g., traumatic brain injury) disorders. MHC is a more encompassing term, and our clinical experience has been that many military members respond more favorably to discussing their "condition" rather than "illness" or "disorder."

with PTSD or depression sought help, and only 43% of those with TBI engaged with care providers (Tanielian & Jaycox, 2008). By 2014, the Institute of Medicine (IOM) had updated estimates of MHCs that were two to three times higher than previously assumed. Specifically, they found that 20% to 23% of military members met criteria for TBI, and up to 24% for PTSD. Additionally, the post-9/11 era saw an increasing awareness of issues disproportionately affecting women (now representing 10% to 15% of total forces). Research indicates that military sexual trauma (MST) is reported by up to 24% of military women compared to 1% of their male counterparts (Gundlapalli et al., 2017). Women who are victims of MST are at nine times the risk for developing PTSD compared to peers with no MST history, and suicide risk is also elevated (Murray-Swank, Dausch, & Ehrnstrom, 2018).

Military Suicide

Any gesture, attempt, or suicide is—clinically—a critical situation. Approximately one in five suicide victims in the United States is a veteran, and veterans may be at slightly elevated risk for taking their own lives compared to civilians (U.S. Department of Veterans Affairs [VA], 2016). However, it is not clear that military suicides have dramatically increased, as is commonly reported. Often, suicide rates in the military are compared directly with civilian rates; however, given the demographics of the military, this is not an appropriate comparison (Ramchand, 2018). Recently, researchers undertook a comprehensive analysis adjusted for demographic and other differences and found that—contrary to popular belief—rates of military suicide, historically, were actually *lower* than that of the civilian population. Something did change in 2005, though: Military suicide rates began to increase *up to* that of the civilian population (Reimann & Mazuchowski, 2018). However, it does not appear that the increase in suicide rates was due to combat exposure or the stress of deployments, as was commonly assumed; in fact, rates for the never-deployed active-duty, Reserve, and Guard components also increased. In the large-scale longitudinal Millennium Cohort Study, factors most strongly associated with military suicide were sex (male), mental disorder (depression, "manic depression"), and substance abuse (alcohol). Combat and other deployment experience did *not* factor into any of the predictive models (LeardMann et al., 2013).

Poverty

Although many military members have a right to access services and assistance, a disturbing percentage of veterans face both food and housing insecurity

(Fargo et al., 2012; *Feeding America*, 2017; U.S. Department of Housing and Urban Development [HUD], 2018). In 2017, for example, *Feeding America* (now partnering with the VA) reported that 20% of households receiving regular food aid contained at least one veteran or military member. Additionally, when compared to civilians, male veterans are at 1.3 times the risk of homelessness and women veterans are at 3.6 times the risk of homelessness. Fortunately, this problem has been addressed aggressively, and numbers are continuing to drop from a high of 200,000 homeless veterans in 2003 to 40,000 in 2017 (HUD, 2018).

Family Problems

On average, military members marry and have children earlier than their civilian counterparts; not only must military members adjust to a potentially high-risk career, they also bear the responsibility of engaging their family in this lifestyle (Clever & Segal, 2013). As might be expected given the unique stressors of military life, the families of military members evidence a slightly higher risk of behavioral and mental health problems compared to the civilian population; military children sometimes manifest anxiety/mood problems as well as difficulties in school (Siegel & Davis, 2013). Military spouses often struggle to cope with the responsibilities of both parental roles while the military member is away (Lewy, Oliver, & McFarland, 2014).

Considerations for the Clinician

Although anywhere from 15% to 30% of military members live with a MHC, given the demands of military life, it could be argued that most military members and their families evidence a remarkable degree of resilience. This reminder is offered as a caution against perceiving veterans as a "broken" or "disabled" population as they are often portrayed in media representations. Therapeutically, it is more helpful to adopt a strengths-based approach with military members; not only is it less stigmatizing, but such an approach is similar to military culture and values familiar to the client.

Barriers to Service Delivery

Systems of Care

None of the major systems of care serving military members are designed to collaborate or share information, and eligibility criteria can vary. Demand routinely exceeds capacity, and there are longstanding calls for broad reforms and improved solutions. Not surprisingly, from the veteran's perspective, finding treatment can seem like a daunting task.

Private Sector

Although federal agencies provide care to a vast number of veterans, the need is greater. To address this gap, thousands of nonprofit, faith-based, and community-based organizations sprung up post-9/11 to offer free services to veterans (Tanielian, Batka, & Meredith, 2017). Philanthropic contributions for these initiatives were strong in the early years of the conflicts; however, donor support has declined steadily over the past decade. Furthermore, although many organizations provide excellent care, because most are free from federal oversight there is no way to ensure quality or consistency of care. Additionally, the fact that veteran information is not shared between private and federal entities can be problematic when attempting to coordinate care for the veteran (especially those in crisis).

Government

It may be surprising to learn that less than half of the nation's 22 million veterans are enrolled in federally supported systems of care (Tanielian et al., 2017). The enrollment rate for post-9/11 veterans is higher (62%) than the average, with nearly six in 10 enrolled veterans carrying a mental health diagnosis (VA, 2017). Military members receive health care primarily from two federal systems: The Military Health System (MHS) within the DoD serves active-duty and retired veterans and the Veterans Health Administration (VHA) within the VA primarily serves veterans. Eligibility requirements vary, and not all veterans qualify for VA care; however, the VHA provides health care to approximately 40% of all veterans and some active-duty service members. With more than 1,200 health care facilities and programs, the VHA is the largest integrated health care system in the United States; currently, more than 9 million veterans are enrolled in VA programs (VA, 2018).

The MHS and the VHA provide a wide range of specialized and cutting-edge mental health care programs and clinics for military members; indeed, they are often on the forefront of state-of-the-art treatment approaches such as virtual reality exposure therapy for PTSD (Rizzo, Hartholt, Grimani, Leeds, & Liewer, 2014). Nonetheless—as might be expected within systems of care serving millions of military members—barriers remain.

Access to Care

Recently, attention has been paid to long wait lists and other issues for veterans receiving care at the VA (e.g., Government Accountability Office [GAO], 2016).

In 2014, Congress created the Veterans Access, Choice, and Accountability Act of 2014 (Veterans' Choice program), which authorized a $10 billion fund in an effort to ensure speedy access to a civilian doctor for veterans who (a) live 40 miles or more from a facility or (b) cannot see a VA doctor within the mandated 30-day consultation window. The Veterans' Choice program was widely applauded but rapidly drew down funds and soon approached bankruptcy, forcing the government to face the specter of another debilitating scandal and potential shutdown of services. In an effort to avoid this, the VA Choice and Quality Employment Act of 2017 was signed into existence and an additional $2.1 billion was authorized to provide for continued service provision, hiring and training of even more providers, and research and development initiatives.

Wait Times

The VA has implemented improvements, and wait times generally have decreased steadily, according to data posted publicly (VA, 2018). Wait time is measured as the amount of time before a veteran is seen, relative to the preferred appointment date. For example, if a veteran is due to be seen by October 10 but the first available appointment is October 15, the wait time would be five days. Fortunately, according to available data, the average wait time for a VA mental health appointment is currently only 5.74 days; however, veterans may wait longer depending on a number of variables, such as the type of treatment required, specialized services available (e.g., polytrauma, PTSD clinics), and regional issues (e.g., ratio of providers to veterans). In addition to other measures, the VA has responded to criticism by expanding capacity, hiring thousands of additional providers, and offering high-quality training in evidence-based practice to clinicians. The VA has also improved transparency by offering online access to view average wait times at local facilities as well as quality ratings of the care provided. These efforts appear to be slowly paying off; some recent studies have found strong support for and satisfaction with VA-based care (Brunner et al., 2018; Kimerling et al., 2015).

Priority Ranking System

In the VA health care system, veterans are enrolled based on an eight-tier scheme that gives preference to those with low income and service-connected disability ratings (e.g., conditions rated 50% or more disabling are given first priority; Purple Heart recipients and prisoners of war are ranked in the third tier). This system was intended to ensure that the most in-need veterans receive attention first; however, especially if other barriers are present (e.g., distance), this type of priority scheduling may deter those veterans with MHCs who have not yet been evaluated for service connection and/or are not considered to be significantly disabled (both of which would fall into priority tier 5).

Distance

Although most VA facilities are located in urban settings, approximately one in four veterans live in rural communities. A specialized office was created in 2007 to address health issues present in the 2.8 million veterans in rural communities across America (VHA Office of Rural Health [ORH], 2016). For rural veterans, the long distances from urban centers limit timely and routine access to many kinds of services, including mental health care. The majority of rural residents are men, but the isolation also negatively impacts women veterans' access to care (up to one third of women veterans reside in rural locales), especially for those who have a history of MST (Brunner et al., 2018; Murray-Swank et al., 2018). Of gravest concern, rural veterans appear to be at higher risk of suicide than their urban counterparts (ORH, 2016), and nearly twice as likely (60%) as urban veterans (35%) to own personal firearms (Cleveland, Azrael, Simonetti, & Miller, 2017), a factor that greatly increases the risk of suicide completion.

Considerations for the Clinician

Clinicians are encouraged to appreciate the significant barriers that many veterans must overcome to access mental health care. Not only may they have waited a long time to qualify for service, they may have traveled a great distance or at great inconvenience to keep an appointment. Respect for their time is shown by adhering to an established schedule and booking appointment times well in advance and at the veteran's convenience if possible. If telehealth treatment options are available and appropriate, this approach may be advantageous for some.

Reluctance to Seek Treatment

Surveys of military members show that concern about the impact of seeking and receiving mental health care is intimately tied to stigma (Bovin et al., 2018; Brown & Bruce, 2016; DeViva et al., 2016; Hoge et al., 2004). Over the past two decades, service members appear to be *slightly* more likely to seek mental health care; however, more than half of those with problems still do *not* seek help, suggesting that destigmatizing efforts must continue (Quartana et al., 2014).

Negative Career Impact

Willingness to seek treatment has been linked to concerns about public shaming, self-stigma, and concern about the impact on career trajectory. In fact, worry about negative career impact is consistently rated as the first (Brown & Bruce, 2016) or second (Tanielian & Jaycox, 2008) most important reason for refusing to seek help for mental health problems. These results suggest that while stigmatization in general is problematic, the culture within military institutions may be even more so. Service members with a MHC may struggle with valid concerns about the potential for a denied promotion, or retracted security clearance, should they request help for MHCs. Acknowledging the cultural stigma as well as concern about military suicide, military leaders have begun to speak openly about MHCs and the need to seek help early (Acosta et al., 2014).

Self-Stigma

Even discussing a condition such as PTSD can be difficult for veterans. For example, the word "disorder" in *post-traumatic stress disorder* is so objectionable to many military members that they have either dropped the word entirely (referring instead to "PTS") or have advocated for changing it to "injury" (or *PTSI*). This latter proposition was considered so important that the cause was taken up by (now retired) Army General Chiarelli, who brought his request to the American Psychiatric Association as it planned the fifth revision of its *Diagnostic and Statistical Manual for Mental Disorders* (DSM) in 2012. Ultimately, the status quo prevailed; however, this brief foray into the highly charged and political realm of disorder-naming revealed that there are sensitivities on all sides. To effectively address stigma means acknowledging its existence at the public, institutional, and individual levels.

Considerations for the Clinician

As authors have noted previously, words matter. Simply choosing language that allows veterans to engage in discussion about psychological injuries without feeling "broken" or "weak" may serve to increase their engagement. Use of the more general term "mental health condition" in conversation is both accurate and less stigmatizing than mental "illness" or "disorder." If the client prefers "PTS" to "PTSD," there is no harm in reflecting it back to them. By mirroring their use of language, mental health providers not only allow the client to feel "heard" but are also protecting their dignity and demonstrating sensitivity around their psychological wounds.

Creating Military Cultural Competence

Although it has gained more currency recently, efforts to promote military cultural competence are not new (Carrola & Corbin-Burdick, 2015; Luby, 2012; Meyer, Writer, & Brim, 2016; Strom et al., 2012). One of the more thoughtful, relevant, and comprehensive reviews of the subject is offered by Reger et al. (2008). They note that "to the extent that a culture includes a language, a code of manners, norms of behavior, belief systems, dress, and rituals, it is clear that the

Army represents a unique cultural group" (p. 22). In fact, these aspects of culture apply equally well to each of the five branches of the U.S. Armed Forces. As clinicians, the importance of cultural competence is reinforced by the American Psychological Association's Ethics Code (2017):

> Where scientific or professional knowledge in the discipline of psychology establishes that an understanding of factors associated with age, gender, gender identity, race, ethnicity, culture, national origin, religion, sexual orientation, disability, language, or socioeconomic status is essential for effective implementation of their branches or research, psychologists have, or obtain the training, experience, consultation, or supervision necessary to ensure the competence of their branches, or they make appropriate referrals, except as provided in Standard 2.02, Providing Services in Emergencies. (pp. 4–5)

To be successful working with military members, clinicians must have an overall appreciation for military culture as well as the impact of that culture on the formation of its members' identity. For many Americans, the terms *mission, teamwork*, and *service* are words that are used loosely in the workplace and peppered throughout human resource presentations. For military members, though, these words have a significance far beyond the way in which they are used in civilian settings. Veterans may have comrades who gave their lives in support of *the mission* and being part of a *team* meant being willing to literally place the life and welfare of your soldiers above your own. It is critical therefore that clinicians first learn to listen carefully and respectfully to the language used by military members; common terms can have a different meaning and valence.

There are many differences between the five branches of service (and even within each branch, subcultures exist); however, a common military culture is woven throughout. Values like honor, duty, obedience, and sacrifice are forged into a core ethos that helps to create a cohesive and strong fighting unit. Understanding military values and principles is essential to forming effective therapeutic relationships with military members. Following is a brief discussion of a few core themes.

Collectivism: The Importance of the Group Over Self

Perhaps the most significant difference between civilian and military cultures is how the military places great emphasis on the importance of the group over the individual; this style is termed *collectivism*. Collectivism is the expression of a cultural value system that emphasizes group cohesiveness, interdependence, common values, and subjugation of self-interest in favor of group benefit

(Christian, Stivers, & Sammons, 2009). On the other hand, in American society, *individualism* is both promoted and valued. As a result, it can be difficult for civilians to understand and respect the mindset that is required in a truly collectivistic organization such as the military. Specifically, collectivism demands (a) acceptance that one's value is only as part of the larger group, (b) an engagement with and commitment to the group on an emotional level, and (c) a singular focus on the goals of the group over one's own agenda (McGurk, Cotting, Britt, & Adler, 2006). This ethos is inculcated in military members from the first day of basic training. Eventually, such values permeate all aspects of a service member's worldview and lifestyle.

Collectivism is the model for militaries worldwide primarily for the purpose of getting things done. In order to accomplish group goals (referred to as the *mission*), service members must work together as a cohesive team with a single vision. In the military, few goals can be accomplished by a solitary individual. The complex and high-stakes nature of military assignments is not conducive to solitary viewpoints, perspectives, or efforts. The mission often requires many highly trained and educated professionals working together toward a common goal. In the civilian world, although teamwork is considered important, a premium is placed on individual accomplishments and self-promotion. In the military, it is just the opposite: Only when the team succeeds does the individual succeed.

As discussed by Moore (2019), collectivism is also important for maintaining unit morale. In my (B.A.M.) experience as an Army psychologist consulting on behavioral health issues with commanders and other senior military leaders in Iraq, lack of unit cohesion and low morale were almost always at the center of a poorly functioning unit. Invariably, these poorly functioning units had senior leaders who put their own needs before the needs of their soldiers, in sharp contrast to core military values. Although this style is often a byproduct of poor training or deficient leadership abilities and not intentional, the lack of a collectivistic unit culture created tension, strife, and hostility between team members. In turn, this led to poor decision making, reduced compassion and empathy, and loss of purpose and meaning.

Considerations for the Clinician

To work effectively with military members, the clinician must understand the central and overarching importance of collectivism. Even after separating from the military, many veterans continue to be influenced by and live their lives in accordance with the values and principles inculcated during military service. If a clinician promotes and urges autonomy and independence within the therapeutic relationship too early, it is possible that a breakdown in communication and trust may occur. Moreover, clinicians should be careful not to view some values—such as a need for strong structure and order—as inherently dysfunctional. Clinicians should become intimately aware of their own value system; as with any client, the psychotherapist's own value system can have a significant impact on treatment outcomes.

Solution-Focused: Adapt and Overcome

The phrase "adapt and overcome" is commonly used in the military. It is used to convey the high value placed on personal characteristics of determination, grit, and problem solving. This philosophy is taught to service members from the first day of basic training and emphasized throughout their careers. Service members are taught that problems are merely obstacles that must be overcome in order to achieve a goal; resilience and dogged refusal to give up on a problem are highly praised. This philosophy also reminds the service member that flexibility and adaptability are critical characteristics that must be practiced and applied.

Considerations for the Clinician

The focus of psychotherapy over the past few decades has shifted from passivity and exploration to one of activity and awareness. Cognitive-behavioral therapy, the most commonly employed and highly researched approach, has broad applicability here. Although every client is unique, the clinician who is comfortable with a more directive and prescriptive approach to treatment will likely find a receptive client in many veterans. As noted, service members are taught early to be solution-focused (as opposed to problem-oriented). This action orientation can pay dividends for the clinician who is able to capitalize on a veteran's training and skill set. In our experience, veterans are more likely than civilian clients to reliably complete homework assignments and follow guidance given. They are generally comfortable with identifying negative cognitions and behaviors and willing to implement strategies to correct them. However, those clinicians who take a more passive and explorative approach to psychotherapy may find that some military clients become impatient, frustrated, or resistant. As a result, difficulty establishing and maintaining rapport or early termination may occur. Clinicians are encouraged to reflect upon their own style and to engage in a discussion with the client about therapeutic orientation and "fit" early in the process.

Show No Weakness

The prototypical military member reflects strength, resolve, and stoicism (Sherman, 2005). These are highly adaptive traits while in service, especially during combat deployment. Display of emotion is seen as weakness and reserved for times with loved ones, if at all. Unfortunately, for the clinician, attempts to avoid being seen as "weak" by displaying emotion will spill over into the therapeutic process (assuming the veteran even gets to that point). Clinicians are reminded that stoicism is closely linked to stigma, which prevents many veterans from seeking care (Hoge et al., 2004); as such, this topic itself may bear discussion early in the therapeutic process.

Considerations for the Clinician

Clinicians must appreciate the fact that stoicism is an adaptive and reinforced trait in the military. The clinician unfamiliar with military culture and values may mistakenly interpret the veteran's stoicism as resistance or disinterest. This may lead to feelings of frustration and inadequacy on the part of the psychotherapist. In our experience, dealing with issues of stigma and stoicism early in treatment is important. Not only does it reduce the chance of misinterpreting the veteran's presentation and the therapeutic relationship, it also demonstrates interest in the client and savvy about military culture. This, in turn, can strengthen the working alliance.

A Military Tradition: Families

Unlike most jobs in the civilian sector, when a person signs a contract with a branch of the armed forces, they are also "signing" on behalf of their family, who instantly become part of the larger "military family." Military family members (or "dependents") are provided services and benefits, receive training and support, and soon learn how the needs of the *mission* and the *team* supersede personal priorities. Families are such an integral part of military culture that family data are included in the annual demographic report on military members (DoD, 2017).

Children often follow in the footsteps of their parents with regard to career choices. This is true in both civilian and military families (Bachman, Segal, Freedman-Doan, & O'Malley, 2000; Dietrich & Kracke, 2009). However, the pattern appears to be even stronger for those with military ties (Gegax & Thomas, 2005). In our work with veterans, we have come to appreciate that the military is more than just an organization; it is also a lifestyle. Growing up as a *military brat*[5] can be a source of strength. This role is connected to a unique subculture of people who possess a remarkable amount of pride, connectedness, and grit. Repeatedly adjusting to new cities, neighborhoods, schools, and friends can

[5] *Military brat* is a non-pejorative term used to describe children of service members.

produce children who are more tolerant, culturally savvy, resourceful, adaptable, and willing to befriend others who are "different" (Park, 2011). However, it can also cause disrupted schooling and behavioral problems in a minority of military children. Although the psychosocial effects of this cultural affiliation are mostly positive, there is a heightened risk of some stress-related problems in military family members (Siegel & Davis, 2013).

Despite the many challenges of military life, there is a strong tradition of service in military families. Those who have grown up in a military family are much more likely than civilians to enter the service themselves; in fact, approximately 60% to 80% of new recruits have a military member in the family, and up to half of new recruits are children of a career military parent. For example, researchers have found that children of Navy veterans are eight to 10 times more likely than civilians to volunteer for military service (Stander & Merrill, 2000). This commitment is remarkable given how disruptive a military lifestyle can be. However, there may be other reasons children follow in their parent's footsteps. Growing up in the insular culture of the military may cause a child to develop a fear or even distrust of the "civilian world." Worldview, values, customs, and rules for living can differ widely between these two realms, which can lead to uncertainty and anxiety. Continuing to work within the "family business" may be the most comfortable and logical choice for some military children (Hall, 2016).

Considerations for the Clinician

Individuals enter the military for many reasons. For many veterans and their families, military service is a source of great pride; they often think of and describe this time as the best years of their lives. Clinicians should avoid assuming that military service was the veteran's only career option, or that they were unequipped for other endeavors. In our experience, there is a prevalent and inaccurate notion that military service is a lesser alternative, chosen only because there were no other career or educational opportunities. To assume such can be deeply insulting to a veteran. Instead, clinicians are encouraged to invite clients to share their own stories and reasons for joining the military. Such a narrative can be very illuminating and contribute to the development of the therapeutic alliance.

Training Resources

Increasing awareness and familiarity with any foreign culture is never a "one-and-done" effort. The best way to gain military cultural competence is to serve within the military; however, we assume that most reading this chapter have not had that opportunity. As such, there are a number of high-quality training resources offered online and in face-to-face workshops. The Center for Deployment

Psychology (www.deploymentpsych.org) offers a variety of cultural competency as well as evidence-based intervention courses for clinicians who work with military members. Another valuable resource is the Tragedy Assistance Program for Survivors (www.taps.org); this material is particularly helpful for clinicians working with family members who have lost a military family member. Lastly, the National Center for PTSD (https://www.ptsd.va.gov/) is a VA program that provides a comprehensive database on information related to PTSD.

Effective Strategies and Empirically-Supported Treatments

The recent wars in Iraq and Afghanistan have led to a tremendous amount of research on the psychological consequences of what is now more than 18 years of sustained operations. Fortunately, a wide range of evidence-based treatments are available for clinicians to learn and implement.

PTSD

A number of treatments are available that are effective for treating PTSD in veterans (see Moore & Penk, 2019). Two of the most popular and widely researched approaches are prolonged exposure (PE) and cognitive processing therapy (CPT). PE is a manualized, trauma-focused intervention based on cognitive behavioral principles and comprises four primary components: (a) imaginal exposure, (b) in vivo exposure, (c) psychoeducation about trauma, and (d) relaxation training (Foa & Kozak, 1986). The typical treatment protocol consists of 60- and 90-minute sessions over the course of 12 weeks (Foa, Hembree, & Rothbaum, 2007). Research supports the use of PE with veterans, and it has been shown to achieve remission rates of more than 50% in some groups (see Peterson, Foa, & Riggs, 2019, for a comprehensive review).

A comparable treatment, in regard to efficacy and relative ease of learning and application, is CPT, which has been shown to be effective in both civilian and military populations (Resick, Monson, & Chard, 2008, 2017; Resick & Schnicke, 1992). Based on the premise that faulty cognitive schemas impair the client's ability to function, CPT helps the client challenge maladaptive beliefs, particularly as they relate to safety, trust, power, esteem, and intimacy. The client is given regular homework assignments that promote awareness of faulty cognitions, and those cognitions are challenged and modified in psychotherapy sessions. Similar to PE, CPT is an intervention lasting 12 to 16 weeks and can be used effectively with the veteran population (see Williams, Galovski, & Resick, 2019, for a comprehensive review).

Based on our experiences, both PE and CPT can be very effective. However, early termination may be a problem for some military clients who are not prepared to confront traumatic memories or complete challenging homework assignments between sessions. Since both approaches are trauma-focused interventions, some level of engagement with the trauma is required. Early termination may be more of an issue with PE as its active ingredients are imaginal and in vivo exposure. On the other hand, CPT requires a significant amount of homework between sessions; for the less motivated client, this may present a problem.

Other Disorders

Depression, generalized anxiety disorder, and panic disorder are highly comorbid with PTSD in the veteran population. Our clinical work has shown that unless addressed specifically, other untreated disorders lead to poorer rates of PTSD remission and overall reduced quality of life. To our knowledge, there are no specific treatments tailored to address these as comorbid conditions. Therefore, standard cognitive and behavioral treatments for panic disorder and generalized anxiety disorder are first-line interventions. Depression is commonly comorbid with PTSD in veteran populations, and although treatments specific to PTSD like PE and CPT can alleviate depressive symptoms (as a side effect), they generally do not lead to remission of depression. Consequently, depression often requires separate psychological and pharmacological interventions. Regarding the former, interventions gaining popularity include acceptance and commitment therapy (ACT) (Hayes, 2004) and mindfulness-based cognitive therapy (MBCT) (Segal, Williams, & Teasdale, 2013). In our experience, like PE and CPT, the ACT and MBCT interventions are relatively easy to learn and apply, and have been found to be effective.

Finally, as noted earlier, suicidality remains one of the more critical and challenging mental health issues to manage. Recall that recent research has shown the top three risk factors for suicide in service members are being male, having depression, and alcohol abuse. Combat and other deployment experiences or trauma did not factor into any of the predictive models (LeardMann et al., 2013). Accordingly, clinicians are encouraged not to make assumptions about suicide risk, but rather to ask about it, sensitively and with respect, after building a degree of therapeutic trust. If suicidality is determined to be a factor, two suicide risk mitigation interventions that have shown some success are the collaborative assessment and management of suicidality (Jobes, 2016) and brief cognitive-behavioral therapy for suicide prevention (Bryan & Rudd, 2018; Rudd et al., 2015). Both interventions are rooted in cognitive-behavioral principles and incorporate practical strategies for minimizing and eliminating risk in treatment planning. Research on these treatments specific to the veteran population is limited; however, in our clinical experience, these interventions have been effective at reducing suicidal ideation in military members. Furthermore, they are well tolerated and relatively easy to administer by clinicians with education and training in cognitive and behavioral therapy.

Future Steps

For us and many of those drawn to working with military members, the motivation can be summed up simply: *to serve well those who have served.* The most important first step to improving care for military members is to create greater awareness and opportunity for training in military cultural competence; such courses are becoming widely available and clinicians are strongly urged to utilize them. Next, clinicians must be aware of and actively confront stigma surrounding mental health treatment; addressing these issues early can help to build a stronger and more effective working alliance. Also, because many veterans may not be willing or able to engage directly with the VA, other models for service delivery should be expanded. By embedding mental health in primary care or community-based outreach centers, veterans are more likely to utilize services as well as less likely to worry about issues related to stigma (Cigrang et al., 2017; Shiner et al., 2009).

Finally, advances in technology over the past two decades have allowed for a range of telehealth services. A recent study of PE therapy comparing in-person versus telehealth-delivered services found equal outcomes in terms of veteran improvement and satisfaction (Gros, Lancaster, López, & Acierno, 2018). Our experience is that post-9/11 veterans (the millennial cohort) generally report satisfaction with tele-mental health services, especially as it can reduce wait times and improve accessibility. To this end, we believe expanded efforts to research and implement new and proven tele-mental health services are needed. This modern approach may be the most practical solution given the numbers of military members needing services and the comfort level with technology of the millennial cohort.

Ultimately, telehealth delivery is also likely to reflect the best cost-to-benefit ratio; however, it is not without risk. The care of clients in active crisis and knowledge of governing law are among the many issues that clinicians must carefully prepare for and think through. In addition to a host of clinical issues, consideration should be given to training in technology, cybersecurity and related competencies, as well as potential liability. One veteran recently reported to the first author (K.C.K.) that tele-mental health "works well, but *only* in a controlled setting." Consistent with VA policy, veterans must attend a VA clinic or Veterans' Center to connect with a telehealth provider; if the veteran is in crisis or suicidal, the clinician can immediately alert local staff or emergency responders. For this reason, it may be unwise for private practitioners to engage veterans in the same telehealth format as civilian clients (i.e., located in their homes) who may not have the same trauma or risk profiles as do veterans. Clinicians interested in telemental health service delivery should seek out training (often offered as continuing education courses) and ensure they clearly understand the practical, legal, ethical, and therapeutic implications of engaging in this 21st-century approach to the provision of mental health treatment.

In closing, clinicians are encouraged to remember that successfully reducing barriers to mental health treatment for military members depends upon a combination of (a) increasing military cultural competency in providers, (b) decreasing stigmatizing beliefs in the military and its members, while (c) expanding nontraditional systems of service delivery. Only when all of these options have been fully exhausted can we truly say that we have fulfilled our nation's obligation to serve well those who have served in our nation's armed forces.

Acknowledgment

The authors wish to thank research assistant Randee Schmitt for her unrelenting work ethic, commitment, and dedication in the researching and preparation of this chapter.

References

Acosta, J. D., Becker, A., Cerully, J. L., Fisher, M. P., Martin, L. T., Vardavas, R., . . . Schell, T. L. (2014). *Mental health stigma in the military*. Retrieved from http://www.dtic.mil/dtic/tr/fulltext/u2/a610275.pdf

American Psychological Association. (2017). Ethical principles of psychologists and code of conduct. Retrieved from https://www.apa.org/ethics/code/

Bachman, J., Segal, D., Freedman-Doan, P., & O'Malley, P. (2000). Who chooses military service? Correlates of propensity and enlistment in the U.S. Armed Forces. *Military Psychology, 12*(1), 1–30.

Bovin, M. J., Miller, C. J., Koenig, C. J., Lipschitz, J. M., Zamora, K. A., Wright, P. B., . . . Burgess, J. F., Jr. (2018). Veterans' experiences initiating VA-based mental health care. *Psychological Services* [E-pub before print: doi:10.1037/ser0000233]

Brenner, L., Gutierrez, P., Cornette, M., Betthauser, L., Bahraini, N., & Staves, P. (2008). A qualitative study of potential suicide risk factors in returning combat veterans. *Journal of Mental Health Counseling, 30*(3), 211–225.

Brown, N. B., & Bruce, S. E. (2016). Stigma, career worry, and mental illness symptomatology: Factors influencing treatment-seeking for Operation Enduring Freedom and Operation Iraqi Freedom soldiers and veterans. *Psychological Trauma: Theory, Research, Practice, and Policy, 8*(3), 276–283.

Brunner, J., Schweizer, C. A., Canelo, I. A., Leung, L. B., Strauss, J. L., & Yano, E. M. (2018). Timely access to mental health care among women veterans. *Psychological Services* [E-pub before print: doi:10.1037/ser0000226]

Bryan, C. J., & Rudd, M. D. (2018). *Brief cognitive-behavioral therapy for suicide prevention*. New York, NY: Guilford Press.

Carrola, P., & Corbin-Burdick, M. F. (2015). Counseling military veterans: Advocating for culturally competent and holistic interventions. *Journal of Mental Health Counseling, 37*(1), 1–14.

Christian, J., Stivers, J., & Sammons, M. (2009). Training to the warrior ethos: Implications for clinicians treating military members and their families. In S. Morgillo-Freeman, B. A. Moore, & A. Freeman (Eds.), *Living and surviving in harm's way: A psychological treatment handbook for pre- and postdeployment of military personnel* (pp. 27–49). New York, NY: Routledge/Taylor & Francis.

Cigrang, J. A., Rauch, S. A., Mintz, J., Mitchell, J. A., Najera, E., Litz, B. T., . . . Peterson, A. L. (2017). Moving effective treatment for posttraumatic stress disorder to primary care: A randomized controlled trial with active duty military. *Families, Systems, & Health, 35*(4), 450–462.

Cleveland, E. C., Azrael, D., Simonetti, J. A., & Miller, M. (2017). Firearm ownership among American veterans: Findings from the 2015 National Firearm Survey. *Injury Epidemiology, 4*(33), 1–10.

Clever, M., & Segal, D. R. (2013). The demographics of military children and families. *The Future of Children, 23*(2), 13–39.

Deployment Health Clinical Center. (2017). *Mental health disorder prevalence among active duty service members in the military health system, fiscal years 2005–2016*. Retrieved from http://www.pdhealth.mil

DeViva, J. C., Sheerin, C. M., Southwick, S. M., Roy, A. M., Pietrzak, R. H., & Harpaz-Rotem, I. (2016). Correlates of VA mental health treatment utilization among OEF/OIF/OND veterans: Resilience, stigma, social support, personality, and beliefs about treatment. *Psychological Trauma: Theory, Research, Practice, and Policy, 8*(3), 310–318.

Dietrich, J., & Kracke, B. (2009). Career-specific parental behaviors in adolescents' development. *Journal of Vocational Behavior, 75*(2), 109–119.

Fargo, J., Metraux, S., Byrne, T., Munley, E., Montgomery, A. A., Jones, H., . . . Culhane, D. (2012). Prevalence and risk of homelessness among US veterans. *Preventing Chronic Disease, 9*, E45.

Feeding America. (2017, June 29). New partnership with U.S. Department of Veterans Affairs: Veterans pantry pilot establishes mobile or on-site food assistance for veterans. Retrieved from https://www.feedingamerica.org/about-us/press-room/veterans-affairs

Foa, E. B., Hembree, E. A., & Rothbaum, B. O. (2007). *Prolonged exposure therapy for PTSD: Emotional processing of traumatic experiences therapist guide*. New York, NY: Oxford University Press.

Foa, E. B., & Kozak, M. J. (1986). Emotional processing of fear: Exposure to corrective information. *Psychological Bulletin, 99*, 20–35.

Gegax, T. T., & Thomas, E. (2005, June 20). The family business. *Newsweek, 145*(25), 24–31.

Gros, D. F., Lancaster, C. L., López, C. M., & Acierno, R. (2018). Treatment satisfaction of home-based telehealth versus in-person delivery of prolonged exposure for combat-related PTSD in veterans. *Journal of Telemedicine and Telecare, 24*(1), 51–55.

Gundlapalli, A. V., Brignone, E., Divita, G., Jones, A. L., Redd, A., Suo, Y., . . . Fargo, J. D. (2017). Using structured and unstructured data to refine estimates of military sexual trauma status among US military veterans. *Studies in Health Technology and Informatics, 238*, 128–131.

Hall, L. (2016). *Counseling military families: What mental health professionals need to know* (2d ed.). New York, NY: Routledge/Taylor & Francis.

Hayes, S. C. (2004). Acceptance and commitment therapy, relational frame theory, and the third wave of behavioral and cognitive therapies. *Behavior Therapy, 35*, 639–665.

Hoge, C. W., Castro, C. A., Messer, S. C., McGurk, D., Cotting, D. I., & Koffman, R. L. (2004). Combat duty in Iraq and Afghanistan, mental health problems, and barriers to care. *New England Journal of Medicine, 351*(1), 13–22.

Institute of Medicine. (2014). *Treatment for posttraumatic stress disorder in military and veteran populations: Final assessment.* Washington, DC: National Academies Press.

Jobes, D. A. (2016). *Managing suicide risk: A collaborative approach.* New York, NY: Guilford Press.

Kimerling, R., Pavao, J., Greene, L., Karpenko, J., Rodriguez, A., Sawekis, M., & Washington, D. L. (2015). Access to mental health care among women veterans: Is VA meeting women's needs? *Medical Care, 53*(4, Suppl. 1), S97–S104.

LeardMann, C. A., Powell, T. M., Smith, T. C., Bell, M. R., Smith, B., Boyko, E. J., . . . Hoge, C. W. (2013). Risk factors associated with suicide in current and former US military personnel. *Journal of the American Medical Association, 310*(5), 496–506.

Lewy, C. S., Oliver, C. M., & McFarland, B. H. (2014). Barriers to mental health treatment for military wives. *Psychiatric Services, 65*(9), 1170–1173.

Luby, C. D. (2012). Promoting military cultural awareness in an off-post community of behavioral health and social support service providers. *Advances in Social Work, 13*, 67–82.

McGurk, D., Cotting, D., Britt, T., & Adler, A. (2006). Joining the ranks: The role of indoctrination in transforming civilians to service members. In T. W. Britt, A. B. Adler, & C. A. Castro (Eds.), *Military life: The psychology of service in peace and combat: Vol. 2. Operational stress* (pp. 13–31). Westport, CT: Praeger.

Meyer, E., Writer, B. W., & Brim, W. (2016). The Importance of Military Cultural Competence. *Current Psychiatry Reports, 18*(3), 26–32.

Moore, B. A. (2019). Understanding and working within the military culture. In B. A. Moore & W. E. Penk (Eds.), *Treating PTSD in military personnel: A clinical handbook* (2nd ed., pp. 9–21). New York, NY: Guilford Press.

Moore, B. A., & Penk, W. E. (Eds.). (2019). *Treating PTSD in military personnel: A clinical handbook* (2nd ed.). New York, NY: Guilford Press.

Murray-Swank, N. A., Dausch, B. M., & Ehrnstrom, C. (2018). Mental health status and barriers to seeking care in rural women veterans. *Journal of Rural Mental Health, 42*(2), 102–115.

Park, N. (2011). Military children and families: Strengths and challenges during peace and war. *American Psychologist, 66*(1), 65–72. doi:10.1037/a0021249

Peterson, A. L., Foa, E. B., & Riggs, D. S. (2019). Prolonged exposure therapy. In B. A. Moore & W. E. Penk (Eds.), *Treating PTSD in military personnel: A clinical handbook* (2nd ed., pp. 46–62). New York, NY: Guilford Press.

Quartana, P. J., Wilk, J. E., Thomas, J. L., Bray, R. M., Rae Olmstead, K. L., Brown, J. M., . . . Hoge, C. W. (2014). Trends in mental health services utilization and stigma in US soldiers from 2002 to 2011. *American Journal of Public Health, 104*(9), 1671–1679.

Ramchand, R. (2018). *Comparing suicide rates: Making an apples-to-apples comparison.* Retrieved from https://www.rand.org

Reger, M., Etherage, J., Reger, G., & Gahm, G. (2008). Civilian psychologists in an Army culture: The ethical challenge of cultural competence. *Military Psychology, 20*(1), 21–35.

Reimann, C. A., & Mazuchowski, E. L. (2018). Suicide rates among active duty service members compared with civilian counterparts, 2005–2014. *Military Medicine, 138*(1), 396–402.

Resick, P. A., Monson, C. M., & Chard, K. M. (2008). *Cognitive processing therapy: Veteran/military version*. Washington, DC: Department of Veterans Affairs.

Resick, P. A., Monson, C. M., & Chard, K. M. (2017). *Cognitive processing therapy for PTSD: A comprehensive manual.* New York, NY: Guilford Press.

Resick, P. A., & Schnicke, M. K. (1992). Cognitive processing therapy for sexual assault victims. *Journal of Consulting and Clinical Psychology, 60*, 748–756.

Rizzo, A., Hartholt, A., Grimani, M., Leeds, A., & Liewer, M. (2014). Virtual reality exposure therapy for combat-related posttraumatic stress disorder. *IEEE Computer Society, 47*(7), 31–37.

Rudd, M. D., Bryan, C. J., Wertenberger, E. G., Peterson, A. L., Young-McCaughan, S., Mintz, J., & Bruce, T. O. (2015). Brief cognitive-behavioral therapy effects on post-treatment suicide attempts in a military sample: Results of a randomized clinical trial with 2-year follow-up. *American Journal of Psychiatry, 172*(5), 441–449.

Segal, Z., Williams, M., & Teasdale, J. (2013). *Mindfulness-based cognitive therapy for depression* (2nd ed.). New York, NY: Guilford Press.

Sherman, N. (2005). *Stoic Warriors. The Ancient Philosophy behind the Military Mind.* Oxford: Oxford University Press.

Shiner, B., Watts, B. V., Pomerantz, A., Groft, A., Scott, D., Street, B., & Young-Xu, Y. (2009). Access to what? An evaluation of the key ingredients to effective advanced mental health access at a VA medical center and its affiliated community-based outreach clinics. *Military Medicine, 174*, 1024–1032.

Siegel, B. S., & Davis, B. E. (2013). Health and mental health needs of children in US military families. *American Academy of Pediatrics, 131*(6), e2002–e2015.

Stander, V., & Merrill, L. (2000). *The relationship of parental military background to the demographic characteristics of 11,195 Navy recruits* (Report No. 00-14). Retrieved from https://apps.dtic.mil/dtic/tr/fulltext/u2/a432135.pdf

Strom, T. Q., Gavian, M. E., Possis, E., Loughlin, J., Bui, T., Lindardatos, E., & Siegel, W. (2012). Cultural and ethical considerations when working with military personnel and veterans: A primer for VA training programs. *Training and Education in Professional Psychology, 6*(2), 67–75.

Tanielian, T., Batka, C., & Meredith, L. S. (2017). *The changing landscape for veterans' mental health care.* Retrieved from https://www.rand.org/pubs/research_briefs/RB9981z2.html

Tanielian, T., & Jaycox, L. H. (Eds.). (2008). *Invisible wounds of war: Psychological and cognitive injuries, their consequences, and services to assist recovery.* Retrieved from https://www.rand.org/pubs/monographs/MG720.html

U.S. Department of Defense, Office of the Deputy Assistant Secretary of Defense for Military Community and Family Policy. (2017). 2015 demographics: Profile of the military community. Retrieved from http://download.militaryonesource.mil

U.S. Department of Housing and Urban Development. (2018). *2017 AHAR: Part 2—Estimates of homelessness in the U.S.* Retrieved from https://www.hudexchange.info/resources

U.S. Department of Veterans Affairs. (2017). *Analysis of VA health care utilization among Operation Enduring Freedom (OEF), Operation Iraqi Freedom (OIF), and Operation New Dawn (OND) veterans*. Retrieved from https://www.publichealth.va.gov

U.S. Department of Veterans Affairs. (2018). *Pending appointment and electronic wait list summary—National, facility, and division level summaries wait time calculated from preferred date for the period ending: 10/15/2018*. Retrieved from https://www.va.gov

U.S. Government Accountability Office. (2016). *Actions needed to improve newly enrolled veterans' access to primary care*. Retrieved from https://www.gao.gov/products

VA Choice and Quality Employment Act of 2017, 10 U.S.C. § 114 (2017). Retrieved from https://www.congress.gov/bill/115th-congress/senate-bill/114/text/pl?overview=closed

Veterans Access, Choice, & Accountability Act of 2014, Pub.L.No.113-146 §128 Stat.1754. Retrieved from https://www.congress.gov/113/plaws/publ146/PLAW-113publ146.pdf

Veterans Health Administration Office of Rural Health. (2016). *THRIVE 2016 Annual Report*. Retrieved from https://www.ruralhealth.va.gov

Williams, A. M., Galovski, T. E., & Resick, P. A. (2019). Cognitive processing therapy. In B. A. Moore & W. E. Penk (Eds.). *Treating PTSD in military personnel: A clinical handbook* (2nd ed., pp. 63–77). New York, NY: Guilford Press.

3

Delivering Mental Health Assistance in the Wake of Natural and Manmade Disasters

Alec Cecil

These days it seems hard to escape the frequent news of disaster events occurring with ever-greater frequency around our country and across the entire planet. Hurricanes, tornados, cyclones, tsunamis, extreme flooding, and wildfires, along with transportation accidents, mass shootings, and other deliberate hostile and terroristic attacks, are in the news so often that it can be very difficult to see and hear the reports. Just in the U.S. it has been estimated that 60% or more of adults and 40% of children and adolescents will experience some type of traumatic event in their lives (Everly & Mitchell, 2008; Halpern & Vermeulen, 2017; National Institute for Environmental Health Services [NIEHS], 2015).

While there is no one definition of "disaster," the word generally refers to catastrophic events of a certain size and scope that are not typically part of one's ordinary experience. Destruction of property and/or loss of life affecting large numbers of people and even whole communities are generally the hallmarks. The demands of such events, individually and collectively, exceed the usual capacity of personal or local resources. As such, most people would be subject to significant stress and trauma following such an experience. In addition to local response, outside assistance is frequently utilized. Often the media will descend in force. People must deal with their crises in the public domain, so there are personal, collective, and public elements to their suffering and loss. Communities and even larger regions may be devastated and permanently reshaped (Das-Brailsford, 2010; Everly & Mitchell, 2008; Halpern & Vermeulen, 2017; Miller, 2012).

In spite of considerable resources and experience, a variety of barriers exist that impede the timely and effective delivery of sufficient services to address the needs of those affected. This chapter discusses some of these challenges from a mental health perspective. Given the size, scope, and number of disaster events and the effects they have on so many people, meeting the psychological needs of survivors and others affected is a monumental task. Assessing those needs and delivering important mental health interventions can be crucial in facilitating recovery in individuals, families, and communities. Cultural and historical factors that will influence reactions and responses at individual and community levels are also important considerations that must be addressed to improve the delivery and utilization of services. In addition to immediate and short-term response, assisting communities in preparing for potential disasters and following up with their recovery are crucial components.

Professional disaster mental health (DMH) focuses on crisis intervention and enhanced psychological first aid (PFA) delivered in the field. Traditional psychotherapies are not the first line of mental health response. Although they may be indicated and useful for some in the months and even years following a disaster, they are less effective in the immediate aftermath (Everly & Lating, 2017). Certainly most of those affected are not looking for anything resembling "psychotherapy" in the short term; they have pressing concrete social and community concerns to address and will welcome assistance in meeting those needs. Most mental health professionals are not trained in disaster response. Efforts to expand the numbers of, and disaster response training for, mental health providers have been increased in recent years, yet still more needs to be done.

The Scope and Description of the Problem

While generally unpredictable in their timing, during the past 20 years worldwide, over 7,000 natural disasters have occurred, affecting over 4 billion people (Center for Research on the Epidemiology of Disasters [CRED], 2017). 2017 was a record hurricane season, with the three most significant, Harvey, Irma, and Maria, all hitting the United States. They were only three of 93 natural disasters to hit the Americas that year (CRED, 2018). Hurricane Irma alone affected 10 million people in the United States and the Caribbean (CRED, 2018). Mass shootings in Las Vegas; Sutherland Springs, Texas; Parkland, Florida; and Santa Fe, Texas followed, all in less than a year.

Just in the latter half of 2018, the news was full of reports regarding Hurricane Florence (primarily in North and South Carolina) and Hurricane Michael (primarily in the Florida panhandle and Georgia) and the wildfires in northern and southern California. There were also mass casualty shootings at a synagogue in Pittsburgh and a country music club in Thousand Oaks, California, and the crash of a stretch limousine that killed 20 people in a rural small-town area in upstate New York. On a much smaller yet still significant scale, local Red Cross chapters all across the country responded to floods, tornados, transportation accidents, and fires to single- and multiple-family homes.

Research on past disasters has demonstrated that many people affected by disasters will have notable psychological reactions and a significant minority may subsequently meet criteria for a mental health diagnosis (NIEHS, 2015;

University of Albany, 2017). A Centers for Disease Control and Prevention (CDC) poll taken shortly after 9/11 in the New York City metropolitan area reported that 75% of respondents acknowledged problems related to the attacks (Everly & Mitchell, 2008). A study after the Oklahoma City bombing found over 90% of survivors symptomatic to some degree (North, 2017). One study following Hurricane Katrina found that half of the parents in Gulf Coast areas indicated that at least one of their children had psychological problems related to being displaced (Knapp, 2010). Overall, as many as 30% to 40% of direct disaster victims (and 10% to 20% of rescue workers) are likely to exhibit a psychological disorder such as acute stress disorder (ASD), post-traumatic stress disorder (PTSD), depression, anxiety, or substance abuse (National Institutes of Health [NIH]/NIEHS, 2015; Substance Abuse and Mental Health Services Administration [SAMHSA]/American Red Cross [ARC], 2015; Watson, 2017).

The frequency and magnitude of disaster incidents, the huge number of people affected, and the significant breadth of psychological impact all speak to the tremendous need for DMH response capacity. While most disasters elicit major response efforts to assist in basic needs, which are certainly helpful, the demand far exceeds the supply. The need for mental health interventions following disasters is greater than ever (Halpern & Vermeulen, 2017; Knapp, 2010). Even when available, matching resources to need and promoting greater utilization are great challenges. Increasing the availability of sufficient services requires considerable planning and training in many communities and greater collaboration among agencies and providers. More public education and other efforts to expand knowledge and awareness and to encourage people to be more receptive and accepting of interventions are also needed.

This requires attention to expanding awareness of and sensitivity to cultural and historical factors in affected populations. The limited number of providers with appropriate training; lack of sufficient funding to provide free or low-cost treatment; client resistance based on financial, cultural, and historical concerns; and stigma may inhibit sufficiently reaching most of those in need. One study found that six months following Hurricane Katrina, only 6% of people affected had received mental health services (Das-Brailsford, 2010). Greater allocation of financial resources is, of course, necessary to accomplish all of this.

Barriers to Service Delivery

Clearly, meeting the psychological needs of the many people affected by so many disasters requires more available responders from all quarters, with adequate preparation and training. DMH, as an organized, targeted, and comprehensive discipline, is a relatively new phenomenon (Halpern & Tramontin, 2007; Weine et al., 2002). While efforts to address the psychological effects of combat in war go back at least to World War I (Salmon, 1917, cited in Everly & Lating, 2017), and some earlier efforts were made to address some specific public incidents (North, 2017), it was not until the early 1990s that the ARC initiated a specific DMH function, making it the first disaster relief agency to incorporate attention to psychological needs into its mission (Everly & Mitchell, 2008; Halpern & Tramontin, 2007). At first, even this was focused more on addressing the psychological concerns in other responders than on meeting the psychosocial needs of disaster survivors in general.

As formulated by the ARC today, "The mission of Disaster Mental Health is to respond to the psychosocial and emotional needs of people affected by a disaster, including Red Cross disaster workers, across the continuum of disaster preparedness, response and recovery" (ARC, 2018, pp. 1–3).

Since DMH is a relatively new specialty and as it is often difficult to study in the midst of disasters, quality research is limited on immediate and short-term psychosocial responses. Yet there is some empirical support, along with considerable consensus on many aspects of what is typically done (ARC, 2017a; University of Albany Center for Public Preparedness & State University of New York at New Paltz Institute for Disaster Mental Health, 2017; Watson, 2017). Some treatments of the most common diagnoses—ASD, PTSD, depression, and grief—have more solid data (Benedek & Wynn, 2017; Foa et al., 2009). Most survivors of disaster will not reach a level of distress over time to receive a diagnosis and fewer still will receive psychotherapy. Yet we often overlook the broader interventions, both before and after disasters, that are so important in helping individuals and communities heal.

DMH is not psychotherapy, and it can be very demanding work under trying conditions. Specific training is required, and not all clinicians will be interested in doing or prepared to do this work. It takes most psychotherapists out of their typical role, requires much patience (and no "patients"!), considerable flexibility, and a willingness to put the needs of not only the clients but also the organization ahead of one's own. It is important not to push services but rather to be available and reach out as survivors and fellow responders may be open to speaking and to accepting what DMH workers have to offer. Clinicians may become frustrated or disappointed, not feeling fully utilized or appreciated for their professional expertise.

This work requires the emergency mental health professional to follow the incident command system format and table of organization, something many mental health professionals may not find easy to do. "Stay in your lane" is an expression meant to highlight the importance of recognizing and adhering to one's role toward the more efficient and effective operation of a relief response. Not adhering to this precept may create resentments that leave people less open to receiving services and can interfere with the effective delivery of services. Particularly on national deployments, mental health clinicians may be subject to physical hardships, lack of usual comfort or good food, limited sleep, and much stress, along with financial concerns if they are volunteering for the deployment.

Mental health providers unaffiliated with a relief organization are often not wanted on a site, as they may have no expertise in DMH, have not been vetted in any way, and may interfere with the response operation. While undoubtedly well intentioned, such unaffiliated responders are not part of the incident command structure and may disrupt the organized delivery of services and confuse survivors. ARC does have a process, in some situations, for accepting event-based volunteers, which can be used to provide expedited yet partial vetting and training so they may be quickly deployed on a response. Remote DMH work by telephone is sometimes another option for professionals who cannot deploy to assist in the response. However, this is not the same as being there in person and limits situational awareness and the local knowledge base of the provider.

Volunteers do much of the short-term response work, and even people who are employed by response agencies are not likely to be well paid. Volunteers make up 90% of the ARC workforce, for example. It is not easy for someone with a full-time job and a family to find much time to devote to disaster response, especially if it means being away from home for an extended time. The ARC requires at least a 10-day commitment to a national deployment. Local responding may be more feasible for many clinicians but still requires a certain level of commitment and availability. The emotional toll can also be substantial, particularly in mass casualty incidents, so it is important for clinicians to recognize their own realities in deciding whether or not to do this work in general and also in response to any particular disaster. Most DMH responders will attest, however, that the work can be quite rewarding in spite of the difficulties and challenges.

While local clinics and other agencies often make staff available when disasters strike their communities, they are frequently underfunded and already busy, with long waiting lists. There are neither enough of them nor enough mental health staff, and, again, they have rarely engaged in the requisite training or planning. Even though DMH capacity is widely recognized as an important component of public health preparedness, one study found less than one third of public health departments even offer mental health services. Research in New York state following Hurricane Sandy found that a lack of staff trained to offer psychological services was a serious gap in the storm response (University of Albany, 2017). In addition, many local mental health providers may be affected by the disaster themselves, as may be the infrastructure in their area. In rural communities, readily available mental health resources may be few and far between (Everly et al., 2014).

It is also not uncommon for some tension to develop between local agencies and outside DMH responders related to roles and authority during the immediate response. In spite of the desire to assist in the short term and help connect residents to services for when they leave, out-of-area responders may be seen as interlopers trying to displace some local providers who naturally want to help. There may even be tension among the local and national responders within the same organization. However, as the local providers will be around for the long haul and may be affected by the event themselves, the outsiders can offer them a brief respite in the early days and refer clients to see them for the longer term. It is often true, however, that because of their training and extensive experience, major relief organizations and their personnel are more knowledgeable and skilled at the immediate steps and often prefer to exercise greater control of the initial operation. Effective collaboration is essential for optimal delivery of services yet is difficult if the groundwork has not been established beforehand, which is too often the case. Training and collaborating with other responders, such as rescue, health care, and spiritual care professionals, can expand the implementation of basic and early interventions to address psychosocial issues. Not understanding the functions of other disaster workers or coming to some agreements about prioritizing and sharing delivery of services may lead to tension or conflict among responders and confusion among clients, which will interfere with effective and efficient assistance.

Creating Cultural Competency

"Every disaster has a unique social ecology that influences perceptions and experiences before, during and after the disaster" (Miller, 2012, p. 8). Cultural histories, beliefs, and practices; economic infrastructure; dynamics related to status and power; and intra- and inter-group relations all affect reactions and response and even aspects of the event itself. For example, it was not simply an accident or coincidence that the lower Ninth Ward of New Orleans was the most affected area of the city from Hurricane Katrina. With little assistance directed there, at least initially, it has probably been the slowest neighborhood to rebuild. Lower-income residents often inhabit the most vulnerable areas, and civic resources are often arranged to favor the wealthier sections of a city. The residents have fewer sources of assistance to help mitigate and recover from the effects of the storm and often face cultural insensitivity in how aid is provided (Boyd-Franklin, 2010). Internationally, developing countries have more frequent and more destructive disasters than developed countries (CRED, 2017). They may be more vulnerable because poverty leads people to live in more exposed or dangerous areas, environmental planning in development is poor, and fewer warning or protection systems are in place.

Disaster responders tend to be middle-class or upper-middle-class and White (ARC, 2017; New York State Office of Mental Health, 2017), which means there is often a mismatch with people seeking assistance following disasters. In addition to race and socioeconomic status, ethnicity and nationality, language, religion, gender, sexual orientation, age, and developmental and ability functioning are all cultural factors that may influence one's interactions with others. Being aware and respectful of differences (as well as similarities) and being open to examining one's own background and perspectives are ongoing processes necessary to more effectively assist survivors. Responders need to learn more about the populations they will be encountering, through ongoing training and often by listening to survivors or other community members to ensure that services and information are provided in a culturally and linguistically appropriate manner (Boyd-Franklin, 2010; Miller, 2012). This also relates to the importance of planning and training to improve cultural knowledge, sensitivity, and collaboration.

Health and health care disparities, along with stigma regarding psychological disturbance, are often barriers to both provision and utilization of mental health services for many members of lower-income and minority communities. Concern about negative stereotypes regarding aspects of one's culture and about mental illness, histories of inadequate treatment (and worse), and limited knowledge about and expectations of effective treatment lead to mistrust of government and other agencies and resentment of outsiders (Boyd-Franklin, 2010). All of this may contribute to resistance to seeking help. Concerns about cost, including those related to time away from work or transportation and childcare expenses, also impede the ability as well as the inclination to utilize services. The ARC can provide some financial assistance to facilitate mental health services and it tries to make clear that it is independent of any government entities. For immigrants, concerns about the ramifications of speaking with even nongovernmental agencies, along with difficulty finding services in their language, may be real impediments to seeking assistance. In communities that largely consist of immigrants (and if responding in other countries), it is also important for responders to be aware of social and political hierarchies and customs related to culture and religion. In these situations, utilizing cultural intermediaries who speak the language and engender sufficient trust may be crucial (Halpern & Vermeulen, 2017).

For many cultural groups, religion and spirituality play a major role in their lives and may be more relevant in their reactions to disaster. Referring to and collaborating with chaplains or clergy may be more important than traditional psychological interventions at this time. The ARC has disaster spiritual care as a specialty working alongside DMH. Although still in development, this has proven to be a useful alliance in responding to communities where faith is a prominent part of the culture. A focus on extended family and community is often another component of many cultures that differs from the more typical Westernized individual orientation. In addition, many cultures have particular expressions of emotional and psychological distress and a reliance on traditional ways of healing that may appear unsettling to those unfamiliar with those practices (Miller, 2012).

Many disaster relief organizations, along with mental health associations, have guidelines and training on cultural competence and consider it an ethical responsibility for their members to develop (see the list of websites in the reference list). They also make efforts to diversify their workforce and membership and to actively collaborate with the members and leadership of the communities they serve.

Cultural considerations also apply to other populations at risk, including children, frail elderly, and those with disabilities, who may require special attention and consideration in all phases of disaster work (Halpern & Vermeulen, 2017). The ARC, in fact, has recently created a role for a disability integration specialist in disaster response.

First responders also have their own cultures. Not only are they exposed to some of the worst sights and situations imaginable, they may question or lament what they were or were not able to do in terms of rescuing or protecting civilians. In disasters, they often have to work long hours and be away from their families. This can all take a significant psychological toll, particularly in mass casualty incidents and especially if children are victims. Yet the ethos of being strong and stoic may make it hard for them to seek help; so do concerns about stigma, confidentiality, and how their job assignments might be affected. Fortunately, some literature indicates more openness to acknowledging and addressing emotional reactions among these groups. Utilization of trained peers in collaboration with the deployed mental health professionals has been quite helpful in this regard (Everly & Mitchell, 2008).

Effective Strategies and Empirically-Supported Treatments

The Disaster Scene: What to Expect

When disasters occur, aid is mobilized right away. Governmental agencies move to help as soon as they can. First responders are on the scene immediately, engaging in search and rescue, possibly assisted by state and national personnel, depending on the size and scope and type of disaster. Local resources, when and where available and if still functioning, spring into action to provide assistance.

Churches and community groups offer their buildings for shelters or assistance centers. People who can help step up to provide food, clothing, blankets, and other supplies to help take care of those affected and in need.

Regional, national, and even international organizations will deliver supplies and personnel to assist survivors, generally over the immediate and short term. The ARC, for example, will open and/or assist in managing shelters and assistance centers, provide food and supplies, and engage in outreach to the communities to help in any ways they can. This will include health services, mental health, and spiritual care. Services are offered to everyone affected by the incident, including those who respond to assist.

Most of the outside help is relatively short term, weeks, even days, or possibly a few months in situations with more extreme and extensive destruction. It is designed to assist populations in addressing their most significant needs through the most disruptive time period. In addition to material supports, this will include efforts to connect people with family and friends and to local resources, and possibly to help build capacity for communities to continue moving forward in their recovery (Miller, 2012). The aim is to enhance people's natural abilities to cope in the present and future.

Not surprisingly, reactions to disasters cover the range of human functioning—physical, cognitive, emotional, behavioral, and spiritual (Halpern & Tramontin, 2007; Miller, 2012; NIEHS, 2015)—and they will differ among individuals and within individuals over time. Yet many reactions are to be expected. Aside from potential injury, survivors may experience shock and a host of somatic reactions, including palpitations, sweating, shaking, restlessness, fatigue, difficulty breathing, pain, biochemical changes, and weakened immune systems. They may be disoriented or confused and have difficulty with memory, clear thinking, or decision making and problem solving. They may feel fearful and anxious, sad, angry, vulnerable, guilty, overwhelmed, or out of control. Behaviors may be tearful, irritable, hyper-vigilant, isolating, or erratic. Disturbances in appetite, sleep, activity level, substance use, and self-care may be present. People may question their purpose or meaning in life or their religious views (ARC, 2017a&b, 2018).

In spite of strong initial reactions and distress, most people will be quite resilient over time (Bonanno, 2004; NIEHS, 2015), though many will have some long-term effects that may impair functioning, even if they do not constitute a diagnosable disorder. Early interventions are generally designed to help survivors utilize and build upon their natural resources and resilience. They can help people cope more effectively in the immediate aftermath and reduce the likelihood of persistent and more severe sequelae (Fox et al., 2012; SAMHSA/ARC, 2015; Watson, 2017). Yet even a small percentage of survivors with longer-term impairment will mean there will be a significant demand for intervention over time, especially for diagnosed disorders such as ASD, PTSD, depression, anxiety, and sometimes overwhelming grief. It is important to pay attention to and make referrals for these people as well (Halpern & Vermeulen, 2017).

Elements of the disaster combine with personal characteristics and experiences, as well as with aspects of the response itself, to determine the ongoing reactions of any individual survivor (Benedek & Wynn, 2017; Halpern & Vermeulen, 2017; Joshi & Cerda, 2017). One's strengths and vulnerabilities, preexisting conditions and circumstances, history of other disasters or trauma, coping styles and support networks, and education and financial resources are all important. Proximity and level of exposure to the event and the degree of personal loss will also influence post-disaster functioning (ARC, 2017a; Miller, 2012; World Health Organization, 2011).

Regarding the response, relevant issues include the degree of resources and planning that were developed prior to an event, along with the scope and effectiveness of the initial response from municipal, state, and perhaps national governments, as well as from nongovernmental agencies (Halpern & Tramontin, 2007). The extent, intrusiveness, and duration of the media presence may also be a factor (Halpern & Vermeulen, 2017). In some cases, communities will galvanize to protect survivors and mourners from being filmed or photographed in their time of grief. Yet some individuals may want to express their thoughts and feelings publicly (Applebome & Stelter, 2012).

Disasters differ in many respects that are important to consider in responding. The size and scope of the destruction includes the extent of damage and the number of people affected, as well as the length of the disaster itself and of the recovery process. This will determine the number of responders and amount of resources that may be required, as well as the ability to place them in the location and the duration of the response. Whether or not the event was expected and, if so, the period of warning and steps available and taken will also have an impact. These affect the possibility of pre-positioning supplies and personnel, the number of casualties, and the reactions of survivors based on the degree to which they did or did not respond to the warnings. Even the season and the time of day may be quite salient, as related to weather conditions and to where people are located when the disaster strikes (e.g., at school or work, at home, with family members together or apart).

Of great relevance will be the cause or causes. Events caused by human behavior, in whole or in part, are likely to lead to much greater psychological distress over a longer period of time (ARC, 2017b; Halpern & Vermeulen, 2017; Miller, 2012; NIEHS, 2015; although see North, 2017, for an alternative view), as are those in which more people have died. This is especially true of intentional infliction of mass casualties. More intense and extended grief, anger, and blame, as well as ongoing or renewed trauma due to media coverage or if legal proceedings ensue, may all be expected in these cases. The experience of a DMH responder is often quite different—for example, working in shelters for those displaced by hurricanes or flooding as compared to family assistance centers or other settings following a mass shooting or a transportation accident. Not only specific tasks and functions but also the whole emotional overlay of the experience will reflect the nature of the event and the response. Mass casualty incidents will have a much greater proportion of mental health responders than natural disasters.

Today the ARC has some 5,000 DMH volunteers (Halpern & Vermeulen, 2017), and there are many other organizations that provide disaster relief and/or training and information for responders. Quite a few of them incorporate mental health services into their response (e.g., Green Cross, Medical Reserve Corps), as well as education for survivors and responders regarding reactions to disasters and how to address them (these include the International Society for Traumatic Stress Studies, the National Child Traumatic Stress Network, the New York State Office of Mental Health, SAMHSA, and many others). Many local mental health services do exist that will respond to the needs of their communities to the best of their ability, should disaster strike. While a focus on trauma-informed treatment has become fairly widespread, this is not the same thing as knowledge and experience in treating survivors of large-scale disasters (SAMHSA, 2015). It is important to note that while providing a range of psychosocial supports to survivors is certainly valuable, this includes acknowledging and promoting the natural resilience of most people as a crucial element of disaster response (ARC, 2017a, 2018). We are primarily there to help people help themselves.

Interventions and Phases of Disasters

Most discussions of disasters refer to phases—before, during, and after; or threat/warning, impact, rescue, and reconstruction (Das-Brailsford, 2010); or prepare, respond, and recover (ARC, 2018; SAMHSA/ARC, 2015). Following a disaster, reactions and response will vary in the immediate, short term, and longer term. During the event, more dramatic reactions will occur that may both help and hinder one's functioning. In the midst of great shock and horror, some people take heroic actions in the rescue phase. A honeymoon phase often follows in which expressions of gratitude and optimism may be present along with efforts to assist one another. With the recognition that recovery will be long and difficult, this gives way to disillusionment, accompanied by distress, frustration, anger, blame, sadness, and grief. Then comes the long road to recovery, with greater acceptance and integration of the event and its consequences, as well as rebuilding of lives and communities (ARC, 2017a; SAMHSA/ARC, 2015). It will be here that many more serious psychological diagnoses will come to the fore.

While there is not always a clear delineation, interventions are generally related to the phases in the disaster cycle.

Critical Incident Responses

Initial responses focus on addressing basic needs and safety. Food, water, shelter, information, and organization, as well as other forms of assistance that can be provided under difficult circumstances, are crucial first steps. Helping survivors to feel safe and to connect with family members and other social supports and community resources helps them use their natural strengths in service of self and collective empowerment. The ARC, for example, will pre-position people and supplies when possible, and otherwise respond immediately to disasters. Much of the early DMH work involves providing material comfort (often water and blankets) and direction. Simply making contact and being a calm, kind, and compassionate presence helps to stabilize those directly affected. "Water therapy," just handing a bottle of water to someone, can provide an initial connection and possible opening for more conversation. The ARC frequently provides an emergency response vehicle with hot coffee and food to support first responders as well as clients at disaster scenes, vigils, or memorial services. The goal is to provide comfort and to facilitate recovery and healing in disaster survivors and others affected (ARC, 2018).

Surveying the situation, gathering what accurate information is available (and sharing it with survivors if appropriate), making brief assessments, and considering triage when necessary are all vital first steps in implementing mental health interventions, the most basic of which is PFA. This is taught to all ARC volunteers and is a prominent component of education in other organizations as well (e.g., Institute for Disaster Mental Health, National Child Traumatic Stress Network, New York State Office of Mental Health, SAMHSA).

The Interagency Standing Committee of the United Nations (2007) suggests an intervention pyramid for mental health and psychosocial support in emergencies. The base consists of security and basic needs, followed by strengthening family and community supports. Then come focused supports that may be provided individually or in small groups by non-specialized workers who have been trained and supervised. This would include PFA and psychosocial interventions by general health services staff. Given that the great need outstrips the capacity of available mental health professionals, teaching PFA to all responders and even to other community members has become increasingly important. The ARC also collaborates with health service and spiritual care providers. At the top of the pyramid are the specialized services of professional mental health clinicians that may be directly required for the small percentage of people who have significant symptomatology or impairment or who are at greater risk thereof (Interagency Standing Committee, 2007; Miller, 2012).

PFA, as its name implies, is a knowledge base and set of tools (many of which are mentioned above) that responders can use in the early phases of a disaster to assist survivors and first responders in managing and reducing stressful reactions and fostering more effective coping. Often-cited key elements of disaster responding include fostering a sense of safety, calming, facilitating connectedness and self and group efficacy, and instilling hope (Hobfoll et al., 2007; Miller, 2012; Watson, 2017). Such early intervention may also reduce post-disaster symptoms and impairments (Birkhead & Vermeulen, 2018; North, 2017; Watson, 2017). While controlled studies are difficult to conduct in disaster settings, considerable support exists for elements of PFA, including enhancing coping, social support, and problem solving (Foa et al., 2009). In addition, substantial experience and expert opinion lead PFA to be considered an "evidence-informed" intervention (Fox et al., 2012, p. 251). Further support for early intervention comes from research on treating service members in combat zones using the principles of proximity, immediacy, and expectations (Everly & Mitchell, 2008). In those circumstances, the more quickly treatment can be provided close to the front and with expectations of return to duty, the more likely warriors are to do so. While one does not have to be a mental health professional to provide PFA, for other responders, knowing when and how to make a referral to DMH workers is an important component.

The basic skills of PFA, after ensuring safety and basic needs, include empathic listening and attending as survivors talk about their experiences and circumstances; knowing what reactions and risk and resilience factors to look for; staying in the present; providing realistic reassurance and accurate information; and ending conversations so one can move on to assist others. Regulating one's own reactions, remaining calm, and maintaining boundaries are also important, as is knowing what *not* to say or do. Well-meaning responders may want to help survivors feel better and, perhaps unwittingly, to feel better themselves. Efforts to get people to talk about their experience before they are ready, or comments that include unrealistic reassurance or expectations, comparative or self-referenced, and irrelevant diversions are not helpful and may cause harm. One cannot undo the calamities that many survivors are facing. Responders can only help them bear the burdens and let them know they are not alone, buttress their natural strengths, and impart hope.

Mental health professionals offer a higher level of intervention, which includes crisis intervention and psychoeducation components, as well as connections and referrals to local services that will be able to further assess and assist clients over the longer term or for those who need a higher level of immediate assessment and care. They can help survivors recognize that their reactions are typical and to be expected in the face of such events and assist them in understanding and utilizing positive coping skills and techniques. They also provide guidance on dealing with children and family members or with particularly difficult situations.

DMH workers will be active in providing crisis intervention and an enhanced PFA and will assist in other functions as well. Understanding and collaborating in other relief tasks is a good way to make connections with survivors and especially with other responders whom DMH clinicians are also there to serve. Outreach is often an important component as well. Going to community centers, houses of worship, schools, police and fire facilities, small business establishments, and even door to door in hard-hit neighborhoods allows providers to assess and assist a wide range of the affected public and to collaborate with community leaders.

Again, the ARC stresses that DMH workers are not to do psychotherapy or formal psychological assessments or diagnosing in disaster responding. Reasons for this include the difficult conditions and the limits on privacy, time, and number of contacts with clients, which may not allow for sufficient information, informed consent, building an alliance, or ensuring follow-up (ARC, 2018). In fact, establishing too close a relationship with a client might lead to yet another experience of loss when the responder leaves. Disaster mental health professionals are there to provide immediate relief and to assist and collaborate with local agencies, not to stand in their stead.

Preparation and Planning

Too often, communities overlook or lack the resources for building effective capacity to respond to disasters. Just as, sadly, many schools today hold active shooter drills in case such a potential (yet still unlikely) tragedy might occur, preparation can be vital (ARC, 2017a, 2018; Halpern & Tramontin, 2007; Watson, 2017). Mental health professionals have multiple roles to play in planning at every step. Educating responders and the public on likely psychological reactions to various situations and useful steps in addressing them will help promote coping during and after an incident. Printed and online materials can be prepared and disseminated. Integrating mental health considerations and psychoeducation into all components of response will result in more efficient overall management. It can be crucial for emergency managers to consider human factors that often affect what may seem to make sense structurally. A recent example at a county planning meeting was a discussion that parents will quickly become aware from social media of any incident at a school and will flock to see if their children are OK. This must be anticipated to avoid interference with the response by police, firefighters, and emergency medical services.

This is also the stage of trying to ensure that adequate psychological services will be available and effectively allocated when needed. Local health and mental health agencies and providers can collaborate to arrange for training and to create a plan for cooperation in a response. Representatives from relief organizations can assist with this and establish relationships that can be very valuable in the event of a disaster. Tabletop exercises and actual simulation drills are vital components. The ARC sponsors drills in anticipating incidents at airports, schools, public events, and a nuclear facility and general environmental events such as earthquakes and hurricanes. These experiences are realistic and quite helpful when responding to a real disaster.

Recovery

As has been noted, particularly without more extensive disaster mental health interventions, a significant minority of survivors are likely to experience psychological disorders in the weeks and months (and years) following disaster experiences. These include ASD, PTSD, depression, complicated grief, and substance use disorders. While it is beyond the scope of this chapter to discuss these in depth, research has supported a number of effective treatments for these disorders, primarily including cognitive behavioral and interpersonal approaches. Prolonged exposure therapy, cognitive processing therapy, and eye movement desensitization and reprocessing considered evidence-based treatments for ASD and PTSD, as are some medications (particularly serotonin and serotonin/norepinephrine reuptake inhibitors) (Benedek & Wynn, 2017; Foa et al., 2005, 2009; SAMHSA, 2014).

Mind–body techniques (Gordon, 2013; SAMHSA, 2014) have shown utility in treating trauma and may be briefly used in DMH for stress reduction. Group therapy (Dembert & Simmer, 2000; Sloan & Beck, 2016) also has support in treating trauma if particular attention is paid to the composition of the groups, the timing, and the structure of the group process. Critical incident stress debriefing, which was designed to be delivered in the short term following a disaster, remains controversial, as evidence for its efficacy is limited and possible negative effects have been noted (Bisson et al., 2009). At this point, critical incident stress debriefing is generally not recommended in disaster response and is specifically prohibited in ARC interventions. Yet some broader principles of critical incident stress management, employed over a longer term, seem to have more adherents, particularly to work with preexisting or spontaneous groups that have closely shared exposure and experiences (Everly & Mitchell, 2008, Foa et al., 2009; Halpern & Vermeulen, 2017).

Again, these formal treatments are not the province of DMH, as they require multiple and more structured sessions and ongoing relationships with clinicians; however, some elements of these interventions may be helpful in the response phase for people at significant risk of developing disorders. For the most part, cognitive behavioral techniques have empirical support in treating trauma, yet these therapies require more time, and appropriately trained clinicians are in limited supply. Use of cognitive behavioral therapy in acute disaster situations has not been well studied, although some aspects of it are commonly utilized in PFA and DMH, such as psychoeducation, problem solving, and stress reduction. Monitoring people affected by trauma incidents to identify those who may be most in need of more extended follow-up treatment can be an important service (Brymer et al., 2009; Litz & Bryant, 2009).

Grief and mourning may be significant following disasters, especially those involving mass casualties, and those survivors may benefit from more ongoing intervention. Not only have people lost loved ones, but their social support systems and physical environments may also be disrupted. What is usually more private mourning becomes very public. This can all impede some of the typical rituals around death and loss. DMH responders may assist by bearing witness and listening to the stories of the bereaved. They attend vigils and memorials that often arise spontaneously as well as being organized by local community groups and are so important for collective healing. This may also include assistance in planning such events so they may be more healing and inclusive and to increase awareness and attention over the long term, such as anniversary reactions. Clinicians may visit those in mourning and even attend funerals, if invited. Simply being present and providing information and sometimes guidance are much appreciated (ARC, 2017b; Dass-Brailsford, 2010; Halpern & Vermeulen, 2017).

Self-Care for the DMH Responder

As noted earlier, disaster work can take a significant toll on the provider. The ability to assist others is largely based on one's own well-being, so taking care of oneself is a priority stressed by relief organizations. In addition to being potentially subject to some of the same effects of trauma as survivors, DMH workers are at risk of secondary trauma, compassion fatigue, and burnout (Figley, 2005; New York State Office of Mental Health, 2017). Yet they are often not so good at taking their own advice. The desire to be of service to others and the situational pressures on a response, unrealistic beliefs about one's own ability to resist or cope with the stress, concern about how one may be seen by colleagues, and the powerful feeling of being a part of something much larger than oneself may all lead to ignoring or "postponing" sufficient attention to the very human needs of the DMH professional.

Living and working conditions on a response may make it difficult to exercise, eat well, find private space, or engage in recreation. Spending some time with colleagues, away from clients, and having a sense of humor even amidst the difficult circumstances can be helpful. Keeping in touch with friends and family is important to remain grounded and not let the disaster take over one's own life. Some of the same traits important in working with others may be applicable to taking good care of oneself. These include being flexible and genuine, as opposed to rigidly maintaining a "professional" barrier, finding some enjoyment in the work, and being creative about exercise (running laps around a motel parking lot, for example). Many find comfort from the therapy dogs that may be brought by some groups after disasters and also from local spiritual care providers. I believe that relief organizations should pay more active attention to these issues during and after a response. Designating DMH personnel specifically to attend to staff can improve the functioning and well-being of many responders.

Future Steps

Sadly, as both natural and human-caused disasters become more frequent and affect more people, responding to the psychological and social effects on survivors is becoming an ever more important component for the mental health professions. Based on early efforts at research and the accumulation of significant experience at this point, evidence has led to a considerable degree of consensus on what may be helpful. Yet much more remains to be done. The unpredictability and chaotic nature of disasters make well-designed research difficult. Yet, providing advanced training and preparation to arrange for studies and interventions will make them more likely (Brymer et al., 2009). More efforts are underway to do this and to enhance the resilience and recovery of individuals and communities (Birkhead & Vermeulen, 2018). Mental health professionals have much to offer and are committed to assisting others. With greater efforts to make them aware of the opportunities and need related to disaster preparedness and response, and if more training were provided, more would step up to meet the challenge.

The first step is serious and extensive planning and outreach, to include as many potential resources as possible that will agree to play a role and collaborate before, during, and after an incident. Anticipating human factors, maintaining clear lines of communication, educating the public about plans, and disseminating useful, accurate information are also important aspects of preparation as well as in the response and recovery phases of a disaster. Tabletop exercises and practice drills are vital components of effective preparation. This is also the period to offer training in PFA to all those who may respond, as well as to implement training in DMH and in evidence-based, trauma-focused psychotherapies to local mental health professionals.

When a disaster strikes, and in the immediate warning period if there is one, having DMH responders available will allow for quickly assisting the public in anticipating and coping with likely reactions and in marshaling their individual and collective resources and for providing crisis intervention and connections to other services when indicated. Along with addressing physical safety and basic needs, this can be crucial in improving their capacity to manage and to recover. Advocacy on behalf of survivors may also be an important service when needed.

In the longer term, continuing to provide information and access to services in the community remains important, particularly for those who suffered the most significant losses. In addition, having local mental health resources prepared to offer affordable psychotherapy for trauma-related conditions is needed to address those who are experiencing the greatest impairment in recovery. Greater funding is required so more communities have greater access to mental health services in general.

Public education as primary prevention, along with PFA and psychoeducation to survivors, combined with cultural awareness and competence in delivery of all services, can help reduce client barriers to obtaining assistance. The overall reduction of stigma regarding psychological difficulties and the promotion of greater socioeconomic equity are tall orders for society, yet we can each do our part as mental health professionals and as citizens. Disaster response agencies can also do more to promote the importance of DMH services and, not incidentally, to make sure that their DMH responders take care of themselves and one another.

Finally, it is hoped that this chapter may play a small role in promoting the involvement of more mental health providers in this type of work. Acknowledging the sacrifices and challenges, and recognizing that it is not for everyone, this can be a remarkably enriching path.

References

American Red Cross. (2017a). *Psychological first aid instructor manual.* Washington, DC: American Red Cross.

American Red Cross. (2017b). *Reference guide—Supplemental information for the disaster mental health program.* Washington, DC: American Red Cross.

American Red Cross. (2018). *Disaster mental health fundamentals—Part I instructor manual.* Washington, DC: American Red Cross.

Applebome, P., & Stelter, B. (2012, December 16). Media spotlight seen as a blessing, or a curse, in a grieving town. *New York Times.* Retrieved from www.nytimes.com/2012/12/17/business/media/newtown-has-mixed-feelings-about-the-media-horde-in-its-midst.html

Benedek, D. M., & Wynn, G. H. (2017). Acute stress disorder and posttraumatic stress disorder. In R. J. Ursano, C. S. Fullerton, L. Weisaeth, & B. Raphael (Eds.), *Textbook of disaster psychiatry* (2nd ed., pp. 101–123). New York, NY: Cambridge University Press.

Birkhead, G. S., & Vermeulen, K. (2018). Sustainability of psychological first aid training for the disaster workforce. *American Journal of Public Health*, 108(S5), S381–S382.

Bisson, J. I., McFarlane, A. C., Rose, S., Ruzek, J. I., & Watson, P. J. (2009). Psychological debriefing for adults. In E. Foa, E. M. Keane, M. J. Friedman, & J. A. Cohen (Eds.), *Effective treatments for PTSD* (pp. 83–105). New York, NY: Guilford Press.

Bonanno, G. A. (2004). Loss, trauma, and human resilience. *American Psychologist*, *59*(1), 20–28.

Boyd-Franklin, N. (2010). Families affected by Hurricane Katrina and other disasters: Learning from the experiences of African American survivors. In P. Dass-Brailsford (Ed.), *Crisis and disaster counseling: Lessons learned from Hurricane Katrina and other disasters* (pp. 67–82). Los Angeles, CA: Sage.

Brymer, M. J., Steinberg, A. M., Vernberg, E. M., Layne, C. M., Watson, P. J., Jacobs, A., . . . Pynoos, R. S. (2009). Acute interventions for children and adolescents. In E. Foa, E. M. Keane, M. J. Friedman, & J. A. Cohen (Eds.), *Effective treatments for PTSD* (pp. 106–116). New York, NY: Guilford Press.

Center for Research on the Epidemiology of Disasters. (2018). *Natural disasters 2017*. Brussels: CRED.

Center for Research on the Epidemiology of Disasters. (2018). *Economic losses, poverty and disasters 1998–2017*. Brussels: CRED.

Dass-Brailsford, P. (Ed.). (2010). *Crisis and disaster counseling: Lessons learned from Hurricane Katrina and other disasters*. Los Angeles, CA: Sage.

Dembert, M. L., & Simmer, E. D. (2000). When trauma affects a community: Group interventions and support after a disaster. In R. H. Klein & V. L. Schermer (Eds.), *Group psychotherapy for psychological trauma* (pp. 239–264). New York, NY: Guilford Press.

Everly, G. S., & Lating, J. M. (2017). The Johns Hopkins guide to psychological first aid. Baltimore, MD: Johns Hopkins University Press.

Everly, G. S., McCabe, O. L., Semon, N. L., Thompson, C. B., & Links, J. M. (2014). The development of a model of psychological first aid for non-mental health trained public health personnel: The Johns Hopkins RAPID-PFA. *Journal of Public Health Management Practice*, *20*(5), S24–S29.

Everly, G. S., & Mitchell, J. T. (2008). *Integrative crisis intervention and disaster mental health*. Ellicott City, MD: Chevron Publishing Corporation.

Figley, C. R. (2005, Oct. 17). Compassion fatigue: An expert interview with Charles R. Figley. *Medscape*. Retrieved from https://www.medscape.com/viewarticle/513615

Foa, E. B., Cahill, S. P., Boscarino, J. A., Hobfoll, S. E., Lahad, M., McNally, R. J., & Solomon, Z. (2005). Social, psychological, and psychiatric interventions following terrorist attacks: Recommendations for practice and research. *Neuropsychopharmacology*, *30*, 1806–1817.

Foa, E., Keane, T. M., Friedman, M. J., & Cohen, J. A. (2009). *Effective treatments for PTSD*. New York, NY: Guilford Press.

Fox, J. H., Burkle Jr, F. M., Bass, J., Pia, F. A., Epstein, J. L., & Markenson, D. (2012). The effectiveness of psychological first aid as a disaster intervention tool: Research analysis of peer-reviewed literature from 1990-2010. *Disaster Medicine and Public Health Preparedness*, *6*(3), 247–253.

Gordon, J. (2013, April 25). Center for Mind Body Medicine. Presentation at Albert Einstein College of Medicine, New York, NY.

Halpern, J., & Tramontin, M. (2007). *Disaster mental health: Theory and practice*. Belmont, CA: Thompson Brooks/Cole.

Halpern, J., & Vermeulen, K. (2017). *Disaster mental health interventions: Core principles and practices*. New York, NY: Routledge.

Hobfoll, S., Watson, P., Bell, C., Bryant, R., Brymer, M., Friedman, M., . . . Ursano, R. J. (2007). Five essential elements of immediate and mid-term mass trauma intervention: Empirical evidence. *Psychiatry, 70*(4), 283–315.

Inter-Agency Standing Committee. (2007). *IASC guidelines on mental health and psychosocial support in emergency settings*. Geneva: IASC.

Joshi, S., & Cerda, M. (2017). Trajectories of health, resilience, and illness. In R. J. Ursano, C. S. Fullerton, L. Weisaeth, & B. Raphael (Eds.), *Textbook of disaster psychiatry* (2nd ed., pp. 76–86). New York, NY: Cambridge University Press.

Knapp, K. C. (2010). Children and crises. In P. Das-Brailsford (Ed.), *Crisis and disaster counseling: Lessons learned from Hurricane Katrina and other disasters* (pp. 83–98). Los Angeles, CA: Sage.

Litz, B. T., & Bryant, R. A. (2009). Early cognitive-behavioral interventions for adults. In E. Foa, E. M. Keane, M. J. Friedman, & J. A. Cohen (Eds.), *Effective treatments for PTSD* (pp. 117–135). New York, NY: Guilford Press.

Miller, J. L. (2012). *Psychosocial capacity building in response to disasters*. New York, NY: Columbia University Press.

National Institute for Environmental Health Services. (2015). *Care provider's role: Disaster workers behavioral health care*. Washington, DC: NIEHS.

New York State Office of Mental Health. (2017). Long-term impact of disaster response on counselors. *NY DMH Responder*, 22(3), 8–9.

North, C. S. (2017). Epidemiology of disaster mental health: The foundation for disaster mental health response. In R. J. Ursano, C. S. Fullerton, L. Weisaeth, & B. Raphael (Eds.), *Textbook of disaster psychiatry* (2nd ed., pp. 27–43). New York, NY: Cambridge University Press.

Substance Abuse and Mental Health Services Administration. (2014). *Trauma-informed care in behavioral health services*. Treatment improvement protocol (TIP) Series 57. HHS Publication No. (SMA) 13-4801. Rockville, MD: Author.

SAMHSA/ARC. (2015, June 18). A mental health response to disaster. Presentation. Retrieved from https://www.mentalhealthamerica.net/sites/default/files/MHA%20Disaster%20MH%20All.pdf

Sloan, D. M., & Beck, J. G. (2016) Group treatment for PTSD. *PTSD Research Quarterly, 27*(2), 1–4.

University of Albany Center for Public Preparedness & State University of New York, New Paltz, Institute for Disaster Mental Health. (2017). *Psychological first aid training coordinator guide*. Albany, NY: University of Albany.

Watson, P. J. (2017). Early interventions for trauma-related problems. In R. J. Ursano, C. S. Fullerton, L. Weisaeth, & B. Raphael. *Textbook of disaster psychiatry* (2nd ed., pp. 87–100). New York, NY: Cambridge University Press.

Weine, S., Danieli, Y., Silove, D., Van Ommeren, M., Fairbank, J. A., & Saul, J. (2002). Guidelines for international training in mental health and psychosocial interventions for trauma-exposed populations in clinical and community settings. *Psychiatry, 65*(2), 156–164.

World Health Organization. (2011). *Psychological first aid: Guide for field workers*. Geneva: WHO.

Websites with Information and Training Materials on DMH

American Psychiatric Association—www.psychiatry.org
American Psychological Association—www.apa.org
American Red Cross—www.redcross.org
Centers for Disease Control and Prevention—https://emergency.cdc.gov/, https://www.cdc.gov
Center for the Study of Traumatic Stress (part of Uniformed Services University)—https://www.cstsonline.org/
Green Cross—https://greencross.org/International Critical Incident Stress Foundation—https://icisf.org/
International Society for Traumatic Stress Studies—https://www.istss.org/
National Child Traumatic Stress Network—https://www.nctsn.org/
Office of Homeland Security—www.ready.gov
Substance Abuse and Mental Health Services Administration—https://www.samhsa.gov/
U.S. Department of Veterans Affairs—www.ptsd.va.gov
World Health Organization, Interagency Standing Committee—http://www.who.int/mental_health/emergencies/guidelines_iasc_mental_health_psychosocial_june_2007.pdf

SECTION 2

UNDERSERVED DUE TO DISCRIMINATION

4

Serving the Underserved

Delivering Culturally Appropriate Psychotherapy to Racial and Ethnic Minorities

Changming Duan

Much organizational as well as individual effort in the field of psychotherapy has been made toward eliminating racial/ethnic disparities in psychological care and delivering equitable and quality therapeutic services to racial/ethnic minorities in the United States. Over the past few decades, significant progress has been made in understanding the issue at hand and in motivating psychotherapy clinicians to pursue equity, justice, and parity for all people. However, substantial challenges remain, and people of color in the United States are still underserved or inadequately served in mental health (American Psychological Association [APA], 2016).

This state of affairs should alarm and trouble the psychotherapy community and individual psychotherapists, both in our sense of professional responsibility and consciousness as helping professionals. Due to the fact that we are part of the cultural and societal contexts that are less than favorable or even hostile toward racial/ethnic minorities, we should commit to taking actions contributing to the work necessary to change the current situation of disparity. In reality, we either help racial/ethnic minorities by bringing culturally effective services to them or harm them by not attending to their psychological needs. We should understand that either providing no service or delivering harmful service that does not empower them but further marginalizes them is not acceptable.

The links between mental health and individual demographic characteristics, including race and ethnicity, have long been observed (Sue & Sue, 2016). The general stereotypical perception is that people of color are more likely to suffer from mental illness, are more in need of help, and are less likely to receive help. Empirical evidence informs the mental health community that an unhealthy environment tends to lead to unhealthy mental or psychological experiences (Schmidt, 2007), that disordered conditions may lead to disordered behavior (Keizer, Lindenberg, & Steg, 2008), and that "mental illness, diagnoses and associated concepts are social constructions" (Walker, 2006, p. 71). Consequently, it should be clear to all of us who are psychotherapists and mental health professionals that it is not the minority status per se, but the social treatments and conditions associated with people's demographics, that cause those individuals' psychological difficulties and concerns. A number of studies have demonstrated that sociocultural factors play significant roles in mental illness (e.g., Hsieh & Kirk, 2005; Tew, 2011; Vargas, Clemente, & Mayoral, 2016) and in its recovery (Tew et al., 2011; Walker, 2006). However, this knowledge does not seem to have been adequately integrated into clinicians' thinking or psychotherapy theories and practices.

To address how we can help reduce and ideally eliminate racial disparity in mental health care, we have to understand how this disparity exists, why it is challenging to correct this situation, and what our responsibilities as individual psychotherapists are in making changes both in the systems of health care and in how we can provide culturally effective psychotherapy to those who have been marginalized by society. Effective efforts need to be built upon the understanding that psychological problems

> do not exist on their own, nor do they come out of thin air; they are connected to people`s social support, employment status, housing conditions, history of discrimination and overall personal and political power . . . promoting complete health means promoting social justice, for there cannot be health in the absence of justice. (Prilleltensky, 1999, p. 106)

Thus, we need to address broader contextual issues, such as the influence of the system of privilege and oppression, as well as how we can develop and enhance our willingness to serve and our cultural competence in serving ethnic minority clients effectively.

The Scope and Description of the Problem

There is little dispute that racial/ethnic disparities in mental health services, defined as "inequalities in access to good mental health professionals, differences in insurance coverage, or discrimination by health professionals in the clinical encounter" (McGuire & Miranda, 2008, p. 393), exist and are in fact quite common in the United States (Smedley, Stith, & Nelson, 2003). The supplement to the 2001 Report by the U.S. Surgeon General detailed the evidence of unfair treatment of racial/ethnic minorities in *access* and *use* of mental health services (Substance Abuse and Mental Health Services Administration, 2001). In 2012, more than a decade after the Surgeon General's report, a national survey revealed that

> In the decade since the Surgeon General's landmark publication, its basic findings of striking disparities for minorities in mental health services have not changed. . . . Racial/ethnic minorities still have less access to mental health services than whites, and when they receive care, it is more likely to be of poorer quality. (Bussing & Gary, 2012, p. 663)

Most recently, a series of meta-analyses drawing on data from more than 4.7 million clients in 130 studies revealed that racial/ethnic discrepancies are still substantial (Smith & Trimble, 2016). The result of the analysis also provided evidence that confronted the assumption that racial disparity was mainly caused by differences in income and health insurance, and demonstrated that race is an equally independent predictor of disparity in access to mental health treatment.

When individuals' racial/ethnic backgrounds become "reasons" for lack of access to quality mental health service, gross social injustice is present and the society faces serious problems. Both in historical contexts and the current social reality within the United States, legalized (Takaki, 1993) subtle forms of racial/ethnic discrimination (Deitch et al., 2003) have persisted in all areas of life. This presents a disparaging and reproachful environment for racial/ethnic minorities, who are more likely to suffer from stressors such as poverty and violence than are mainstream cultural group members (Reeves, Rodrigue, & Kneebone, 2016). Such harsh conditions weigh heavily in psychological experiences of racial/ethnic minorities, and at the same time deter quality professional service from being delivered to them.

Mental disorders are no more prevalent among ethnic minorities than among whites; in fact, there is evidence that minority groups tend to have lower rates of mental disorders than whites (McGuire & Miranda, 2008). However, as McGuire and Miranda report, "those who become ill tend to have more persistent disorders" (p. 394), "have less access to mental health services," and are "less likely than whites to receive the best available treatments" (p. 396). Further, when they do receive treatment, "rather than feeling that they have been provided benefits, clients often feel invalidated, abused, misunderstood, and oppressed by their providers" (Sue, 2003, p. 5). Using financial input as an indicator, McGuire and Miranda report that the available data from the Institute of Medicine showed that the overall spending for outpatient mental health care for blacks and Latinos is "about 60% and 75% of spending rates for whites, respectively, after taking into account need for care" (p. 396).

Various mechanisms contributing to such mental health disparity have been identified and discussed, including systemic, financial, therapist, client, community, and other factors. At the systemic level, the nation's policies in economic structures and health insurance have a significant role in keeping people who are in poverty from receiving needed psychological services.

American poverty is still primarily among people of color. As reported by the National Poverty Center at the University of Michigan (2009), one of every three African American children and one of every four Latino children live in poverty; residents of a predominately black or Hispanic neighborhood have access to roughly half as many social services as those in predominately white neighborhoods; and states with more Blacks and Hispanics on welfare are more likely to impose lifetime limits, family caps on benefits, and stricter sanctions for noncompliance.

The financial disadvantages led to the high uninsured rates among people of color. According to the report by the Henry J. Kaiser Family Foundation (2017), even after activation of the Affordable Care Act, over 27 million people stayed uninsured in 2016. Among them, Hispanics and Blacks have significantly higher uninsured rates (16.9% and 11.7%, respectively) than Whites (7.6%), and the top reason reported for being uninsured was cost. This is an issue that directly relates to the nation's health care policies and structures. This social reality has obviously contributed to psychotherapy services being kept away from racial minorities and raises our awareness that delivering psychotherapy to underserved populations is not exempt from the influence of the nation's politics. Social justice is the foundation for fair distribution of resources, including psychotherapy service.

A noticeable fact directly linked to lack of access by racial/ethnic minorities is that not enough psychotherapists choose or are able to practice in areas where minority groups are concentrated. The National Survey of Psychology Health Service Providers (APA, 2015) showed that nearly half of practicing psychologists (44.8%) worked in private-practice settings and most frequently saw White/Caucasian clients (96%) in a one-on-one format. There are safety, financial feasibility, and other reasons for this situation, because the social, cultural, and economic stratification in society has created and sustained segregation along various visible and invisible lines, including race/ethnicity and poverty. Further, there has been significant underrepresentation of people of color in the psychology workforce as well as an unbalanced distribution of these professionals in terms of geographic locations (APA, 2015). What these situations translate to is that access to mental health care varies and disadvantages people of color and those who live in poor neighborhoods.

Barriers to Service Delivery

Besides the systemic and financial obstacles, the underutilization of psychotherapy by racial/ethnic minorities is a significant barrier to mental health racial parity. To address this aspect of the disparity, psychotherapists have much to learn and reflect on. Research has shown a low acceptance level of psychotherapy, as it is practiced in our society, among the racial/ethnic diverse groups. In the United States, stigma and negative attitudes toward psychotherapy exist in all ethnic minorities (Gary, 2006). There is no question that some of these cultural obstacles toward professional help seeking may be due to cultural beliefs and values that seeking help is viewed as a sign of being weak, crazy, or incapable.

However, minority groups' cultural beliefs do not account for all the reasons that they underutilize psychological services. If we consider the fact that racial/ethnic minority members had been recipients of abusive, inadequate, and unfair treatment by society, including the scientific and psychological communities, such as being viewed as less intelligent (Roth, Bevier, Bobko, Switzer, & Tyler, 2001) and more sick (Snowden, Hastings, & Alvidrez, 2009) than their white counterparts, and being more likely than Whites to receive psychotherapy that left long-lasting negative results (Crawford et al., 2016), we may see psychotherapist factors contributing to the underutilization of mental health services by minority clients. As noted, those minority clients who do enter psychotherapy treatment tend to prematurely withdraw or report poorer therapeutic results or experiences (Davidson, Yakushka, & Sandord-Martens, 2004; Meyer & Zane, 2013; Swift & Greenberg, 2012).

One area of concern is psychotherapist cultural competence, the lack of which could be a barrier to service utilization by the minorities. Due to the fact that racial/ethnic minorities have suffered from negative consequences of racism, discrimination, and other undeserved stressors in life, it is critically important that psychotherapists understand the negative influence of this social context on ethnic minority clients. Psychotherapy should be a place for clients to obtain corrective experience from social oppression, which psychotherapists won't be able to deliver without recognizing negative impacts of the social privilege/oppression system and their own roles in clients' experience. As Sue (2003) pointed out, "Clinicians are not immune from inheriting the biases, stereotypes, and values of the larger society. They often unintentionally act out these biases in the treatment of their clients of color" (p. 5). For example, a hard-working psychotherapist may value the ideals of meritocracy in a culture- or setting-neutral manner, and automatically apply them, without considering the role of social injustice, in viewing "lack of life success" of some ethnic minority clients. Such an unintentional, even automatic, application of socially biased ideology may retraumatize some clients emotionally in psychotherapy. Thus, psychotherapists must make deliberate efforts to develop cultural competence if they are to offer help and avoid harm through psychotherapy to the racially/ethnically diverse.

The multicultural scholar Paul Pedersen (2002) described culturally competent psychotherapists as needing to be "accurately aware of culturally learned assumptions by themselves and their clients, comprehend the culturally relevant facts and information about a client's culture and are able to intervene skillfully to bring about positive change through counseling" (p. 2). It is apparent that psychotherapists have to do self-work to become aware of their learned biases and assumptions about the racially diverse, which involves unlearning racism and discrimination, learning social justice and racial equality, and developing their own racial/ethnic/cultural identity (Duan & Brown, 2015). Otherwise, it is impossible to understand clients of color accurately and do no harm by applying culturally appropriate therapeutic interventions. Empirical evidence has shown that psychotherapist bias and stereotyping, often embedded in the conventional clinical wisdom and interventions, has contributed to racial disparity (McGuire & Miranda, 2008). Without any ill intent, unexamined discriminative beliefs about certain minority groups can translate into the clinician's impression of the patient and treatment decisions regarding the patient's clinical situation (Van Ryn & Burke, 2000). As revealed, "Patient race was associated with physicians' assessment of patient intelligence, feelings of affiliation toward the patient, and beliefs about patient's likelihood of risk behavior and adherence with medical advice" (p. 813). For instance, White psychotherapists who do not recognize that their perception of the world reflects their own social reality and cultural values may evaluate clients of color according to what they believe to be abnormal versus normal, intrapersonal versus interpersonal, or pathological versus functional. Such evaluations, biased by a lack of understanding of the client's social reality, can be costly for clients of color in terms of their sense of normalcy and ability to heal from the pain that brought them to psychotherapy.

In serving racial/ethnic minority clients, psychotherapists often face the challenge of not having culturally valid theories and/or appropriate intervention tools, because the existing system of care is by and large monocultural and ethnocentric in assessment, diagnosis, and treatment (Comas-Diaz, 2011). As a result, unquestioned conventional wisdom of psychotherapies leads to overlooking the impact of clients' social and cultural experience, which could cause harm. One example is "statistical discrimination" (McGuire & Miranda, 2008, p. 397), which refers to the application of clinical standards that are culturally biased in evaluating and treating the culturally diverse in psychotherapy. For instance, the use of the *Diagnostic and Statistical Manual of Mental Disorders*, which is currently in its fifth edition (American Psychiatric Association, 2013), may lead to inappropriate diagnosis of mental disorders among ethnic minorities because the majority norms are viewed as normal and used as criteria for identifying disorders. Most likely the potential problem of this practice is also compounded by clinicians' biases toward clients of color. A relatively recent review of 24 years of empirical literature (Schwartz & Blankenship, 2014) uncovered "a clear and pervasive pattern" (p. 133) that psychotic disorder diagnosis was assigned to African American/Black clients three to four times more often, and to Latino/Hispanic clients three times more often, than to European American/White clients. In a study of psychiatric hospitals in Indiana involving 2,404 clients, Barnes (2008) documented that African Americans were almost five times more likely to be diagnosed with schizophrenia than European Americans in state hospitals, constituting a longstanding problem and critical racial disparity. This overdiagnosis tendency not only hurts the individuals being diagnosed but also negatively damages the public perceptions of the groups. In turn, this bias may cycle back to influence the psychotherapist's clinical impression of African American clients and increase fear, distrust, and stigma about psychotherapy service among racial minorities.

Indirectly, the lack of cultural competence among psychotherapists and the exclusion of cultural diversity in psychotherapy theories and methods have also been important reasons why racial/ethnic minority clients tend to avoid using psychotherapy treatment. With years of multicultural research, we now know that "[t]raditional mental health care is often inappropriate and antagonistic to the cultural values and life experiences of populations of color" (Sue, 2003, p. 5). It has been, and should be, a sobering and motivating process in which clinicians recognize that due to lack of cultural competence we may have unintentionally done harm to our culturally diverse clients, without our awareness. The harm could be shown in our viewing cultural or contextual behavior as pathological, seeing minority clients as sicker than they actually are, feeling less confidence in their recovery, making internal attributions for emotional reactions to unfair external stressors and social injustice, and encouraging culturally unhelpful and even harmful coping behaviors.

We may use some recent empirical findings to illustrate potential consequences when practicing psychotherapists lack cultural competence and our theories and methods lack cultural relevance. An extensive qualitative study on African Americans' perceptions of psychotherapy and psychotherapists (Thompson, Bazile, & Akbar, 2004) reported that in addition to stigma, lack of knowledge, and lack of affordability, psychotherapists' impersonal style and lack of cultural sensitivity to and understanding of client experiences also discourage use of psychotherapy. Suite, La Bril, Primm, and Harrison-Ross (2007) demonstrated that psychotherapists' failure to acknowledge and recognize the role of larger historical and social contexts in client life and health contributes to the underutilization of mental health services among people of color. Further, the research on microaggression by Constantine (2007) demonstrated that African American clients' perceived microaggressions committed by their white psychotherapists significantly influenced their psychotherapy experience, such as working alliance and satisfaction. These findings seem to suggest that knowledge of ethnic minorities' cultures and their experiences of systematic discrimination and social oppression have not been adequately reflected in current psychotherapy systems and principles or in psychotherapist training. Thus, psychotherapists often do not have the ability and/or tools needed to provide racial/ethnic minorities with effective clinical services.

Creating Cultural Competency

The past several decades have witnessed significant effort and volumes of research examining factors that present problems for psychotherapy with ethnic minorities and/or facilitate transforming psychotherapy to become culturally congruent and racially relevant for ethnic minorities (Sue & Sue, 2016). It has become more than clear that increasing the access to and improving the use of psychotherapy among racial/ethnic minorities rely heavily on our professional community's efforts to address how we (a) facilitate social/political change toward racial equality using psychological science and advocacy, (b) increase diversity among psychotherapists, (c) promote multicultural views of self and others to understand client social reality and experience as relevant to therapy, and (d) enhance our ability to deliver culturally appropriate and effective interventions.

Addressing these needs requires us to invest effort in professional activities both in and out of our psychotherapy offices as well as personal development in becoming multiculturally competent. Engagement in and supporting the advocacy work that aims to educate and convince the public and lawmakers to consider the issue of inequality in access to mental health services is an important step in reducing the disparity. Most practicing psychotherapists acquire this competency through continuous learning as most graduate programs did not provide sufficient training in this area (Pieterse, Evans, Risner-Rutner, Collins, & Mason, 2009). One practical way for psychotherapists to start doing such advocacy work is through involvement in professional organizations, through which one can find role models and collegial support for engagement and service toward making psychotherapy available for racial/ethnic minorities who have been unfairly restricted in access to care. For instance, the APA has a Federal Action Network (APA, 2019) that updates clinicians on legislative issues impacting psychology and provides research and service opportunities for action.

Training and mentoring psychotherapists of color continues to be an important task for the profession. As shown in APA's Center for Workforce Studies (APA, 2018), racial/ethnic minorities represented 16% of the psychology workforce in 2016, a 92% increase from 2007. Considering the current demographics of the United States and changing trends, White Americans will represent less than 50% of the population in the next 35 years (World Population Review, 2018). Increasing the proportion of practitioners of color is becoming more and more important. Lack of diversity among mental health care professionals has long been identified as one barrier to care for the racially/ethnically diverse (Substance Abuse and Mental Health Services Administration, 2001). Thus, developing interest, commitment, and competence in training and mentoring psychotherapists of color is a concrete action that practicing psychotherapists and training programs can take.

In the effort to enhance psychotherapists' ability to provide culturally appropriate and effective interventions, cultural competence training and development has been recognized as necessary (Sue, 2003). There have been a number of published theoretical models (e.g., Duan & Brown, 2015; Sue & Sue, 2016) and practical multicultural guidelines (e.g., APA, 2003, 2017) aimed at increasing clinicians' cultural competence. A careful review of these models and guidelines provides a general map for competence development that contains an emphasis on psychotherapists' own multicultural identity (Duan & Brown, 2015); their beliefs, attitudes, and knowledge about their own cultures and those of their clients (Sue & Sue, 2016); and learned skills in culture-centered (Pedersen, 2003) or culturally appropriate psychosocial interventions (Bernal & Sáez-Santiago, 2006). The most recent addition is including a commitment to social justice in clinical work (Vera & Speight, 2003) or offering social justice–oriented interventions (Duan & Brown, 2015).

Psychotherapists' cultural attitudes and beliefs form the foundation of multicultural competence and reflect "an understanding of one's own cultural conditioning that affects personal beliefs, values, and attitudes" (Sue, 2001, p. 798) that can "influence their perceptions of and interactions with others as well as their clinical and empirical conceptualizations" (APA, 2017, p. 4). Various attempts have been made to operationalize and promote the process leading to clinicians' self-awareness of their attitudes and beliefs, including recognizing their learned racism, racial discrimination, prejudice, and biases, and then nurturing respect for the culturally diverse. Considering the diverse cultural contexts of our society and the world and the role individuals play in the interactive nature of these contexts, this process can be challenging and difficult because it often involves unlearning and rediscovering oneself.

Duan and Brown (2015) proposed a process for achieving appropriate attitudes and beliefs and emphasized the necessity of multicultural identity development for psychotherapists, regardless of their race/ethnicity or other cultural backgrounds. Mental health care providers need to see themselves through a multicultural lens because "the diverse makeup of the United States and its international connections automatically makes every resident multicultural, although many have the privilege not to recognize this fact" (p. 135). In interpersonal and social interactions, individuals may consciously or unconsciously contribute to each other's sense of self, social position, and relationships, and psychotherapy is no exception. Those "who are in high social power positions may let their biased attitudes and beliefs influence their perceptions of others who are in lower social power positions" (p. 134). Thus, it is extremely important that psychotherapists develop a multicultural identity so that they can "view clients within cultural contexts in which both the counselor and the client play a role" (p. 136). A multicultural identity involves one seeing oneself as a cultural being with unearned privileges and/or disadvantages, and striving toward being a non- and anti-"ist" (racist, sexist, heterosexist, ableist, etc.) and supporting social justice.

When working with ethnic minority clients, psychotherapists need to be able to see when and where their own personal, cultural, and social reality differs from that of their clients, and when and where their own identities may represent oppression to clients. With a multicultural identity, psychotherapists can see how the system of oppression and privilege plays out in society and enters clinical situations, and the role they play in clients' lives. Further, psychotherapists' multicultural identity may bring them awareness about the ways in which their clinical judgment and interventions reflect their own cultural perspectives due to their social locations. For instance, White psychotherapists may feel comfortable using conventional psychological theories in clinical assessment and intervention, but a multicultural identity may help them recognize potential lack of fit or possibility of harm when applying certain theories noncritically with ethnic minority clients.

Psychotherapy involves therapeutic connection with clients. Psychotherapists with a multicultural identity would enter therapeutic relationships with humility and respect for their ethnic minority clients, allow themselves to be emotionally affected by the social reality our society has unfairly designated to ethnic minority members, and avoid using the lenses entrenched in our own social reality to evaluate client experiences. These are basic conditions for healthy and effective therapeutic relationships with clients who have experienced social marginalization, and for accurate understanding of their experiences in their cultural contexts. Moreover, these are also the necessary conditions for providing clients with corrective experience in relation to their experience of discrimination and oppression. For example, with a good understanding of one's own multicultural identity and that of a stressed and depressed Latina American client in poverty, a White male psychotherapist may choose to pay more attention to listening to the client's stories, validating her experience, and empathizing with her at a deeper and positive level than to quickly fixing her problems by offering specific treatments. Considering "not being heard" or "being told what to do" by White people is a common experience of Latinx Americans with low socioeconomic status in society, hearing and validating her experience effectively in psychotherapy can be a corrective experience for the client. With a multicultural identity, psychotherapists can avoid blind use of the golden rule "treating others as you would want to be treated" with ethnic minority clients, and instead treat the client as the client would want to be treated.

Appropriate and effective interventions for ethnic minority clients have to be free of cultural biases against them and must contain empowering and supportive messages. It is often under-recognized that our nation's racial/ethnic minority groups have experienced significant racial trauma or race-based trauma rooted in cultural and historical trauma caused by racism (Williams, Ching, Printz, & Wetterneck, 2018). Thus, conducting psychotherapy with them in a business-as-usual manner without special attention to the cultural fit of our interventions may lead to unintentional harm such as invalidating them, minimizing their experience, reinforcing negative clinical symptoms, and even retraumatizing them by having them re-experience oppression in therapeutic settings. To prevent such practice, the APA's (2017) Multicultural Guidelines specify that psychotherapists need to "aspire to recognize and understand historical and contemporary experiences with power, privilege, and oppression" (p. 4) to ensure provision of culturally adaptive interventions and preventions.

Meanwhile, we also need to recognize that many of our existing therapeutic systems and practices are inadequate or problematic because they were developed mainly based on psychological knowledge of human experience by and for "people from Western, Educated, Industrialized, Rich, and Democratic . . . societies" (Henrich, Heine, & Norenzayan, 2010, p. 61). Thus, psychology and psychotherapy as we know have by and large left culture, its meaning, and its role in people's life out of the picture. For instance, Christopher, Wendt, Marecek. and Goodman (2014) described how U.S.-trained psychologists offered good-willed assistance to Sri Lanka during the 2004 Indian Ocean tsunami that imposed "pathologized views of suffering" over "local ways of being and behaving, folk psychologies, and moral visions" (p. 646) and popularized post-traumatic stress disorder (PTSD) for the region. People from different cultures have different psychology and would need psychotherapists to offer different and culturally appropriate interventions. Another example Christopher et al. presented was that the *Diagnostic and Statistical Manual of Mental Disorders* (American Psychiatric Association, 2013) provides a medicalized view of suicidal behavior as an expression of psychiatric disorder and overlooks large cultural variations; for instance, sometimes Indians with low social status would use it to protest, or some Chinese would use it to blame wrongdoers or avoid shame to their family.

Psychotherapy is and should be a cultural phenomenon, reflecting the view of mental health, therapeutic goals identified, clinical case conceptualized, change process pursued and evaluated, and communication practice (Duan & Brown, 2015). However, Western mainstream cultural values have dominated the field and ethnocentric monoculturalism has been embedded in the mental health delivery systems and psychotherapy theories (Comas-Diaz, 2011) in the United States. Cultural universality is often assumed or implied in the traditional wisdom of psychotherapy as practiced in the Western cultures. We need to take the challenge of continuously seeking new knowledge and skills that are culturally relevant and effective for the clients we serve. Recognizing that the differences between the dominant culture in the United States and that of racial and ethnic groups exist, permeate psychotherapy, and are often sources of biases, prejudices, and disadvantages for minority clients, we need to involve "assessment of cross-cultural relations, vigilance toward the dynamics that result from cultural differences, expansion of cultural knowledge, and adaptation of interventions to meet culturally unique needs at all levels of service" (Whaley & Davis, 2007, p. 564). Otherwise it is easy to mechanically see an African American male's "black rage" as an intrapsychic issue, a Latino's low test score as reflecting low intelligence, a Chinese client's suicidal ideation as an indication of mental illness, and a Native American's distrust of psychotherapy as resistance, among other stereotypes.

In terms of intervention skills, culturally sensitive and effective methods and strategies should prioritize validating ethnic minority clients' experience and supporting their being, even when their stress and suffering are expressed through "psychopathology" on the surface. All client symptoms have to be understood in the context of social and cultural influences, including those from social injustice and racial discrimination. To avoid blaming the victim, psychotherapists need to recognize those minority clients' cultural strengths, respect their cultural worldviews and perspectives, support their way of healing through traditions, and advocate for social justice at system levels for them. Symptoms are often clients' ways of dealing with the world around them, and psychotherapists' cultural empathy can help prevent harm of inappropriately pathologizing them and provide healing with understanding and respect.

Effective Strategies and Empirically-Supported Treatments

Psychotherapy is a "socially situated healing practice" (Wampold & Imel, 2015, p. 47). However, the efficacy discussion via the evidence-based treatment movement in recent decades has yet to sufficiently address the role of psychotherapists and their cultural competencies as well as therapeutic effectiveness with racial/ethnic minority clients in their cultures and contexts. The APA's 2006 Presidential Task Force on Evidence-Based Practice described the goal of evidence-based practice as "applying empirically supported principles of psychological assessment, case formulation, therapeutic relationship, and interventions" (p. 271). Although the therapeutic relationship is included, no explicit expectations are emphasized concerning the competence of psychotherapists (Norcross, 2011) or non-mainstream cultural contexts (Morales & Norcross, 2010). With the limited research tools available (e.g., randomly controlled trial or meta-analysis), the EBP movement seems to have focused mostly on "the particular examination, identification, and classification of specific treatments which have been shown to be effective in experimental settings for generally recognized psychopathologies" (Casterlnuovo, 2010, p. 27). Considering the complexity of both psychotherapists' and clients' cultural contexts, application of specific evidence-based treatments could potentially lead to "evidence-biased" (p. 27) practice in clinical settings when clients are ethnic minorities and their ethnicity was not considered in the empirical validation process.

There has been recent encouraging advancement in the area that provides empirically supported arguments pointing out promising directions for therapists to take in offering effective psychotherapy for all, including the culturally diverse. These directions involve theoretical integration, technical eclecticism, and emphasis on common factors (Wampold & Imel, 2015) and useful therapeutic relationships (Norcross & Lambert, 2018), as well as promotion of provider cultural competence (Sue & Sue, 2016) and cultural humility (Owen et al., 2016). Below several "good practices" are identified with direct and indirect research evidence and clinical observations as reflective of these promising directions, which exemplify ways to achieve effective therapeutic outcome with diverse clients.

Developing and Exercising Cultural Humility to Overcome Ethnocentric Views

One of the recent discoveries about effective psychotherapist factors is that health care providers' cultural humility, referred to as "ability to maintain an interpersonal stance that is other-oriented (or open to the other) in relation to aspects of cultural identity that are most important to the [person]" (Hook, Davis, Owen, Worthington, & Utsey, 2013, p. 353), facilitates establishing a therapeutic relationship with ethnic minority clients (Owen et al., 2016). Using clients' retrospective ratings of therapist cultural humility and therapy outcomes, Owen et al. discovered that "clients who rated their therapist as being more culturally humble also reported better therapy outcomes. . . . [C]lients who perceived that their therapist missed cultural opportunities [in sessions] reported worse therapy outcomes" (p. 13).

Cultural humility allows psychotherapists to effectively bridge social distance and share power with the powerless and show respect to clients who have been socially neglected or marginalized (Ramanathan, 2014). According to Tervalon and Murray-Garcia (1998), who coined the term, "[c]ultural humility incorporates a lifelong commitment to self-evaluation and self-critique, to redressing the power imbalances in the patient–physician dynamic, and to developing mutually beneficial and non-paternalistic clinical and advocacy partnerships with communities on behalf of individuals and defined populations" (p. 117). The National Association of Social Workers (2015) also promotes psychotherapist cultural humility, referring to "the attitude and practice of working with clients at the micro, mezzo, and macro levels with a presence of humility while learning, communicating, offering help, and making decisions in professional practice and settings" (p. 16).

The development of cultural humility and cultural competence should be pursued simultaneously, involving both self-focused and other-focused learning processes. Cultural humility is only possible for clinicians who have cultural competence in understanding the impact of the system of oppression and privilege, acknowledging their own biases and the ethnocentric biases of psychotherapy theories, being comfortable with cultural differences in a variety of areas of life, and having the psychological and cultural knowledge and skills in therapeutic interventions. By being culturally humble the psychotherapist shows openness to learning from and about clients with diverse social and cultural backgrounds and realities and "relinquishes the role of *expert* to the patient, becoming the *student* of the patient with a conviction and explicit expression of the patient's potential to be a capable and full partner in the therapeutic alliance" (Tervalon & Murray-Garcia 1998, p. 121). With this therapist quality, the therapeutically desired egalitarian, liberatory, empowering, and genuinely empathic therapeutic relationships (Brown, 2018) with minority clients can be achieved.

In the practice of psychotherapy, "trusting your instinct" is often practiced and sometimes given as advice by experienced practitioners. Similarly, theory-driven practice is also highly valued. However, if we reflect on how our psychotherapy theories and our training as psychotherapists have been mostly rooted in uncritical application of European values, traditions, and theories (Duan, 2018), the danger of using such a rule of thumb or wisdom becomes apparent because it allows practitioners to blindly follow ethnocentric views of the person, the issue, and the psychological processes involved in psychotherapy with those whose life experiences were not included in the traditional theories. Only cultural humility can stop practitioners from making ethnocentric judgments about ethnic minority clients' experiences. It is time for us to recognize that "psychopathology" is socially/culturally constructed (Walker, 2006) and for us to be humble in learning from our clients about their views and experiences.

Focusing on Working with and Relating to the Person, Not Curing Disorders

Although the definition of psychotherapy implies treatment of mental disorders, we all know that the medical model for dealing with psychological issues may be problematic and psychological health is not simply being "without symptoms" (World Health Organization, 2014). Further, psychological science has informed us that making changes can be challenging and its success relies on the person's self-motivation and self-efficacy. Thus, it should be clear that what psychotherapists can do—and do well—is helping clients to feel motivated and confident to pursue changes. Psychotherapy that focuses on curing disorders without sufficient attention to the person can be misleading, ineffective, and even harmful, especially when clients are from ethnic minority groups.

The most confirming outcome of years of psychotherapy research is probably the constructive and facilitative functions of the therapeutic working alliance in therapy outcomes, displayed in both symptom reduction and life satisfaction (Wampold & Imel, 2015). Most recently, the Third Interdivisional APA Task Force on Evidence-Based Relationships and Responsiveness provided convincing meta-analytical evidence showing the robustness of the connection between the therapeutic alliance and psychotherapy outcome (Norcross & Lambert, 2018). The conclusion of the task force aligns well with and embodies the evidence-based practice in psychotherapy. Although the research on the importance of the working alliance with ethnic minority clients specifically is limited, there is reason to believe that therapist expertise expressed in ability to show understanding, acceptance, respect, empathy, and trust can be particularly important (Lambert & Barley, 2001) with ethnic minorities, especially when the therapist is not a minority member (Sue, 2003). A strong working alliance with a White therapist may lead ethnic minority clients to "corrective" experience because they can't escape racism and discrimination in social and life settings. Further, a relationship orientation is generally more salient in many minority ethnic cultures than in the dominant Western culture (e.g., Triandis, 1995), and relationship building can be culture syntonic for them.

Empirical evidence has also identified some discredited psychotherapist behaviors, such as using a confrontational style, making frequent interpretations, making/showing assumptions about the client, and displaying therapist-centricity (Norcross & Lambert, 2018). These seem to be descriptors of psychotherapists who adopt the theory-driven mentality and pathology-focused attitude but are unaware of their ethnocentric views or their client's culture and social reality. These practices may be unhelpful to any clients, but the harm may be much greater for the culturally diverse clients, especially when the psychotherapist is not a member of the ethnic minority group. Being confronted constantly due to having different cultural values, being seen as sick or abnormal due to cultural behavior, being assumed to be "less than" others, and being marginalized are too familiar to ethnic minority clients. Psychotherapist confirmation or replication of these conditions may be retraumatizing to clients who are already vulnerable due to these factors.

Therefore, in clinical operation, psychotherapists may want to intentionally avoid being taken away by symptoms and be reminded not to be overly occupied by the need to solve client problems, but to see the person and understand the person in his or her contexts instead. Working on the relationship is worthwhile because the "development and maintenance of the therapeutic relationship is a primary curative component of therapy" (Lambert & Barley, 2001, p. 359). Even if the goal is reducing symptoms (which has to be in the context of improving life quality), having a good therapeutic relationship is the path leading the client to feel understood and therefore motivated to make necessary changes. Exclusive focus on correcting disordered symptoms may reduce the space for relationship development and increase the chance of harm. After all, a positive therapeutic outcome depends more upon the relationship than particular treatment methods, which has been proved by years of psychotherapy outcome research (Norcross & Lambert, 2018).

Adopting Context-Rooted Conceptualization/Understanding of Clinical Symptoms to Avoid Pitfalls of Loyalty to Theories

Theory-based practice is highly valued in our profession, and automatically using and defending our existing knowledge is probably human nature. However, when working with ethnic minority clients in psychotherapy, we need to be willing to challenge any theories that are likely not reflective of our clients' lives and their social reality, and we must allow our thinking to be outside of the theoretical box in which we were trained. Research has informed us that there are numerous environmental and external contributing factors to influence one's mental health problems (Prilleltensky, 1999), and many of these contributors are not integrated into the reasoning of our existing psychotherapy theories. When client social realities deviate from that of the theory, a psychotherapist using the theory blindly tends to generate misconceptions, victim blaming, and pathologizing when confronted with unfamiliar cultural behaviors or coping actions. That is why conducting psychotherapy in a "business-as-usual" fashion under the guidance of traditional theories may cause harm for ethnic minority clients, because those theories tend to overemphasize factors internal to the client while discounting the influence of external factors that could be the cause of client maladaptive behaviors. This caution against using culturally biased therapeutic theories should be exercised in psychotherapy with all marginalized and underserved populations to account for client suffering due to an oppressive social environment.

In practice, an ecological perspective may be helpful to guide clinicians' evaluation of client concerns. Cook (2012) presented convincing empirical evidence supporting the notion that behavior is personal, contextual, relational, meaningful, and changeable. Based on this empirically supported view, it is unthinkable that psychotherapy conceptualization is not more context-based than intrinsic-psyche–based or therapeutic theory–based, and many psychotherapists will not allow themselves to think outside their theoretical boxes. It is important to note and remember that an ecosystem, referring to "the sum total of interactive influences operating within an individual's life in varying degrees of proximity, ranging from his or her biologically determined characteristics to the broader sociocultural context structuring human interactions," exists for all individuals, and what happened to them "rarely occurs in a vacuum but rather is shaped by the confluence of events, propensities, relationships, memories and other features of a life elaborated over time and across settings." (pp. 7–8). Thus, a context-driven conceptualization is needed to reflect the social and clinical reality of clients of color.

To conceptualize or understand the psychological symptoms of ethnic minority clients or other oppressed people, "the value of attending to how disempowerment has led people into a therapist's office cannot be underestimated" (Brown, 2018, p. 38). There are various forms of internalized racism or social oppression that led or contribute to psychological symptoms, and these should not be conceptualized as reflecting personal weakness or intrapsychic defects. For instance, seemingly extreme or disproportional anxiety symptoms associated with finding a job by a Latino immigrant probably should not be readily viewed as neurotic as it often would be; inability to trust anyone by an African American person in a primarily White environment may not necessarily reflect weak ego or emotional insecurity; and having difficulty expressing oneself by an Asian American may not be evidence of low self-esteem or self-efficacy. Psychotherapy can only be empowering for ethnic minorities when it recognizes the impact of oppression on client experiences, including clinical symptoms.

Using Strength-Based Interventions to Maximize Gains and Minimize Potential Harm

It may not have been most clinicians' intuitive response to view clients and client presenting problems in a positive light in psychotherapy. After all, clients are seeking help for their problems, and it is natural that clinicians want to help with elimination of symptoms. However, directly focusing on problems by applying medical or disease models in psychotherapy has turned out to be more problematic than effective (Elkins, 2007), and due to low levels of cultural fit, the medical or disease model has been more of a problem to ethnic minority clients (Sue & Sue, 2016). Knowing that client motivation, self-concept, and self-efficacy as well as the therapeutic alliance are key factors in client change, using strength-based approaches in conceptualization and intervention is critically important in working with ethnic minority clients. At the very least it can minimize harm and, at its best, it can help promote positive self-concept and emotions to motivate clients to make necessary changes even in aversive life circumstances.

Strength-based interventions are based on the belief that people have abilities and internal resources that they can use to deal with life challenges and difficulties. Empirical evidence has shown that by focusing on client strengths that are often embedded in their symptoms, psychotherapists may help clients with "cultivating positive feelings, positive behaviors, or positive cognitions" (Sin & Lyubomirsky, 2009, p. 467). As suggested by Fredrickson's (2004) broaden-and-build theory, positive emotions broaden one's repertoire of action and thought toward well-being. When working with ethnic minority clients, this approach has the additional advantage of preventing harm caused by possible therapist misunderstanding of client cultural behavior.

As one example, goal-focused positive psychotherapy (GFPP) developed by Conoley and Scheel (2018), "promotes client strengths, hope and positive emotions in order to assist clients in accomplishing what they desire in life" (p. 1). This theory diverges from most currently practiced psychotherapy methods. Although there is still room for improvement for diverse clients, GFPP illustrates the power of human strength, focuses on promoting well-being, and aims at producing positive outcomes for clients beyond reduction of symptoms. There is reason to believe that this approach will be more appropriate than deficits-based or disease-based treatment approaches for all clients, including the culturally diverse. In operation, GFPP is delivered via various therapeutic skills and interventions that are generally designed toward establishing and strengthening therapeutic relationship and fostering clients' "strength to access positive emotions as a result of feeling cared about and valuable" (pp. 44–45). To offer quality service of psychotherapy to ethnic minorities, therapists may consider adopting parts or all of this approach to maximize the gain and minimize potential harm.

Cultural Adaptations of Empirically Supported Practice

An empirical-based treatment or evidence-based practice approach has tended to achieve uniformity or systematization in providing care to clients (Bernal, Jiménez-Chafey, & Domenech Rodríguez, 2009), while the APA Presidential Task Force on Evidence-Based Practice (2006) promotes "the integration of the best available research with clinical expertise in the context of patient characteristics, culture, and preferences" (p. 273). Scholars and practitioners have made efforts to address the distance between empirical/evidence-based treatment and the cultural contexts of ethnic minority clients. Focusing on specific cultural groups with specific psychological issues, researchers explored effectiveness of modified empirical/evidence-based treatment with added attention to specific contextual factors (see Morales & Norcross, 2010). For instance, Aguilera, Garza, and Muñoz (2010) reported positive results using a modified cognitive behavioral therapy group manual for treating depression among Latino clients. The modification involved adding culturally sensitive topics in group discussion, paying special attention to each group member's socioeconomic status when picking group activities, using Spanish in communication, for example. Such efforts resulted in the development of general theoretical frameworks that can be used to guide the adaptation of existing empirical/evidence-based methods when serving ethnic minority clients (Mendes, 2015). Currently several such cultural frameworks have been recognized, including "(1) Ecological Validity Framework, and (2) Cultural Sensitivity Framework, (3) the Heuristic Framework, and (4) Planned Intervention Adaptation" (Mendes, 2015, p. 159).

There has been clinical operationalization of and empirical evidence for these frameworks. For instance, using some of the eight dimensions of intervention (language, persons, metaphors, content, concepts, goals, methods, and context) based on the ecological validity model, cognitive behavioral therapy and interpersonal therapy were adapted to help Latino Americans. By adding a focus on *familismo* and *respeto* (content) and encouragement of parent participation (method), the interventions led to positive outcome for Puerto Rican adolescents with depression (Rossello & Bernal, 1999). The meta-analysis by Griner and Smith (2006) revealed that various forms of cultural adaptations have been used under these frameworks that led to positive outcome of empirical/evidence-based methods in helping ethnic minorities reduce depression and anxiety. The most often used cultural adaptations include integrating cultural values and concepts in intervention, matching therapist–client ethnicity, offering psychotherapy in the client's native language, and providing psychotherapists with cultural sensitivity training.

Practically and heuristically, these research findings support the notion of conducting psychotherapy with special attention to client cultures. Culture is the foundation of human behavior, and it shapes personalities (Triandis & Suh, 2002) and permeates human existence (Geertz, 1973). For ethnic minority clients in the United States, both being members of oppressed groups and having different cultural values and worldviews contribute to their psychological experiences, including symptoms and healing. However, our existing psychotherapy diagnostic and intervention theories are mainly rooted in the Western mainstream cultures that often lead to views of different and minority cultural behaviors as unhealthy or abnormal (Duan & Brown, 2015). Thus, it is critical that psychotherapists always wear cultural lenses and use cultural frameworks when applying any existing theories or empirical/evidence-based treatment working with ethnic minorities. Perhaps it can be made a standard practice to always ask questions such as: What roles has culture played in this client's symptoms? Is my reaction to this client's behavior in any way biased by my culture or lack of knowledge of the client's culture? How would this client's behavior be functional, or not, in their culture? What would be the good treatment outcome for this client considering their cultural context? How can I deliver interventions that support, validate, and empower this client in the specific cultural context?

Future Steps

Moving forward, our goal is clear: reducing and, we hope, eliminating racial and ethnic disparity in mental health care as soon and as effectively as possible. There are inspirations as well as challenges in front of us. It is our ethical and professional mandate to meet the challenge by doing what needs to be done to develop ourselves as competent psychotherapists and to deliver service to the underserved ethnic minorities by intervening both at the system and society level and the individual/group psychotherapy practice level.

Development of Competence

In order to serve ethnic minorities effectively, we psychotherapists need to develop an understanding of our own multicultural identity and the impact of the system of privilege and oppression on us and others, above and beyond learning to conduct psychotherapy. We need to view ourselves as cultural beings and recognize the ways in which our identities bring us privileges and/or disadvantages. Our cultural identities will interact with those of ethnic minority clients in therapeutic relationships. The awareness that we may sometimes represent oppressors to them or enjoy privilege at their expense is important and may help us treat relationship issues appropriately. Being responsible professionals, we can gain this awareness by learning and pondering on self-exploration questions such as: What does being a Caucasian (or African, Asian, Latino, Native, etc.) American mean in this society, for me, and for others? Intentional learning about the life experience of others, particularly ethnic minorities, directly or indirectly, through involvement and observation may also be helpful. For instance, paying attention to current social, cultural, and political issues; reading books and watching movies with ethnic minority themes or characters; or doing exercises to reduce our implicit biases about ethnic minorities may increase our sensitivity and understanding.

Engagement in Social Advocacy

Having access to quality mental health care should be not a privilege, but a basic right for all people. The current status quo of racial/ethnic disparity needs to be corrected, and our nation's social and political structure that favors the privileged and disadvantages the oppressed is in great need of change. We have to do what we can, such as providing scientific evidence, professional understanding, and psychological wisdom, as well as devoting our time and energy, to create constructive social changes and promote social justice in mental health policies and systems. This mission is demanding and requires all of us to step out of our comfort zone and develop new skills, including those in public engagement, advocacy, and leadership. The responsibility of working at system levels and being engaged in promoting respect for diversity and social justice in the health care system should be part of our professional responsibility. Taking active social actions beyond serving individuals' or groups' specific psychological needs will be a necessary component of psychotherapy practice in the 21st century to make service available not only for those who can afford it, who have resources, and who share the cultural backgrounds and values of the majority, but also those who do not meet these conditions.

Diversifying the Psychotherapy Workforce

Training and mentoring psychotherapists of color continues to be important and necessary. Diversifying the clinical workforce may help make psychotherapy settings more inviting and reassuring for ethnic minority clients. The cultural knowledge of psychotherapists of color may be helpful not only in helping minority clients but also in helping colleagues learn about minority cultures.

Recruiting diverse students to graduate training programs is an urgent task, and supporting/mentoring them throughout their training and professional careers is an important duty of our field. Enlarging the presence of psychotherapists of color is one of the conditions necessary to ensure that when ethnic minority clients do receive psychotherapy service, they can see role models and feel safe in therapeutic settings. Possible cultural hostility or misunderstanding has to be minimized, which will benefit minority clients in psychotherapy and help reduce the fear and stigma associated with help seeking in their communities.

Continuous Improvement of Interventions

As practicing psychotherapists, we need to be willing to adapt our practice to meet the needs of our diverse clients, communities, and society, and committed to knowledge renewal by integrating new understanding and advancement of theories and interventions into our practice. Learning from emerging new research findings, improved understandings of cultural contexts, new theories and/or methods, or new empirical/evidence-based practices with cultural validity can be beneficial. For instance, we should attend to the recently reported specific psychotherapist relationship behaviors that work, or do not work, as shown by strong empirical evidence (Norcross & Lambert, 2018). One may try to experiment with what have been deemed as probably effective, with possible cultural adaptation, such as strengthening real relationships, repairing alliance ruptures, managing countertransference, cultivating positive expectations, promoting treatment credibility, and being empathic, congruent, and genuine toward the client. Meanwhile, effort is also needed to avoid those discredited relationship behaviors, including using frequent interpretations, being confrontational in relating to the client, and blaming clients for problems. Openness to continuous knowledge and skill renewal is an ethical responsibility of practitioners who seek to be of service to cultural/ethnic/racial minority clients.

Prioritizing Client Needs over Loyalty to Conventional Theories

In psychotherapy communities, a culture of prioritizing client needs over loyalty to psychotherapy theories needs to be promoted, and this should start in graduate training programs. At present, the professional culture of respecting theory-driven practice or the original work of prominent theorists still seems prevalent in graduate training, where traditional theories are taught in traditional ways. The consequence of this tradition may lead to

> presumptive truth evolves into misplaced belief when people become fervently committed to their model; it ceases to be provisional and becomes doctrinaire or dogma instead. Certainty replaces possibility. The imperialist fallacy occurs when people insist that others adopt their belief or model. (Ford & Urban, 1998, p. 35)

Considering the ever-changing cultural contexts of our society, sufficient attention needs to be given to train students to be sensitive to the cultural, social, and political contexts of clients, communities, and society. For practicing psychotherapists, some unlearning and relearning are to be encouraged. Prioritizing ethnic minority clients' needs will challenge us about what we know, were trained in, or had identified with, and will demand that we continuously learn and adopt effective new intervention practices. For instance, the concept and practice of radical healing (Ginwrite, 2010; Neville, 2018) for African Americans has gained recognition and application in recent years. By learning about its theoretical basis and practice, we may better understand how marginalized groups' cultural wounds caused by social, economic, and political oppression underlie many of their symptoms, and they need to heal in supportive communities. As practicing psychotherapists, we have the ethical and professional responsibility to allow, support, and promote such healing practices. Meanwhile, this theoretical perspective gives us more tools to acknowledge and talk about the negative influence of racism and social oppression with our clients in psychotherapy sessions.

Bringing Social Justice to the Center of Psychotherapy

All psychotherapists and students of psychotherapy should gain knowledge about the role of social injustice and culture in human psychology and intervention methods that are based on social justice. In learning and evaluating psychotherapy theories and methods, clinicians and students need to be encouraged to critique and deconstruct them with full consideration of current social and cultural contexts for all people, especially ethnic minorities. To understand ethnic minority clients, clinicians should consider the negative impact of racism and oppression on clients' psychological experiences and avoid pathologizing responsive behaviors to injustice. When offering interventions, reducing, not increasing, the distress caused by societal-level social injustice should be a focus. For instance, to help a minority client overcome social phobia in relating to coworkers, combating irrational beliefs about being "rejected" or desensitizing the client for being "threatened" should be conducted with clinical caution and cultural understanding. Otherwise, therapeutic efforts may feel invalidating and untrusting for the client. What appears irrational from the therapist's perspective may be realistic and functional for the client, and desensitization may reduce reactive symptoms in the lab but does not change the fact that the client is fearful going to work. Social injustice is read in ethnic minorities' reality, and effective therapeutic interventions can't overlook its impact. It is our profession's ethical mandate and professional responsibility to be the change agent toward racial and ethnic parity through offering services that have social justice at the center. Due to lack of training, this is a relatively weak area of practitioners at the present. Thus, continuing education in this area needs to be promoted. Perhaps licensing boards could consider requiring such continuing education credits for license renewal.

Summary

Serving racial/ethnic minority clients in psychotherapy effectively and eliminating racial/ethnic mental health care disparities represent challenging demands for 21st-century psychotherapists in their development of cultural and professional identity and mastering culturally relevant therapeutic knowledge and skills. It is not a choice but a necessity for our profession's sustainability and for our nation's well-being that we stay on the right side of history and reshape our professional practice to meet the challenges of the time and promote racial/ethnic equity and parity in mental health care.

References

Aguilera, A., Garza, M. J., & Muñoz, R. F. (2010). Group cognitive-behavioral therapy for depression in Spanish: culture-sensitive manualized treatment in practice. *Journal of Clinical Psychology: In Session*, *66*, 857–868.

American Psychiatric Association. (2013). *Diagnostic and statistical manual of mental disorders* (5th ed.). Washington, DC: Author.

American Psychological Association. (2003). Guidelines on multicultural education, training, research, practice, and organizational change for psychologists. *American Psychologist*, *58*, 377–402.

American Psychological Association. (2015). *Demographics of the U.S. psychology workforce: Findings from the American Community Survey*. Retrieved from https://www.apa.org/workforce/publications/13-demographics/report.pdf

American Psychological Association. (2016). A new look at racial and ethnic disparities in mental health care. Retrieved from https://www.apa.org/monitor/2016/01/publication-disparities.aspx

American Psychological Association. (2017). Multicultural guidelines: An ecological approach to context, identity, and intersectionality. Retrieved from http://www.apa.org/about/policy/multicultural-guidelines.pdf

American Psychological Association. (2018). *Demographics of the U.S. psychology workforce: Findings from the 2007–16 American Community Survey*. Retrieved from https://www.apa.org/workforce/publications/16-demographics/report.pdf

American Psychological Association (2019). Federal Action Network. Retrieved from http://cqrcengage.com/apapolicy/home

APA Presidential Task Force on Evidence-Based Practice (2006). Evidence-based practice in psychology. *American Psychologist*, *61*, 271–285.

Barnes, A. (2008). Race and hospital diagnoses of schizophrenia and mood disorders. *Social Work*, *53*(1), 77–83.

Bernal, G., & Sáez-Santiago, E. (2006). Culturally centered psychosocial interventions. *Journal of Community Psychology*, *34*(2), 121–132.

Bernal, G., Jiménez-Chafey, M. I., & Domenech Rodríguez, M. M. (2009). Cultural adaptation of treatments: A resource for considering culture in evidence-based practice. *Professional Psychology: Research and Practice*, *40*, 361–368.

Brown, L. (2018). *Feminist therapy* (2nd ed.). Washington, DC: American Psychological Association Press.

Bussing, R., & Gary, F. A. (2012). Eliminating mental health disparities by 2020: Everyone's actions matter. *Journal of the American Academy of Child & Adolescent Psychiatry*, *51*(7), 663–666.

Castelnuovo, G. (2010). Empirically supported treatments in psychotherapy: Towards an evidence-based or evidence-biased psychology in clinical settings? *Frontiers in Psychology*, *1*, 27.

Christopher, J. C., Wendt, D. C., Marecek, J., & Goodman, D. M. (2014). Critical cultural awareness: Contributions to a globalizing psychology. *American Psychologist*, *69*, 645–655.

Comas-Diaz, L. (2011). Multicultural theories of psychotherapy. In R. J. Corsini & D. Wedding (Eds.), *Current psychotherapies* (9th ed., pp. 536–567). Belmont, CA: Brooks/Cole.

Conoley, C., & Scheel, M. (2018). *Goal-focused positive psychotherapy*. New York, NY: Oxford University Press.

Constantine, M. G. (2007). Racial micro-aggressions against African American clients in cross-racial counseling relationships. *Journal of Counseling Psychology*, *54*(1), 1–16.

Cook, E. (2012). *Understanding people in context: The ecological perspective in counseling*. Hoboken, NJ: Wiley.

Crawford, M. Thana, L., Farquharson, L., Palmer, L., Hancock, E., Bassett, P., . . . Parry, G. (2016). Patient experience of negative effects of psychological treatment: Results of a national survey. *British Journal of Psychiatry*, *208*(3), 260–265.

Davidson, M. M., Yakushka, O. F., & Sandord-Martens, T. C. (2004). Racial/ethnic minority clients' utilization of a university counseling center: An archival study. *Journal of Multicultural Counseling and Development*, *32*, 259–271.

Deitch, E. A., Barsky, A., Butz, R. M., Chan, S., Brief, A. P., & Bradley, J. C. (2003). Subtle yet significant: The existence and impact of everyday racial discrimination in the workplace. *Human Relations*, *56*(11), 1299–1324.

Duan, C. (2018). Culture and mental health counseling: A reflective view based on observations in China. *Athens Journal of Social Sciences*, *6*, 71–87.

Duan, C., & Brown, C. (2015). *Becoming a multi-culturally competent counselor*. Thousand Oaks, CA: Sage.

Elkins, D. N. (2007). The medical model in psychotherapy: Its limitations and failures. *Journal of Humanistic Psychology, 49*(1), 66–84.

Ford, D., & Urban, H. D. (1998). *Contemporary models of psychotherapy: A comparative analysis* (2nd ed.). New York, NY: Wiley.

Fredrickson, B. L. (2004). The broaden-and-build theory of positive emotions. *Philosophical Transactions of the Royal Society of London B, Biological Sciences, 359*, 1367–1378.

Gary, G. (2006). Stigma: Barrier to mental health care among ethnic minorities. *Issues in Mental Health Nursing, 26*(10), 979–999.

Geertz, C. (1973). *The interpretation of cultures*. New York, NY: Basic Books.

Ginwright, S. A. (2010). *Black youth rising: Activism and radical healing in urban America*. New York, NY: Teachers College Press.

Griner, D., & Smith, T. B. (2006). Culturally adapted mental health interventions: A meta-analytic review. *Psychotherapy: Theory, Research, Practice, Training, 43*, 531–548.

Henrich, J., Heine, S., & Norenzayan, A. (2010) The weirdest people in the world? *Behavioral and Brain Sciences, 33*(2–3), 61–83.

Henry J. Kaiser Family Foundation. (2017). Key facts about the uninsured population. Retrieved from https://www.kff.org/uninsured/fact-sheet/key-facts-about-the-uninsured-population/

Hsieh, D. K., & Kirk, S. A. (2005). The limits of diagnostic criteria: The role of social context in clinicians' judgments of mental disorder. In S. A. Kirk (Ed.), *Mental disorders in the social environment: Critical perspectives* (pp. 45–61). New York, NY: Columbia University Press.

Hook, J. N., Davis, D. E., Owen, J., Worthington, E. L., Jr., & Utsey, S. O. (2013). Cultural humility: Measuring openness to culturally diverse clients. *Journal of Counseling Psychology, 60*(3), 353–366.

Keizer, K., Lindenberg, S., & Steg, L. (2008). The spreading of disorder. *Science, 322*(5908), 1681–1685.

Lambert, M. J., & Barley, D. E. (2001). Research summary on the therapeutic relationship and psychotherapy outcome. *Psychotherapy: Theory, Research, Practice, Training, 38*(4), 357–361.

McGuire, T. G., & Miranda, J. (2008). New evidence regarding racial and ethnic disparities in mental health: Policy implications. *Health Affairs, 27*(2), 393–403.

Mendes, A. (2015). Cultural adaptations in mental health and behavioral interventions. *Journal of Social & Psychological Sciences, 8*, 159–167.

Meyer, O. L., & Zane, N. (2013). The influence of race and ethnicity in clients' experiences of mental health treatment. *Journal of Community Psychology, 41*(7), 884–901.

Morales, E., & Norcross, J. C. (2010). Evidence-based practices with ethnic minorities: Strange bedfellows no more. *Journal of Clinical Psychology: In Session, 66*, 1–9.

National Association of Social Workers. (2015). *Standards and indicators for cultural competence in social work practice*. Retrieved from https://www.socialworkers.org/LinkClick.aspx?fileticket=PonPTDEBrn4%3d&portalid=0

National Poverty Center at University of Michigan. (2009). The color of poverty: Why racial and ethnic disparities persist. Policy Brief #16. Retrieved from http://www.npc.umich.edu/publications/policy_briefs/brief16/PolicyBrief16.pdf

Neville, H. (2018). Radical healing: A call for an integrative culturally responsive, social justice research agenda. *Focus, 29*, 1–3. Retrieved from http://division45.org/wp-content/uploads/2018/05/FOCUS-Spring-2018.pdf

Norcross, J. C. (Ed.). (2011). *Psychotherapy relationships that work* (2nd ed.). New York, NY: Oxford University Press.

Norcross, J. C., & Lambert, M. J. (2018). Psychotherapy relationships that work. *Psychotherapy, 55*, 303–315.

Owen, J., Tao, K. W., Drinane, J. M., Hook, J., Davis, D., & Kune, N. F. (2016). Client perceptions of therapists' multicultural orientation: Cultural (missed) opportunities and cultural humility. *Professional Psychology: Research and Practice, 47*(1), 30–37.

Pedersen, P. (2002). The making of a culturally competent counselor. *Online Readings in Psychology and Culture, Unit 10 Health/Clinical Psychology and Culture, Subunit 3 Counseling and Psychotherapy in Cultural Context*, 1–13. Retrieved from https://scholarworks.gvsu.edu/cgi/viewcontent.cgi?referer=&httpsredir=1&article=1093&context=orpc

Pedersen, P. D. (2003). Cross-cultural counseling: Developing culture-centered interactions. In G. Bernal, J. E. Trimble, A. K. Burlew, & F. T. L. Leong (Eds.), *Handbook of racial and ethnic minority psychology* (pp. 487–503). Thousand Oaks, CA: Sage.

Pieterse, A. L., Evans, S. A., Risner-Butner, A., Collins, N. M., & Mason, L. B. (2009). Multicultural competence and social justice training in counseling psychology and counselor education. *The Counseling Psychologist, 37*(1), 93–115.

Prilleltensky, I. (1999). Critical psychology foundations for the promotion of mental health. *Annual Review of Critical Psychology, 1*(1), 100–118.

Ramanathan, C. S. (2014, January). What does globalization got to do with cultural competence, social development, and ethics? [Plenary speech]. International Conference on Bounds of Ethics, Christ University, Bangalore, India.

Reeves, R., Rodrigue, E., & Kneebone, E. (2016). *Five evils: Multidimensional poverty and race in America.* Retrieved from https://www.brookings.edu/wp-content/uploads/2016/06/ReevesKneeboneRodrigue_MultidimensionalPoverty_FullPaper.pdf

Rossello, J., & Bernal, G. (1999).The efficacy of cognitive–behavioral and interpersonal treatments for depression in Puerto Rican adolescents. *Journal of Consulting and Clinical Psychology, 67*, 734–745.

Roth, P. L., Bevier, C. A., Bobko, P., Switzer, F. S., III, & Tyler, P. (2001). Ethnic group differences in cognitive ability in employment and educational settings: A meta-analysis. *Personnel Psychology, 54*(2), 297–330.

Schmidt, C. W. (2007). Environmental connections: A deeper look into mental illness. *Environmental Health Perspectives, 115*(8), A404–A410.

Schwartz, R. C., & Blankenship, D. M. (2014). Racial disparities in psychotic disorder diagnosis: A review of empirical literature. *World Journal of Psychiatry, 4*(4), 133–140.

Sin, N. L., & Lyubomirsky, S. (2009). Enhancing well-being and alleviating depressive symptoms with positive psychology interventions: A practice-friendly meta-analysis. *Journal of Clinical Psychology, 65*, 467–487.

Smedley, B. D., Stith, A. Y., & Nelson, A. R. (Eds.). (2003). *Unequal treatment: Confronting racial and ethnic disparities in health care.* Washington, DC: National Academies Press.

Smith, T. B., & Trimble, J. E. (2016). *Foundations of multicultural psychology: Research to inform effective practice.* Washington, DC: American Psychological Association.

Snowden, L. R., Hastings, J., & Alvidrez, J. (2009). Overrepresentation of black Americans in psychiatric inpatient care. *Psychiatric Services, 60*(6), 779–785.

Substance Abuse and Mental Health Services Administration. (2001). *Mental health: Culture, race, and ethnicity—A supplement to Mental Health: A Report of the Surgeon General*. Retrieved from https://www.ncbi.nlm.nih.gov/books/NBK44243/

Sue, D. W. (2001). Multidimensional facets of cultural competence. *The Counseling Psychologist, 29*, 790–821.

Sue, D. W. (2003). Cultural competence in the treatment of ethnic minority populations. In Council of National Psychological Associations for the Advancement of Ethnic Minority Interests (Ed.), *Psychological treatment of ethnic minority populations* (pp. 4–7). Washington, DC: Association of Black Psychologists. Retrieved from http://www.apa.org/pi/oema/resources/brochures/treatment-minority.pdf

Sue, D. W., & Sue, D. (2016). *Counseling the culturally diverse: Theory and practice* (7th ed.). Hoboken, NJ: John Wiley & Sons.

Suite, D. H., La Bril, R., Primm, A., & Harrison-Ross, P. (2007). Beyond misdiagnosis, misunderstanding and mistrust: Relevance of the historical perspective in the medical and mental health treatment of people of color. *Journal of the National Medical Association, 99*(8), 879–888.

Swift, J. K., & Greenberg, R. P. (2012). Premature discontinuation in adult psychotherapy: A meta-analysis. *Journal of Consulting and Clinical Psychology, 80*(4), 547–559.

Takaki, R. (1993). *A different mirror: A history of multicultural America*. Boston, MA: Little, Brown and Company.

Tervalón, M., & Murray-Garcia, J. (1998). Cultural humility versus cultural competence: A critical distinction in defining physician training outcomes in multicultural education. *Journal of Health Care for the Poor and Underserved, 9*(2), 117–125.

Tew, J. (2011). *Social approaches to mental distress*. New York, NY: Palgrave Macmillan.

Tew, J., Ramon, S., Slade, M., Bird, V., Melton, J., & Le Boutillier, C. (2011). Social factors and recovery from mental health difficulties: A review of the evidence. *British Journal of Social Work, 42*(3), 1–18.

Thompson, V. L. S., Bazile, A., & Akbar, M. (2004). African Americans' perceptions of psychotherapy and psychotherapists. *Professional Psychology: Research and Practice, 35*(1), 19–26.

Triandis, H. C. (1995). *Individualism and collectivism*. Boulder, CO: Westview Press.

Triandis, H. C., & Suh, E. M. (2002) Cultural influences on personality. *Annual Review of Psychology, 53*, 133–160.

Van Ryn, M., & Burke, J. (2000) The effect of patient race and socio-economic status on physicians' perceptions of patients. *Social Science and Medicine, 50*(6), 813–828.

Vargas, R. S., Clemente, N. M. J., & Mayoral, A. R. I. (2016). Sociocultural factors in mental illness: Biopsychosocial model. *European Psychiatry, 33*, S612–S613. https://doi.org/10.1016/j.eurpsy.2016.01.1807

Vera, E. M., & Speight, S. L. (2003). Multicultural competence, social justice, and counseling psychology: Expanding our roles. *The Counseling Psychologist, 31*(3), 253–272.

Walker, M. T. (2006). The social construction of mental illness and its implications for the recovery model. *International Journal of Psychosocial Rehabilitation, 10*(1), 71–87.

Wampold, B. E., & Imel, Z. E. (2015). *The great psychotherapy debate: Research evidence for what works in psychotherapy* (2nd ed.). New York, NY: Routledge.

Whaley, A. L., & Davis, K. E. (2007). Cultural competence and evidence-based practice in mental health services: A complementary perspective. *American Psychologist, 62*(6), 563–574.

Williams, M. T., Ching, T. H., Printz, D. M. B., & Wetterneck, T. (2018). Assessing PTSD in ethnic and racial minorities: Trauma and racial trauma. *Directions in Psychiatry, 38*, 179–198.

World Health Organization. (2014). Mental health: A state of well-being. Retrieved from https://www.who.int/features/factfiles/mental_health/en/

World Population Review. (2018). United States population 2018. Retrieved from http://worldpopulationreview.com/countries/united-states-population/

5

Bringing Psychotherapy to People Living in Poverty

Linda F. Campbell and Emily M. Selby-Nelson

People living in poverty continue to be invisible to society, to mental health training and practice, and to diversity initiatives. Researchers and practitioners, albeit small in numbers, have offered a wealth of information about people in poverty who either don't receive psychological services or prematurely terminate. Our understanding of why and how this phenomenon of chronic poverty persists is explained in this chapter. Early stereotypical beliefs about people with lower socioeconomic status (SES) have had a devastating and enduring impact on attitudes toward the poor and view of their "suitability" for mental health services. For example, some common stereotypes are that (a) poor people are hard to empathize with, (b) do not permit appropriate therapeutic procedures, (c) insist exclusively on symptom relief, (d) use unbearably crude language, and (e) are apathetic with regard to treatment (Auld & Myers, 1954). "They are "extrospective . . . relatively unimaginative . . . and have lower estimated intelligence" than their middle- to upper-income counterparts (Brill & Storrow, 1960, p. 343).

Yet, as noted by Lorion (1974), there is no evidence that lower-SES individuals are less able to engage in psychotherapy than any other demographic group, and presumptions to the contrary reflect "therapists' negative bias" (p. 345). Mental health professionals, by virtue of their education and training, may hold privileged worldviews and inadvertently work in an ineffective and oppressive manner with lower-SES individuals (Sue & Sue, 2015). However, "there is ample reason to suspect that people living in poverty stand to benefit from mental health services that are tailored to their experiences and are implemented by clinicians who have been trained to deliver them effectively" (Smith, Li, Dykema, Hamlet, & Shellman, 2013, p. 139).

While some significant changes have occurred since the earlier statements cited above were made, much work remains to be done. Lower SES has been given a place in the list of diversity variables (e.g., culture, language, gender, sexual orientation) but not a place at the table. Many who live in poverty report, through their narratives, the same experiences reported 40 years ago.

This chapter will discuss the invisibility of poverty and the efforts being made to uncloak this elusive problem for the mental health professions. A critical element in removing barriers is the development of cultural competence, specifically class competence. Over recent years, the mental health professions have committed to a transformational level of consciousness raising, standards of training, and reflective practice in correcting longstanding violations of equity, respect, and dignity for all persons with whom we work. It is time for classism to be recognized among the other "isms" on which we are focused. The definitions of classism, poverty, and the poor are offered to provide a shared context for the reader in understanding the frame of reference and worldview that is applicable to this population, those who work with the population, and treatments of choice:

Classism is a form of oppression, which is prejudice plus power. Classism is an intricate system that rests on domination and control of social ideology, institutions, and resources with the intended outcome of privilege for one group and the disenfranchisement of the other (Hardiman & Jackson, 2016).

Poverty is "a human condition characterized by sustained or chronic deprivation of the resources, capabilities, choices, security and power necessary for the enjoyment of an adequate standard of living and other civil, cultural, economic, political, and social rights" (UN Economic and Social Council, 2001, p. 2). Descriptors of those who live in poverty include *low income, lower class, low SES, poor, economically poor, working poor, and disadvantaged* (Smith, 2005).

The poor are people who have been poor all their lives, whose parents were poor, and who have a high probability of remaining poor. It is thus a social, as well as an economic, condition. This definition of "poor" does not have sharp boundaries but includes the unemployed, partially unemployed, and the lower-income members of the working class (Karon & VandenBos, 1977, p. 169).

The Scope and Description of the Problem

Prevalence of Poverty in the United States

The rate of individuals living in poverty in the United States is 13.4% (39.7 million) (U.S. Census Bureau, 2018). Poverty is particularly prevalent among people of color, who already suffer from structural and institutional discrimination. The poverty rate for Whites is 9%, whereas it is 24% for Blacks, 21% for Latinx, and

11% for those of Asian descent. More women than men live in poverty (14% vs. 10%), and the rate of children living in poverty is 19.7%, the second highest in the world. Almost one third (31%) of families with a female head of household live below the poverty line (National Center for Law and Economic Justice, 2014). The poverty level is the metric used by the federal government to determine who is eligible for subsidies, programs, and benefits. The poverty guidelines are updated every January to factor in inflation. In 2018, the official poverty rate in the United States was $12,400 for an individual and $25,100 for a family of four (Fox, 2018).

The functional impact of poverty on marginalized and disadvantaged individuals is staggering. People living in poverty live shorter lives. The life expectancy between the wealthiest 1% and the poorest 1% is 14.6 years, and this percentage has increased over the last 15 years (Chetty et al., 2016).

Poverty and Mental Health Status

Research has demonstrated that those in lower socioeconomic levels have diminished psychological well-being and higher rates of anxiety, depression, and substance abuse than middle-class individuals. The experience of chronic and uncontrollable life events creates a context of stress that is cumulative. Due to increased risk of social determinants of poor health and adverse childhood experiences, individuals living in poverty may be exposed to additionally detrimental levels of stress and adversity, potentially putting them at risk for poor health throughout their lives. Common stressors include inability to meet basic needs, food insecurity, unstable housing, poor transportation availability, obstacles in accessing benefits (e.g., applying for food stamps, Medicaid, job applications), potentially high levels of stress and conflict in the home, and being stigmatized. People in poverty are affected by lack of community resources, lower quality of and access to education, higher crime rates, and greater distance to grocery and supply stores. These multiple complex stressors can adversely impact their ability to work, ability to advance in education, stability in the home, and ability to parent effectively, thereby creating a bidirectional downward spiral that makes high-quality mental health services a necessity. Despite the knowledge that mental health problems most often originate through the stressors of poverty, the mental health professions have done little to develop treatments that are tailored to the poor, resulting in ineffective outcomes and discouragement for clients.

Utilization and Outcomes

People living in poverty are less likely to seek or receive mental health services (Goodman, Smyth, & Banyard, 2010). Stereotypes of the poor (e.g., lack of motivation, intellectual limitations, undependability, assumed responsibility for life issues) persist, and discrepancies between mental health needs, services offered, and lack of preparation by clinicians result in much lower utilization than is needed (Smith, 2005). Patients of lower SES have higher attrition rates and lower improvement rates in psychotherapy than higher-SES clients. Relevant contributing factors may include (a) conventional psychotherapy approaches do not address the needs of those in poverty and (b) biases resulting in distancing (e.g., devaluing, discounting) interfere with psychotherapy (Goodman et al., 2010). The result is underutilization and inadequate mental health services for low-SES individuals.

Research on the psychological effects of poverty suggest that the basic needs categorized as practical/logistical barriers are most frequently noted and are certainly important to survival; however, psychosocial needs are as important for people in poverty as for higher-SES populations. These factors cluster into the following categories (Smith, 2010).

Stress

The inability to provide for oneself and one's family creates an ongoing chronic level of stress. People in poverty may be routinely overwhelmed by stress related to difficulties attaining or maintaining daily needs to sustain life for themselves and their loved ones. Time and resources are often exhausted by daily demands for survival and sustainability. Patients in this type of strenuous situation may not have the ability to consider or prioritize mental health treatment, despite their interest, desire, or motivation to do so. These stressors lead to ongoing negative affective states such as hopelessness, anger, and fear, and responses such as chronic vigilance given community violence, attributions of negative intent, and isolation (Chen & Matthews, 2003). Bureaucratic systems introduce obstacles and complexities that often pose hurdles too high to jump, such as applications for food stamps or housing, the SNAP program, and unemployment procedures. These power imbalances are often not acknowledged by authority figures but are keenly evident to those whose lives can be manipulated by powerful others. These imbalances can lead to feelings of disempowerment, alienation, hopelessness, and helplessness.

Social Isolation and Social Exclusion

Paradoxically, even in urban areas, people living in poverty can feel distanced and isolated and can experience an absence of the social connection that is a major element in protection against stress and serves as a predictor of emotional well-being. Views of the poor often attribute poverty to personal deficits and negative traits such as being unmotivated and lazy (Kunstman, Plant, & Deska, 2016). Poor people of color are doubly stigmatized with stereotypes of classism and racism through pejoratives such as violent, immoral, and abusive. Negative attitudes prevail toward people of all ethnicities regarding public assistance (Cozzarelli, Wilkinson, & Tagler, 2001). In essence, attitudes about the poor continue to suggest that the poor are inferior to others (Lott & Bullock, 2007). Even when low-SES individuals live in populated areas and have access to middle-class experiences, they remain isolated and excluded in the near presence of others. This dynamic occurs by the exclusion of the poor from mainstream opportunities, events, and experiences that others would take for granted and that contribute to a sense of community engagement and belonging. Some activities, such as cultural events, entertainment, and sports, are not affordable; others, such as community, school, and church events, still find low-SES individuals excluded and often invisible from being accepted as either volunteers or participants.

Powerlessness

The inherent power imbalances between people living in poverty and authority representatives who make decisions about them represent ongoing sources of stress and are often traumatic when individuals are blamed, shamed, or abused for being poor (e.g., fear that the wrong answer will result in loss of housing, children, or access to food) (Pajak, Ahmad, Jenney, Fisher, & Chan, 2014). These experiences over time can become internalized as part of one's identity, further disempowering and contributing to mental health difficulties (Goodman, Pugach, Skolnik, & Smith, 2013). Patients' sense of powerlessness can lead to a sense of alienation, distrust, and distancing from professionals and can compromise engagement and rapport in psychotherapy. As Thompson, Cole, and Nitzarim (2012) noted in a participant interview, "There is a huge stigma out there . . . You must be poor for a reason because that's a punishment for a crime you didn't even commit. . . . If you're down and out, you're already thinking that the world hates you because for whatever reason you worked hard enough, but you still didn't make it" (p. 215). Thompson et al. further report a participant stating, "You have to cater to them [therapists] and jump over their hoops because their analysis can mean taking away your kids, stopping or starting Social Security, and other stuff" (p. 215).

Interpersonal and cognitive distancing from the poor (Lott & Bullock, 2007) has, to a significant extent, become ingrained in our professional treatment of those in poverty, which may represent overt classist attitudes or may be inadvertent avoidance of seemingly despairing and entrenched individuals. This phenomenon is thought to occur because, unlike many other diversity variables that have positive attributes, no one wants to be poor, not those who were poor at one time nor those who have never been poor. People tend to avoid those who have what is stereotyped to have no positive attributes. As a result, interpersonal distancing from any social or civic association occurs and cognitive distancing results in not aligning with frame of reference or attempts at empathy. If we listen with respect to the voices of the poor, as we do in service to middle-class clients, we can break the silence of poverty in the treatment room and thereby "meet the clients where they are," which is our empathic goal with all other clients.

Barriers to Service Delivery

Logistical or practical barriers are often the default explanation given as the reason why people living in poverty do not seek mental health services. Very little attention is given to the questions of why there are few if any mental health awareness programs publicly announced for this population, and why few public health efforts are made to increase health education and decrease health disparity for people living in poverty. Awareness of the other equally impactful and harmful barriers to mental health services within the research and practice communities has not been well developed. The research on non-logistical barriers is sparse; however, qualitative researchers in particular have identified variables that can be clustered and defined as the following.

Client Variables

Practical Barriers

Cost of treatment is a barrier for individuals who may not be able to pay or who may be embarrassed to have the financial conversation about ability to pay. Transportation may be unavailable or unreliable (e.g., limited access to reliable vehicles or gas/bus money). Patients without reliable transportation often rely on family or neighbors to take them to appointments. This reliance on others to access care often leads to no shows or an inability to plan for and adhere to regular follow-up treatment. Childcare is tenuous and often means asking favors of others, for which individuals may or may not be able to reciprocate. Poor individuals often have low-wage jobs that entail changing shifts; this makes planning for appointments difficult, and taking time off work can place their job in jeopardy; poor people may have no personal time for appointments; they may have to deal with other inflexible conditions; and they are likely to be challenged by the cost and time involved in public transportation (Beeber et al., 2007). People in poverty may have difficulty adhering to treatment recommendations that require financial expense and or may struggle to follow recommendations to engage in behavioral activation due to inability to afford activities or access transportation to leave the home. As noted, other barriers are critically important to access of care; however, practice barriers must be resolved or at least recognized before other barriers can be addressed.

Even if individuals in poverty can access psychotherapy services, they may still be faced with barriers that prohibit them from following through on the prescribed treatment plan. For example, a typical intervention like behavioral activation may include the encouragement of pleasurable activities. However, patients in poverty may not have the financial means to support that recommendation or treatment goal. Similarly, patients with chronic illnesses, such as diabetes, are often encouraged by a behavioral health provider to purchase healthier foods such as fresh fruits, vegetables, and lean protein. However, individuals in poverty may be living in areas where fresh food is scarce and may rely on gas stations or convenience stores as their food source. These patients are likely unable to go to the store frequently enough to purchase fresh foods and may not be able to afford those foods at all, so they buy less expensive, less healthy processed foods that are typically high in sugar, salt, and carbohydrates. This inability to access healthier food options prevents these patients from adhering to medical recommendations that promote health and wellness. Patients in poverty may be unable to follow through on a therapist's recommendation to increase exercise, as they may not live in an area where it is safe to walk outside or may not be able to afford or access a gym. They may not have access to the internet, a television, or a computer on which to watch exercise videos.

Attitudinal Barriers

The stigma of mental health treatment is held by many in lower-SES positions based on family bias, cultural beliefs, societal stereotyping, and self-blaming/criticism. Ethnic minorities may be suspicious of treatment given historical exploitation and persecution. People in poverty may fear that their pursuit of services could jeopardize their parental status in that saying "the wrong thing" to a psychotherapist can result in their children being taken away, their disability being questioned, and their access to resources (e.g., food stamps, Medicaid) being brought under examination beyond their control (Copeland & Snyder, 2011).

Social and Psychological Barriers

Low-income people primarily hold jobs in which authority figures (e.g., managers, supervisors) oversee their work and have considerable control over their work conditions. People living in poverty have experienced so many negative encounters and dismissive treatment that any interaction with those with authority and power in decision-making positions can engender fear, anxiety, and a filtering of information. Given that psychotherapists are viewed as authority figures, it is understandable that clients would anticipate negative consequences and the possibility of demeaning attitudes, devaluation, and inability to empathize.

Psychotherapist Variables

The mental health field has consistently misplaced the rationale for lower participation, as well as lower successful outcome rates, for lower-SES individuals on stereotype bias by psychotherapists and/or actual barriers of clients and has neglected the role of psychotherapists. "Modalities of care suggested as appropriate for the lower classes may turn out to be inadvertent discrimination in disguise" (Siassi & Messer, 1976, p. 32). Although alternatives to conventional therapeutic interventions are, in fact, suggested, the recommendations for "shortcuts" and brief services is not the adaptation needed to serve the poor.

Classism

Occupation and education are among the most defining characteristics of class. Mental health professionals have attained the status of middle or upper middle class by virtue of education, even if they began their lives in working-class or poor families. Psychotherapists can fall prey to implicit bias or to overt classism, communicating distance and devaluation to patients (Appio, Chambers, & Mao, 2013; Smith, 2005). "Psychotherapists' willingness and ability to work with the poor is compromised by persistent, unexamined classist attitudes" (Smith, 2005, p. 687). As Sue and Lam (2011) emphasize, "Despite the important influence of socioeconomic status on an individual's life, this variable has been widely ignored. It seems that there are still biases and stereotypes that psychologists have with regard to this population" (p. 414).

People who live in poverty are keenly aware of the factors that separate them from others around them, such as clothing, jewelry, vocabulary, and the décor and furnishings displayed in the office. Appio et al. (2012) cite examples taken from participant narratives. One participant noted that even though she and her psychotherapist "got along," she could not help but notice that all of the books on the shelves were "way over my head." Another client noted that her counselor had pictures of her vacations all over the office and pictures of her playing tennis. These symbols communicated to this client that they lived in two different worlds. The participant reported, "I like vacations, too, but I will never be able to go on one."

These examples can be reasonably attributed to implicit bias; however, psychotherapists also have expressed overt classism through beliefs that the poor as a group are disorganized; they aren't motivated (as evidenced by not being prompt for appointments, for example); or they are cognitively limited and not able to fully participate (Appio et al., 2013). The failure to recognize the contextual and environmental barriers of the poor perpetuates a trait rather than state causal view of the problem, thereby creating additional barriers to treatment. The inherent privilege of the psychotherapist, contrasted with that of a lower-SES patient, is not typically acknowledged, discussed, or utilized as part of the therapeutic situation or relationship; however, this factor often acts as a treatment barrier.

Adherence to Conventional Psychotherapy and Inflexibility

Treatment outcomes are not as successful for lower-SES clients as others principally because of the aforementioned barriers. But when treatment plans are adapted for the context and the barriers of people living in poverty, significant improvements in retention rates as well as symptomatology are evidenced (Grote, Zuckoff, Swartz, Bledsoe, & Geibel, 2009). The adherence to conventional psychotherapy precludes meeting after business hours, accommodating walk-in appointments, meeting elsewhere than the office, allowing children in the office, eliminating no-show and cancellation policies, and assisting in making calls to agencies regarding resources and benefits. These are activities that are not typically viewed as within the scope of practice of mental health professionals but are key elements in the access of mental health services for the poor (Goodman et al., 2013).

Silence

The failure to initiate and then allow an ongoing discussion about class has the same deleterious effect as the failure to bring into psychotherapy ethnic, cultural, gender, or other diversity variables that could impact psychotherapy. Clients rely on the knowledge and skills of the clinician and think that if social class is not at least recognized, then the psychotherapist is either biased, unknowledgeable, and potentially ineffective; is distancing from the client; or is unable to align and empathize with the patient. Avoidance of open discussions about class differences also heightens the anxiety of clients, for fear of judgment engendering shame and humiliation over their plight (Appio et al., 2013). Paradoxically, psychotherapists may fear drawing attention to social class as though if they don't speak about it, the clients won't notice the contrast.

Competency

Multicultural competence is now a mainstay of graduate education and a standard requirement for accreditation. Poverty and class, however, have yet to be included in curriculum requirements and clinical training for most doctoral programs (Stabb & Reimers, 2013). Class competency should not be confused with the classism heretofore described. Competency is measured by knowledge, skills, and attitudes (i.e., interpersonal competence) that are learned through didactic education and supervised experience while in training and through consultation, continuing education, and professional development as a practicing mental health professional. Incompetency is not characterized by prejudice, bias, and discrimination that is inherent in classism; however, incompetency can also be damaging to clients when the contextual understanding necessary to be effective in working with people in poverty is not a mastered skill.

Despite years of multicultural research, practice innovations, and inclusion in the training and accreditation of graduate programs, the factors of conventional treatment applicability, classism, and the stereotypical attributions and bias against people living in poverty have not been investigated in any meaningful way (Smith et al., 2013).

Systems Variables

Local, state, and national governmental agencies as well as other nonprofit and nongovernmental systems (e.g., hospitals, health clinics, educational systems) are central to the basic needs and availability of resources for people living in poverty. These entities have extraordinary decision-making authority and control over the lives of the poor. These power imbalances, coupled with the survival need to be compliant with these systems, are primary stressors. In addition, the pursuit of these resources can be extraordinarily difficult: (a) clients may not understand the system, (b) the multistep process in applying for food stamps requires a set of appointments, (c) applying for subsidized housing can take several years, and (d) just finding the entitlements for which one is eligible can be challenging. These are just a few examples of the impact of the power imbalance (Pajak et al., 2014). Medical and mental health services rarely have sufficient bilingual and ethnic minority psychotherapists. Often professional as well as support staff who lack training in working with low-income individuals aren't aware of relevant barriers to compliance and are unaware of the community resources available, which then often go underutilized (Green, Kaltman, Frank, Glennie, Subramanian, & Fritts-Wilson, 2011).

When individuals are already economically disadvantaged, they can experience uniquely complicated hardship following challenging events like community-based or natural disasters, exacerbating their preexisting adversity. This population has an increased chance of living in subpar housing or in homes that have become devalued due to the financial inability to maintain and restore them. When a disaster occurs at a magnitude where homes and other buildings are damaged or destroyed, people in poverty struggle significantly when disaster recovery funds are awarded based on the pre-disaster value of one's destroyed assets. These families are required to downsize and move into homes or alternative living that is supported by their low recovery funds.

Creating Cultural Competency

Awareness and knowledge of classism are foundational components of multiculturally competent practice (Zalaquett & Chambers, 2017). Cultural competency, as has been noted here, is an essential component in training and professional practice standards of care. More typically a competency section would include several diversity variables; however, competence in this chapter will focus on class and socioeconomic competence. As has been noted, class has not been reliably embedded in diversity training and has not been a focus of continued skill development in standards of practice, and research in this area has not advanced significantly beyond what has been known for 25 years. Further, institutional practice has not incorporated training or practice policies for wide dissemination throughout the profession. As a result of these deficits in training and practice preparation to work with this population, attaining a level of cultural competence often falls on individual psychotherapists to pursue. An organized developmental approach to cultural competence for practitioners who did not receive such training is an imperative for continuing education and professional development offerings. Actions that can promote cultural competence for individual practitioners are identified below.

Self-Awareness and Personal Beliefs

Practitioners should engage in self-reflection regarding their own experiences with low-SES individuals related to their own social class, noting their emotional and psychological reactions. They should endeavor to identify the occasions in which they interact with low-SES individuals, the quality of those interactions, and any stereotypical beliefs that emerge. They may believe that (a) people living in poverty have too many basic life problems to focus on mental health needs; (b) given their other problems, the practitioner cannot even make a dent in their situation; (c) mental illness is an expected life condition for these individuals

(Smith et al., 2013); and (d) in some way, poverty is the fault of the individuals living in those conditions, and they must help themselves first (Liu, 2012).

Case Consultation

Peer consultation, particularly group supervision, enables practitioners to go beyond their own self-reflective assessment of their cultural competence. Implicit bias is the influence of stereotyped and biased attitudes and beliefs outside of our conscious awareness or knowledge and is much more nuanced than overt classism. Peer consultation regarding the treatment of low-SES clients gives practitioners the opportunity to explore their awareness, treatment choices, the clinical relationship, and other case dynamics in an open and supportive environment.

Introduction of Class into the Psychotherapy Session

Intuitively, practitioners may not address the subject of class if clients do not include the topic in working issues for psychotherapy. They may perceive that clients aren't aware of class differences, that drawing attention to class might make the client uncomfortable, or that psychotherapists themselves will be uncomfortable. Practitioners should know that if they notice a class difference clients surely will, and furthermore will likely be uncertain about how to express their observations. Practitioners may introduce the topic through immediacy and the here and now of the session just as they would other session variables that are obvious but unrecognized (Smith, 2005). Experiential psychotherapists might call this action "making overt the covert." Practitioners would explore how clients feel about any perceived differences, how they think these differences could affect their psychotherapy, and what the psychotherapist can do to respect and respond to class factors.

Working Alliance

The psychotherapy relationship is a central component in effective treatment and outcome across modalities, diagnostic classifications, and client and psychotherapist variables. Formation of a working alliance is particularly valuable with low-SES clients given their skepticism about services, self-doubts, and anticipation of emotional barriers. Development of collaboration that conveys equality and promotes trust encourages disclosures that might otherwise be seen as too risky (Appio et al., 2013). Attention to social class cues is a skill that can significantly advance cultural competence awareness and enhance the working alliance (Thompson et al., 2012). Just like other basic psychotherapy skills such as attending to nonverbal cues of clients and clinicians, practitioners should be alert to social class cues exhibited by clients and those that can be interpreted by clients as defining characteristics of the clinician. Social class cues from clients can include nuanced expressions of anxiety, self-consciousness, uncertainty, or embarrassment about transportation or tardiness, or a restricted range of conversation topics. Social class cue interpretations by clients of their clinicians, as noted previously, can include the décor of the office, personal photos, jewelry, conversation about free time or travel, and vocabulary. Psychotherapists' professional surroundings typically reflect their educational and professional status. These same symbols of comfort and validation to psychotherapists can signify class privilege and "not belonging" to the poor. Psychotherapists who become aware of these inadvertent messages can begin to have authentic conversations with clients about their perceptions and how these may affect their willingness to accept services.

Advocacy

Advocacy has not been viewed as part of conventionally delivered psychotherapy. However, qualitative studies have demonstrated that taking an advocacy stance significantly enhances the psychotherapy experience for low-SES individuals. An advocacy stance may include strategies that support and train clients to effectively represent and assert their needs, navigate the systems around them, utilize resources, and promote community engagement. Examples of advocacy engagement include teaching life skills (e.g., assertiveness, insurance coverage negotiations), financial information (e.g., compound interest impact on loans), accessing resources (e.g., housing subsidies, Social Security Disability Income, training opportunities), and communicating directly with other health professionals (Thompson et al., 2012).

Language and Client Literacy

Practitioners will want to become familiar with colloquialisms, metaphors, and idioms that are characteristic of the regional culture of low-SES clients. For example, Appalachian people may say they feel like "a lost ball in the high weeds," or they feel "fair to middlin." Psychotherapists may feel ambivalent about altering their own language use in that they don't want to "talk down" to clients, yet it is important to avoid language that laypeople may not know, such as "operant conditioning," "cognitive dissonance," "countertransference," or "behavioral reinforcement schedules." In terms of literacy, the 2018 adult literacy level was determined to be an eighth-grade level of reading (U.S. Department of Health and Human Services, 2019). Practitioners often provide or recommend reading material for clients and will want to be aware of the level of difficulty both for paper documents and online recommendations. Online services are available through which materials can be evaluated for reading level.

In addition to being alert to reading literacy, practitioners will want to be aware of their clients' health literacy, which is the ability to obtain, process, and understand health information well enough to make health-related decisions (Centers for Disease Control and Prevention, 2018). Education on how to read prescription labels, understand the importance of dosage, know what medications must be taken regularly and which should be taken as needed, how to access financial assistance for annual physical exams, and other health literacy factors should be part of health discussions with low-SES clients.

Access to Integrated Settings

When working with low-SES clients, practitioners in independent, group, integrated, or other settings can collaborate with interdisciplinary settings that would include access to social work, pharmacy, public health, and medical professionals to engage with whole-person care for their clients. Low or no-cost primary care clinics committed to serving those below the poverty line often welcome collaboration with practitioners whose clients receive medical care at these clinics. Mental health practitioners are welcomed at clinics serving low-income patients such as for conducting presentations to staff, providing pro bono services to other patients, collaborating with medical professionals, helping to improve adherence to treatment plans for patients (e.g., hepatitis C programs), and offering other behavioral health expertise that mental health practitioners bring to primary care settings. A secondary advantage of affiliation with integrated care settings is the reduction of stigma for low-income patients (Shim & Rust, 2013) in that individuals may be willing to seek primary care at an accessible and available clinic but not be willing to go to a second site for behavioral health.

Effective Strategies and Empirically-Supported Treatments

Methods and techniques that contribute to improved outcome in providing psychological services to the poor can be clustered as (a) quantitative studies on treatment outcome, (b) flexible evidence-based treatments, (c) qualitative studies identifying factors that make a difference to clients, and (d) recommendations for therapeutic approaches that depart from conventional psychotherapy.

Quantitative Studies

Miranda et al. (2006) compared the effectiveness of cognitive behavioral therapy (CBT) versus medication in the treatment of depressed, low-income White and ethnic minority women. At a one-year follow-up, decreases in depression were found for both groups (50.9% for antidepressants and 56.9% for CBT). In a related study (Roy-Byrne et al., 2006), the effectiveness of evidence-based care across income lines was compared. Primary care patients diagnosed with panic disorder were given either CBT or pharmacotherapy, and the patient groups were divided into those living above the poverty line and those below. Initially, those living below the poverty line had much more symptom severity and comorbidity. However, reduction of symptoms was similar across the two groups, and poor individuals were just as responsive to psychotherapy as other income groups. The significance of these findings is that they further support the usefulness of psychotherapy for the poor and challenge assumptions that individuals in poverty may be less able to participate effectively and remain engaged in treatment.

Two studies examined the effects of interpersonal psychotherapy (IPT) for low-income women. The first recruited individuals with trauma histories and diagnoses of post-traumatic stress disorder (PTSD) and randomly assigned them to IPT or wait list group. At the one-year follow-up, participants in the IPT group not only demonstrated significant reductions in PTSD compared to the wait list group but also showed improved interpersonal functioning. A second study investigated the effect of IPT on women with depression. A culturally relevant version of IPT was conducted, and the participants receiving enhanced IPT-B, compared with those in enhanced usual care, demonstrated significant reductions in depression across three months and at six months showed significant improvement in social functioning (Grote et al., 2009).

Multiple studies on collaborative care treatment for depression among low-income Latino adults have been conducted. When collaborative services are engaged and patients receive medical care, medication, symptom monitoring, and relapse prevention, their depression significantly improved (Ell, et al., 2011). These and other quantitative studies demonstrate the applicability of psychotherapy to the poor, begin to dispel the longstanding stereotypes of intractability of low-income people in resistance to psychotherapy, and offer suggestions for interventions and culturally sensitive approaches to treatment that may yield outcomes for individuals in poverty.

Flexible, Evidence-Based Treatments

Conventional treatment interventions have not proven effective with low-SES individuals; however, evidence-based treatments that have implemented intensive outreach, transportation, flexible scheduling, convenience locations, and childcare remove many of the barriers that prevent people in poverty from a fair playing field in access to mental health services. Santiago, Kaltman, and Miranda (2013) identified the following key recommendations from their experience working with people of poverty. *Flexibility* in treatment schedules may vary by session given shift employment, childcare, and other barriers; flexibility should be built into the treatment plan rather than being an exception made occasionally. *Tailoring* treatments (e.g., flexible hours, meeting outside the office, bringing family members) to the specific needs of clients, even though it may represent a departure from standard practice, greatly contributes to overcoming the physical and logistical barriers. Substantial *outreach for engagement and retention* is a key element to provision of services. Many low-SES individuals are not familiar with mental health services and are not aware of the applicability or accessibility to them. Training of staff in class culture and awareness of classism changes the contextual experiences of clients coming into the therapeutic environment as well as their expectations for services. Commensurate with ongoing outreach is telephone engagement, which can be time intensive initially but has been shown (Miranda, Lawson, & Escobar, 2002) to significantly improve retention and subsequent outcome. In the same study, those who were skeptical of psychotherapy were offered an educational session that was meant to increase understanding of what psychotherapy would be like and would thereby demystify the process. All of these efforts contribute to building trust and communicating respect and transparency, which are prerequisites for successful outcomes.

Qualitative Studies

Perspectives from the Poor

Given the higher dropout rate for low-income people, Pugach and Goodman (2015) studied the experiences of ten low-income women through a qualitative descriptive model. The data characterized the individuals' responses as follows:

1. Awareness therapy was meaningful when the psychotherapist was aware of the nature of poverty and had direct exposure to poverty.
2. Practice—psychotherapy was useful when the psychotherapist was flexible, provided support, and focused on strengths rather than deficits.
3. Relational factors were important and were demonstrated by the psychotherapist listening, sharing power, and showing authenticity.

Enhancing the 50-Minute Hour

Thompson et al. (2012) examined the process of psychotherapy with low-income clients after completing six months of treatment to capture the clients' experiences of social class in psychotherapy. The rich and insightful narratives of these interviewees illuminated several themes:

1. The psychotherapist's ability and willingness to manage and to acknowledge social class within the room significantly shifted the balance of power and reinforced respect toward the client.
2. Social class was acknowledged as a contextual characteristic that influences the psychotherapy process. These methods include deliberate conversations regarding social class differences between psychotherapist and client.
3. Social class content was integrated into psychotherapy. Mental health treatment with people who live in poverty specifically needs to address social class-related complexities (Goodman et al., 2010).

The most important single characteristic noted by interviewees was willingness to extend the 50-minute hour in terms of flexibility, support, advocacy, and relationship building. The psychotherapist treated clients as whole persons rather than attending only to decreasing mental health symptoms. Individual acts of caring included checking up by phone between sessions (e.g., calling on the first anniversary of the death of the client's father), expressing sympathy upon the loss of a family member, engaging in appropriate self-disclosure, giving the client small gifts symbolic of progress, informing the client of financial literacy resources or resources for reduced cost of medication, and supporting clients in filling out applications.

Some patients in poverty express appreciation for other types of flexibility in service delivery. Being rigid in no-show and lateness policies falls short of meeting these patients where they are in in their lives. Scheduling policies that allow more flexibility in absences, late attendance, and same-day work-in appointments offer the flexibility needed to support these patients, who face numerous and unexpected stressors in their daily life outside of treatment. Accessibility to individuals who are transient or experiencing homelessness is relevant to this population and should be integrated into the psychotherapist's practice by developing alternate locations for sessions (e.g., arrangements with shelters, service agencies, and free or low-cost clinics for space). The level of life stress, unpredictability in daily routine, and barriers to care are significantly more complex and severe for these underserved populations and warrant extra sensitivity and consideration.

Modified Therapeutic Modalities

The Relationship-Centered Model

Goodman et al. (2007) developed the relationship-centered advocacy (RCA) model, in which mental health professionals and clients collaborate on setting goals and overcoming any barriers to achieving them. Meeting times and locations are flexible and require travel to local agencies. The psychotherapy therefore involves both psychological and systemic concerns and barriers. The RCA model entails practitioners and clients (often termed "partners" to emphasize collaboration) working together for a given number of hours per week and focusing on the immediate needs and issues of the clients. Meetings are typically at the client's home or another preferred location. The pair work together for an agreed-upon number of weeks or months (Weintraub & Goodman, 2010). Goodman et al. offered the example that when a client felt ashamed when a store manager spoke loudly to her about items her food stamps didn't cover, the psychotherapist could work with the client on her feelings of shame, but also collaboratively identified a way the patient could return to the store and speak to the manager about his manner to people using food stamps.

Feminist Therapy

Psychotherapy must extend beyond the walls of the treatment room and beyond the focus on symptom reduction to a contextual level of awareness and advocacy. Recognition of power, who has it, and how it can be negotiated are important components of the therapeutic dialogue with lower-income clients. Reconceptualizing boundaries, selective self-disclosure, showing emotion, and other unconventional stances that are among basic tenets of feminist theory are also among the key elements of psychotherapy with people in poverty (Brown, 2009).

Relational-Cultural Therapy (RCT)

Although RCT was born out of the recognition that traditional psychotherapies did not represent women's experiences and were often not effective with women, the modality has been equally applied to many groups who are marginalized by more powerful societal forces. The concept of disconnection, which is expressed in the writings of poverty as distancing, is a central dynamic in RCT. Disconnections are invalidations of those in the lower classes that give rise to shame, particularly in the presence of silence about social class (Jordan, 2010). RCT promotes awareness of power imbalances and societal and institutional systems that perpetuate oppression and link these concepts to the psychotherapy in the room. Naming and discussing client experiences and putting them in a cultural and societal context is instrumental to the tenets of RCT, feminist therapy, and effective treatment of people living in poverty.

Future Steps

The rise of diversity and its role in our society's developing moral compass is relatively new. Steps forward can be viewed through the lens of training, practice, research, and settings.

Training

Class competency is not a designated curriculum component of graduate training and with few exceptions (e.g., social work) is not taught at all. Specific didactic and clinical training experiences need to be embedded in the multicultural curriculum or taught as a separate emphasis. That is, specific course content and specific practicum experience in working with people in poverty should be clearly identified. Such curriculum should also operationalize the unique struggles of people living in poverty in urban versus rural areas. Practicum and other clinical training experiences that take place in the poor communities ensure integration of skills and healthy attitudes. *Resources for Inclusion of Social Class in Psychology Curriculum* (American Psychological Association, 2008) provides useful educational material, but the resources in this book do not reflect recent work. Supervision of practitioners working with people in poverty should focus on class competency, encourage awareness of and address provider privilege, and promote provider self-care and continued development in professional flexibility and patient-centered care. Supervisors also should have received formal training or continuing education, consultation, and professional development to ensure competence to supervise.

Greater attention by continuing education and professional development sponsors (e.g., American Psychological Association, National Association of Social Workers, American Counseling Association, American Association for Marriage and Family Therapy, and the American Psychiatric Association) to the teaching of classism, stereotyping, and prejudicial treatment is essential so that practitioners have the knowledge and skills to develop these class competencies.

Research

Treatment research through quantitative methods continues to be vital to the area; however, increased utilization of qualitative approaches will illuminate the need for investigation into psychotherapist and client variables that impact psychotherapy usage and outcome. Effective research in the future will need to consider making the same flexibility modifications that practitioners have made (e.g., transportation, childcare, and time flexibility) if applicable and meaningful research is to be done in this area (Miranda et al., 2002). Future researchers in this area are also encouraged to study the unique experiences and treatment needs of individuals from varied levels and types of poverty and disadvantaged situations.

Practice

Successful practice with lower-SES populations will involve practitioners' awareness of their own specific cultural identity and effort to understand the differences between themselves and their lower-SES patients.

Recognition of the importance of emotional and psychological support for mental health professionals in this work is important for the avoidance of burnout. Practitioners need access to materials and methods that promote the sustainability of this service while supporting the whole-person health and well-being of practitioners. Additionally, interprofessional alliances will promote ongoing development of clinicians while also contributing to interpersonal connectedness and the increase of the value of work with people in poverty by others.

Creative contextual and flexible mental health practices will involve becoming collaborators rather than experts with clients and require flexibility in thinking about ethical frameworks and possible reconsideration of traditional practice. Advocacy for clients on a practical clinical level and on the institutional and policy levels is important for any progress in the treatment of poor people. Advocacy on any level can be a valuable activity for providers as it allows for new challenges, learning, and diversity in professional activity and factors found to reduce burnout risk.

Settings and Systems

A true challenge in promoting psychotherapists' interest in working with people living in poverty is motivation and incentive. Those who have written about, and practice with, this population are primarily motivated by values of service, compassion for the poor, and the creed "To whom much is given, much is expected." Other than pro bono commitments, practitioners are not likely to engage with marketing and recruitment for this population. Two developments in mental health practice of recent years are changing the landscape favorably toward greater potential for services to this population.

In recent years, advocacy has become not only an accepted but an expected component of advancing mental health services. Advocacy is now a standard among many accreditation requirements, benchmark competency models, and multiple diversity guidelines. Grassroots, as well as systems, efforts to enhance Medicaid, SNAP, welfare or Temporary Assistance for Needy Families (TANF), and the Children's Health Insurance Program (CHIP) are among the vehicles for supporting the basic needs of the poor. Such safety nets elevate the poor and bring within reach mental health services for psychological and emotional needs.

Second, integrated behavioral health care in this country has taken a transformative trajectory. Not long ago, mental health professionals faced barriers to accessing employment and integrating into medical settings and primary care facilities. For several reasons, including successful advocacy, strategic initiative, and interprofessional engagement, behavioral health is becoming a mainstay in integrated and primary care settings. Psychotherapists, as behavioral health professionals or consultants, are now part of an integrated team in which low-SES clients are seen for medical treatment, with the psychological services offered as a companion service and adjunct to medical services. This collaborative care approach opens up opportunities for clinicians that were not previously possible. In underserved rural and remote areas, rural hospitals and community health centers are more often providing integrated primary care services to patients who may have not previously had access to care in that some of these facilities treat underinsured and uninsured patients. These medical settings often provide services in a whole-patient care model by including integrated behavioral health services, resulting in improved access to mental health care for patients who would otherwise go untreated. People living in poverty in these underserved communities are now more likely to have access to much-needed treatment and resources. These clinics also may employ health care professionals such as care coordinators and patient representatives, who are trained to assist patients in overcoming barriers to care and resolving practical lifestyle and financial issues, such as housing, job insecurity, transportation, and food insecurity, and referring them to other resources and services (e.g., legal assistance) (Stabb & Remiers, 2013).

Training programs are beginning to affiliate with low-cost or free clinics that serve only those living under the poverty line. As an example, the first author of this chapter maintains a doctoral practicum site at a free clinic in which low-SES patients who receive medical services at the clinic are, for the first time, offered behavioral health treatment. The students and supervisors work directly with the medical staff on integrated treatment plans that greatly enhance the whole-person care of the low-SES patients.

This chapter has attempted to review the myriad problems, complex barriers, and possibilities for advancement in the welfare of those living in poverty. The invisibility of this population is profound and, once realized, cannot be forgotten. We knew 40 years ago what we know now. We only hope it is not another 40 years before we as a society, and people of conscience, will act to lift the oppression that represents the life of people in poverty.

References

American Psychological Association. (2008). *Report of the APA task force on socioeconomic status.* Washington, DC: Author.

Appio, L., Chambers, D. A., & Mao, S. (2013). Listening to the voices of the poor and disrupting the silence about class issues in psychotherapy. *Journal of Clinical Psychology: In Session, 69*(2), 152–161.

Auld, F., & Myers, J. K. (1954). Contributions to a theory for selecting psychotherapy patients. *Journal of Clinical Psychology, 10,* 56–60.

Beeber, L. S., Cooper, C., Van Noy, B. E., Schwartz, T. A., Blanchard, H. C., Canuso, R., . . . Emory, S. L. (2007). Flying under the radar. *Advances in Nursing Science, 30,* 221–234.

Brill, N. Q., & Storrow, H. A. (1960). Social class and psychiatric treatment. *Archives of General Psychiatry, 3*(4), 340–344.

Brown, L. S. (2009). *Feminist therapy.* Washington, DC: American Psychological Association.

Centers for Disease Control and Prevention. (2018). Health literacy. Retrieved from https://www.cdc.gov/healthliteracy/index.html

Chen, E., & Matthews, K. A. (2003). Development of the cognitive appraisal and understanding of social events (CAUSE) videos. *Health Psychology, 22*(1), 106–110.

Chetty, R., Stepner, J., Abraham, S., Lin, S., Scuderi, B., Turner, N., . . . Cutler, D. (2016). The association between income and life expectancy in the United States, 2001–2014. *Journal of the American Medical Association, 315,* 1750–1766.

Copeland, V. C., & Snyder, K. (2011). Barriers to mental health treatment services for low-income African American women whose children receive behavioral health services: An ethnographic investigation. *Social Work in Public Health, 26,* 78–95.

Cozzarelli, C., Wilkinson, A., & Tagler, M. (2001). Attitudes toward the poor and attributions for poverty. *Journal of Social Issues, 57,* 207–227.

Ell, K., Xie, B., Kapetanovic, S., Quinn, D., Lee, P.-J., Wells, A., & Chou, C. (2011). One-year follow-up of collaborative depression care for low-income, predominantly Hispanic patients with cancer. *Psychiatric Services*, *62*(2), 162–170.

Frank, J. D. (1961). *Persuasion and healing: A comparative study of psychotherapy*. New York, NY: Schocken Books.

Fox, L. (2018). The Supplemental Poverty Measure: 2017: Current population reports. U.S. Census Bureau report # P60-265. Retrieved from https://www.census.gov/content/dam/Census/library/publications/2018/demo/p60-265.pdf

Goodman, L., Litwin, A., Bohlig, A., Weintraub, S., Green, A., Walker, J., . . . & Ryan, N. (2007). Applying feminist theory to community practice: A multilevel empowerment intervention for low-income women with depression. In E. Aldarondo (Ed.). *Advancing social justice through clinical practice* (pp. 265–290). New York: Lawrence Erbaum.

Goodman, L., Pugach, M., Skolnik, A., & Smith, L. (2013). Poverty and mental health practice: Within and beyond the 50-minute hour. *Journal of Clinical Psychology: In Session*, *69*(2), 182–190.

Goodman, L. A., Smyth, K., & Banyard, V. (2010). Beyond the 50-minute hour: Increasing control, choice, and connections in the lives of low-income women. *American Journal of Orthopsychiatry*, *80*, 3–11. doi:10.1111/j.1939-0025.2010.01002.x

Green, B., Kaltman, S., Frank, L., Glennie, M., Subramanian, A., & Fritts-Wilson, J. (2011). Primary care providers' experiences with trauma patients: A qualitative study. *Psychological Trauma: Theory, Research, Practice, and Policy*, *3*, 37–41.

Grote, N., Zuckoff, A., Swartz, H., Bledsoe, S., & Geibel, S. (2009). Engaging women who are depressed and economically disadvantaged in mental health treatment. *Social Work*, *52*, 295–308.

Hardiman, R., & Jackson, B. (2016). Conceptual foundations for social justice courses. In M. Adams, L. A. Bell, & P. Griffin (Eds.), *Teaching for diversity and social justice* (pp. 16–29). New York, NY: Routledge.

Jordan, J. V. (2010). *Relational-cultural therapy*. Washington, DC: American Psychological Association.

Karon, B. P., & VandenBos, G. R. (1977). Psychotherapeutic technique and the economically poor patient. *Psychotherapy: Theory, Research and Practice*, *14*, 169–180.

Kunstman, J., Plant, F., & Deska, J. (2016). White ≠ poor: Whites distance, derogate, and deny low-status ingroup members. *Personality and Social Psychology Bulletin*, *42*, 230–243.

Liu, W. M. (2012). *Social class and classism in the helping professions: Research, theory, and practice*. Washington, DC: Sage Publications.

Lorion, R. P. (1974). Patient and therapist variable in the treatment of low-income patients. *Psychological Bulletin*, *81*, 344–354.

Lott, B., & Bullock, H. (2007). *Psychology and economic injustice: Personal, professional, and political intersections*. Washington, DC: American Psychological Association.

Miranda, J., Green, B., Krupnick, J., Chung, J., Siddique, J., Belin, T., & Revicki, D. (2006). One-year outcomes of a randomized clinical trial treating depression in low-income minority women. *Journal of Consulting and Clinical Psychology*, *74*(1), 99–111.

Miranda, J., Lawson, W., & Escobar, J. (2002). Ethnic minorities. *Mental Health Services*, *4*, 231–337.

National Center for Law and Economic Justice. (2014). *Poverty in the United States: A snapshot* (Fact sheet). Retrieved from http://www.nclej.org/poverty-in-the-us.php

Pajak, C., Ahmad, F., Jenney, A., Fisher, P., & Chan, L. (2014). Survivor's costs of saying no: Exploring the experience of accessing services for intimate partner violence. *Journal of Interpersonal Violence, 29*, 257–259.

Pugach, M. R., & Goodman, L. A. (2015). Low-income women's experiences in outpatient psychotherapy: A qualitative descriptive analysis. *Counselling Psychology Quarterly, 28*(4), 403–426.

Roy-Byrne, P., Sherbourne, C., Miranda, J., Stein, M., Craske, M., Golinelli, D., & Sullivan, G. (2006). Poverty and response to treatment among panic disorder patients in primary care. *American Journal of Psychiatry, 163*(8), 1–7.

Santiago, C., Kaltman, S., & Miranda, J. (2013). Poverty and mental health: How do low-income adults and children fare in psychotherapy? *Journal of Clinical Psychology: In Session, 69*(2), 115–126.

Shim, R., & Rust, G. (2013). Primary care, behavioral health, and public health: Partners in reducing mental health stigma. *American Journal of Public Health, 103*(5), 774–776.

Siassi, L., & Messer, S. B. (1976). Psychotherapy with patients from lower socioeconomic groups. *American Journal of Psychotherapy, 30*, 29–40.

Smith, L. (2005). Psychotherapy, classism, and the poor: Conspicuous by their absence. *American Psychologist, 60*(70), 687–696.

Smith, L. (2010). *Psychology, poverty, and the end of social exclusion*. New York, NY: Teachers College Press.

Smith, L., Li, V., Dykema, S., Hamlet, D., & Shellman, A. (2013). "Honoring somebody that society doesn't honor": Therapists working in the context of poverty. *Journal of Clinical Psychology, 69*(2), 138–151.

Stabb, S., & Reimers, F. (2013). Competent poverty training. *Journal of Clinical Psychology, 69*, 172–181.

Sue, D. W., & Sue, S. (2015). *Counseling the culturally diverse: Theory and practice* (5th ed.). New York, NY: Wiley.

Sue, S., & Lam, A. G. (2011). Cultural and demographic diversity. In J. C. Norcross (Ed.), *Psychotherapy relationships that work: Therapist contributions and responsiveness to patients* (pp. 401–422). New York, NY: Oxford University Press.

Thompson, M. N., Cole, O. D., & Nitzarim, R. S. (2012). Recognizing social class in the psychotherapy relationship grounded theory exploration of low-income clients. *Journal of Counseling Psychology, 59*, 208–221.

United Nations Economic and Social Council (UNESC), Committee on Economic, Social and Cultural Rights. (2001). *Substantive issues arising in the implementation of the International Covenant on Economic, Social and Cultural Rights: Poverty and the International Covenant on Economic, Social and Cultural Rights.* Retrieved from http://www2.ohchr.org/english/bodies/cescr/docs/statements/E.C.12.2001.10Poverty-2001.pdf

U.S. Department of Health and Human Services. (2018, January). Poverty guidelines. Retrieved from https://aspe.hhs.gov/poverty-guidelines

U.S. Census Bureau. (2018). Poverty thresholds. Retrieved from https://www.census.gov/topics/income-poverty/poverty.html.

Weintraub, S. R., & Goodman, L. A. (2010). Working with and for: Student advocates' experience of relationship-centered advocacy with low-income women. *American Journal of Orthopsychiatry, 80*(1), 46–60.

Zalaquett, C. P., & Chambers, A. L. (2017). Counseling individuals living in poverty. *Journal of Multicultural Counseling and Development, 45*, 152–161.

Additional Resources

Hays, P. A. (2016). *Addressing cultural complexities in practice.* Washington, DC: American Psychological Association.

Hook, J. N., Davis, D. D., Owne, J., & DeBlaere, C. (2017). *Cultural humility: Engaging diverse identities in therapy.* Washington, DC: American Psychological Association.

Smith, L. (2013). *Psychology, poverty, and the end of social exclusion: Putting our practice to work.* New York, NY: Teachers College Press.

6

Out of the Shadows

Improving Health Care for Sexual Minority and Gender Diverse Individuals

Douglas C. Haldeman

> I have lived my life in terror. I come from a small town in rural Wyoming, where I may have been the only gay person trying to come out. There was no gay community. I struggled for years with alcohol and prescription drug abuse; I developed an eating disorder; and nothing relieved my depression. I started therapy a couple of times, but the first time was with someone who tried to refer me for conversion therapy. I didn't want that; I just wanted to be able to live with myself—and maybe, someday, another man. After that, I drank and snorted vikes (Vicodin) until I was numb to it all.
>
> When I woke up in a pool of my own puke, I decided I'd better try therapy again—but this time, I was too afraid to come out to the therapist after what had happened with the last one. So I quit after two visits. If I couldn't be honest about what was really bothering me, what was the point? That's when I decided to pack up and leave home. I am hoping it might be easier here [a large West Coast city]—and in some ways it is. It's certainly easier to meet guys. But it's harder, in a different way: I don't really know anyone here, and I'm afraid. Afraid of the city, afraid of the [LGBTQ] community—and afraid of myself. I'm going back into the same bad habits [alcohol/prescription drugs] that I had back home. And I'm so homesick. Right now, I'm just trying to hang on, but I'm having a hard time. And you know? I know that you [referring to the therapist] are gay too, but I'm just not sure I can really trust you.

At his intake, this was the commentary of "Scott," a 26-year-old White, low-socioeconomic-status (SES) gay male from a rural area. His remarks illustrate how disparities in access to appropriate care can exacerbate issues common to non-heterosexually identified and gender diverse individuals. There may be psychotherapists available, as in the above case, but—at least for Scott—lack of access to competent care can make a bad situation worse.

Before going further, a word about the terminology that will be used in this chapter. The term *sexual orientation* refers to an individual's internal experience of how sexual and/or romantic attractions are experienced. Therefore, a heterosexually oriented person would primarily or exclusively experience sexual attraction (as determined by fantasy, autoerotic practice, etc.) to those of the opposite sex. Conversely, a homosexually oriented person experiences those attractions to members of the same sex—regardless of the person's actual sexual behavior. A related term, *sexual identity*, describes the several ways in which persons may claim an internal understanding of the self and present themselves to the outside world: as heterosexual, gay, lesbian, bisexual, asexual, pansexual, questioning, queer, and so forth. *Gender identity* refers to the way in which people understand and express their gender: as male, female, gender fluid, nonbinary, and so forth. When one's gender identity corresponds to the sex assigned at birth, one is said to be *cisgender*. When that identity is different from one's natal sex, the individual may be said to be *transgender*. The myriad options of letters and acronyms that would be required to accurately include all of the possible permutations of these variables is somewhat cumbersome. Words coined to capture these variables, such as *queer* or *genderqueer*, invariably exclude some and may lack resonance with some generational cohorts. Therefore, in this chapter, persons of non-heterosexual orientation will be referred to as *sexual minorities* (SM) and transgender or gender-nonconforming individuals will be referred to as *gender diverse* (GD), except in those cases where the literature refers only to some subgroups of the SM/GD world.

Designating SM/GD persons in the aggregate as an underserved group is a bit like the old adage of the blind men and the elephant. Just how underserved various groups in the SM/GD community may be depends upon a variety of factors other than sexual orientation or gender identity: age, SES, ethnic/racial identity, geographic location, and ability status. Since the 1970s and even earlier, SM/GD persons have clustered in larger cities and communities. The same is true for SM/GD psychotherapists. So, for a privileged few—principally, affluent White urbanites—access to competent care may or may not necessarily be a challenging issue. However, for the rest of this very diverse community comprising a number of subgroups, health disparities, differential treatment needs, and access to competent care can indeed be a significant challenge. In this chapter, I will first address the health disparities and impediments to care affecting SM/GD people. Subsequently, I will discuss how barriers to care might be reduced, along with pro-health programs that can be developed to serve this population.

The Scope and Description of the Problem

The mental health needs of SM/GD persons have historically been greater than that of the heterosexual population. This has been documented for decades (Gilman, Cochran, & Mays, 2001). In context, however, research starting with the pioneering work of Evelyn Hooker (1957) has consistently shown that there is no inherent difference in mental health functioning between non-clinical, matched samples of lesbian, gay, and bisexual (LGB) and heterosexual people. Studies such as this served as the evidentiary basis for eliminating "homosexuality" from the American Psychiatric Association's *Diagnostic and Statistical Manual of Mental Disorders*. How to account for this apparent contradiction? The answer is that social forces—from family systems to social, cultural, and religious institutions—have, by virtue of anti-gay policies, positions, and expressions of prejudice and discrimination, adversely affected the mental health and well-being of otherwise normal SM/GD persons. The internalization of negative effects due to hostile and discriminatory practices contaminates the mental health landscape for many LGBT persons, as explained below in greater detail.

Gilman et al. (2001) found that adult gay men were 1.3 more times likely to suffer from anxiety disorders than their heterosexual counterparts, 1.7 times more likely to experience mood disorders, and 1.5 times more likely to have substance use disorders. For lesbians, the picture is even more serious: they are 1.8 times more likely than heterosexual women to have anxiety disorders, 2 times more likely to suffer from mood disorders, and 2.4 times more likely to have a substance use disorder than heterosexual women. Gay men are 2.4 times more likely to have attempted suicide than heterosexual men, and lesbians 1.5 times more likely to have attempted suicide than heterosexual women. These data are seen as robust, having been derived from the population-based National Comorbidity Study (Gilman et al., 2001). At the same time, it is possible that these data are on the conservative side, given that many SM/GD respondents minimize or conceal sensitive information—including their identities—in random national samples such as this.

For SM/GD youth, the picture is even more disturbing. Huygen (2006) found that LGB youth were significantly more likely than non-LGB youth to have attempted suicide. These data have been replicated numerous times, including in the largest study to date of transgender and gender-nonconforming youth, which found that 41% had attempted suicide (Grant, Mottet, & Tanis, 2011). The reasons for this are shown to be both internal and external stressors. Internally, trans and gender-nonconforming youth report an inability to cope with the daily stress involved with the dissonance of being socially obliged to present as a different gender than that which is appropriate to the individual's identity. Externally, transgender and gender-nonconforming youth face bullying, victimization, and violence at the hands of peers—and worse, in the context of their families, leaving no safe refuge in the young person's life. In fact, Ryan, Russell, and Heubner (2010) found that LGB and gender-nonconforming youth from rejecting families were three times more likely to have attempted suicide than LGB/gender-nonconforming youth from low- or non-rejecting families. A recent study went on to indicate that youth who are forced into so-called conversion therapy by their families are up to three times more likely to experience depression and to attempt suicide (Ryan, Toomey, Diaz, & Russell, 2018).

Historically, the internalization of stigma and trauma associated with experiences of discrimination, harassment, and violence has been viewed as the primary factor implicated in the higher rate of mental health and substance use issues among SN/GD persons. That trend remains unchanged today and is in fact in greater evidence at present (Office of Disease Prevention and Health Promotion, 2016; Ward, Dahlhamer, Galinsky & Joestl, 2014)—due, perhaps, to improved statistical tracking of LGBT health issues in general. More recent studies reveal the same pattern, relatively unchanged and unmitigated by advances in pro-LGBTQ social policy (e.g., same-sex marriage, the end of the "don't ask, don't tell" policy in the armed forces). A major longitudinal study found that experiences of discrimination and harassment that may begin in youth as bullying and escalate from there to discrimination in housing and/or employment, to physical/sexual assault, are implicated in the greater prevalence of mental health and substance use disorders among SM/GD persons (Balsam, Rothblum, & Beauchaine, 2005).

These disturbing statistics serve as the basis from which the Fenway Institute (2014), an SM/GD health care organization in Boston, called on the U.S. Department of Social and Health Services (USDSHS) to designate SN/GD persons as a medically underserved population (MUP), many of whom inhabit a health professional shortage area (HPSA). MUPs are defined as groups that do not receive adequate care. HPSAs are defined as shortages in primary, dental, or mental health care by geographic area, population, or facility. In the case of SM/GD individuals, these designations are appropriate due to two factors: health disparities and barriers to competent care.

Barriers to Service Delivery

Disparities in health care have long been documented for SM/GD individuals, due to access issues as well as competent care (de Vries, 2014), with particular concerns identified among older SM/GD persons (Fredriksen-Goldsen, Kim, Barkan, Balsam, & Mincer, 2010). One study points to the role societal stigma plays "as a pre-disposing and perpetuating factor in many aspects of ill-health" (Williamson, 2000, p. 105). Hatzenbuehler, McLaughlin, Keyes, and Hasin (2010) found that, when compared with prevalence rates for mood disorders among LGB people living in more progressive, tolerant areas, LGB persons in jurisdictions that passed anti–same-sex marriage referenda in 2006 showed a 36% greater rate of any mood disorder, a 41% greater incidence of alcohol use disorder, and an astronomical 248% increase for generalized anxiety disorder.

Conversely, another study found that medical care and mental health care visits dropped significantly among gay men in Massachusetts in the year following the adoption of same-sex marriage in that state (Hatzenbuehler et al., 2012), irrespective of marital or partnered status. These studies demonstrate the significance of sociopolitical ecology and its effect on the health of LGB people. In short, anti-gay laws and policies can make us sick; pro-gay policies can reduce health care costs and improve overall well-being—at least for gay men. More research in this area is needed to verify results for other subgroups within the SM/GD communities.

It is essential, therefore, to acknowledge the interplay between psychosocial context and the health and well-being of SM/GD people. Understanding barriers to care for SM/GD persons requires an examination of the institutional, systemic, political, and unique sociocultural factors that can affect their health. In 2011, the Institute of Medicine issued a report that cited a variety of factors implicated in SM/GD health disparities. It is a lengthy list but includes the following disparities in health for lesbians: significantly greater incidence of breast cancer, obesity, cardiovascular issues, and substance use disorders than heterosexual and cisgender women (Haldeman & Hancock, 2017). Gay men are disproportionately affected by the obvious issue of HIV/AIDS and other sexually transmitted diseases (STDs; Halkitis, 2013), as well as significantly greater rates of smoking and substance use disorders, including methamphetamine addiction, than heterosexual men (Centers for Disease Control and Prevention [CDC], 2012).

For these reasons, a recent study (Klein, 2017) called upon the USDSHS to designate SM/GD persons as stigmatized and underserved. This report explains that SM/GD health disparities are, for many in these groups, exacerbated by economic, social, and environmental disadvantages. The health-related concerns of SM/GD persons must necessarily be viewed in the context of the complex interplay among stigma, minority stress, and health. It is clear that mental well-being has a significant impact on physical health, and vice versa. Stressors internalized from a hostile environment—in one's workplace, community, or home—adversely impact a number of factors that lead to the above-identified health concerns.

Social, political, and environmental stress and acts of prejudice, discrimination, and violence all take a toll on an individual's health and well-being. For many SM/GD persons, this stress may be derived from external sources (e.g., actual events of discrimination) as well as internalized impact from past events. For lesbians, for example, this stress may manifest in mistrust of health care professionals, leading to an avoidance of medical care. This decision, in turn, augments the increased propensity for undiagnosed cancer and cardiac-related issues (Haldeman & Hancock, 2017). For gay men, HIV/AIDS—and in particular prevention of STD transmission—remains a significant issue that elicits stigma, even from health care professionals. In general, HIV transmission rates have diminished among gay men taken as a whole; however, alarming rates of new HIV infection continue to be a significant concern among young gay men of color, and older gay men of the baby boomer generation who survived the initial wave of HIV-related deaths in their generational cohort (CDC, 2012).

Further, both groups are susceptible to substance use disorders and smoking, owing to the development of unhealthy strategies for coping with both enacted and internalized stress. The issues that have the greatest negative effect on the health of SM/GD persons are primarily behavioral in nature. It can be argued that obesity, higher rates of smoking and substance use, and sexual risk-taking (leading to STD transmission) all have their origins in unhealthy stress coping patterns. Taken together, it is clear that environmental and internalized stressors have an adverse impact on the health and well-being of SM/GD persons; in turn, this affects mental and emotional functioning.

A difference in prevalence rates of mental health issues between SM/GD people and their heterosexual/cisgender counterparts has been noted for decades (Ward et al., 2014). Estimates have historically suggested that SM/GD persons experience depression and suicidality at rates three to four times that of heterosexuals. At present, this picture remains unchanged—if anything, it is worse. A recent survey by the National Alliance on Mental Illness (2018) reports that suicide is the leading cause of death among SM/GD teenagers, and that all generational cohorts of these groups experience depression at a rate three to four times that of the general population. This study echoes the disparity in prevalence rates of other mental health and substance use issues described earlier.

How do we explain this, when it may appear to the dominant culture that public opinion about SM/GD people has shifted dramatically over the past 40 years? This change in public opinion, along with judicial rulings and sociopolitical activism, has resulted in advances for SM/GD individuals that were but dreams at the dawn of the gay rights era: same-sex marriage, protections against discrimination based on sexual orientation and gender identity, ability of SM/GD people to serve openly in the military, and so forth. SM/GD visibility in the media—from news to entertainment—was once a rarity but is now commonplace. Fortune 500 corporations take seriously the notion of providing safe workplaces for their SM/GD employees. Pride celebrations all over the country are attended by heterosexual nuclear families alongside SM/GD participants. Many schools now offer variations (from heteronormative/cisgender norms) on sexuality and gender identity and expression in sex education classes; "gay/straight" student groups—unheard of even 20 years ago—are now commonplace. Health care organizations from medicine to nursing—and, of course, mental health—promote SN/GD-inclusive policies. In the eyes of many, this progress in such a relatively short time is astonishing. Sadly, though, the incidence of serious mental health concerns among SM/GD people may simply indicate that things—at least for many, especially those who are disadvantaged by low SES, age, ethnic/racial identity, or ability status—are not better.

Vulnerability Factors

Age

SM/GD teens, for example, report that bullying, especially cyberbullying, is a serious issue. A large study reveals that SM/GD youth are three times more likely than their heterosexual siblings to have experienced bullying, including physical assault (Balsam et al., 2005). These data are verified by a recent report from the Suicide Prevention Resource Center (2015), which estimates that SM/GD teens attempt suicide at a rate of 1.5% to 3% greater than heterosexual/cisgender teens. Numerous studies in this area all point to one primary cause: The world is still a more difficult place for SM/GD teens to navigate, owing to hostile school and family environments. As to the latter, Ryan et al. (2010) found that rejecting families are responsible for the threefold difference in suicide attempts between SM/GD and heterosexual/cisgender teens. It comes as no surprise that when young people being bullied at school come home to an unsympathetic, rejecting family, they will feel that there is no place to turn. Another recent survey of SM/GD teens supports these findings, indicating a significantly higher level of depression, suicidality, and risky sexual and drug-related behaviors than is found in heterosexual/cisgender teens. The authors further link these findings to hostile environments at school and at home (Hafeetz, Zeshan, Tahir, Jahan, & Naveed, 2017).

SM/GD persons on the other end of the life spectrum face serious issues of their own related to health care disparities. Although no hard data are available about the number of people in this category (or in any generational cohort of SM/GD people), a recent study by UCLA's Williams Institute estimates the U.S. population of SM/GD persons at between 2 and 4 million individuals (Choi & Meyer, 2016). A further study of SM/GD seniors indicates that they are significantly more likely than their heterosexual/cisgender counterparts to avoid or delay medical care (and hence to have a greater incidence of untreated medical problems) and to conceal their sexual orientation/gender identity from their providers; they also experience significantly greater rates of depression and suicidality, as well as risky health behaviors. These issues are exacerbated by financial instability and a greater incidence of low SES among SM/GD seniors (Choi & Meyer, 2016).

Further, senior SM/GD people are more likely to live alone and not to have children to care for them, thus causing them to rely on "families of choice," a common theme among SM/GD persons of all ages—especially those coming from intolerant families of origin. Generationally, many of today's SM/GD seniors came out at a time when it was much safer socially to remain closeted. In addition, many SM/GD seniors report systemic discrimination in the health care system (Choi & Meyer, 2016). As mentioned above, SM/GD seniors are more likely to avoid or delay health care, and perhaps some with good reason to do so. Choi and Meyer found that a significant number of SM/GD elders reported encountering discriminatory behaviors from health care practitioners and institutions as well. These seniors reported that practitioners at a minimum lack understanding about LGBT issues, and at worst display open hostility and prejudicial treatment. Elders are often at the mercy of care facilities, many of which are reported to be systemically homophobic (Choi & Meyer, 2016). It comes as no surprise, then, that the overall mental and physical health picture for SM/GD seniors is worse than for heterosexual/cisgender elders.

Geography

Age is not the only critical factor, however, in assessing health disparities between SM/GD people and their heterosexual counterparts. As with other sociocultural and economic factors that affect SM/GD individuals, geography plays a key role in both their mental well-being and access to care. In its recent report on its Behavioral Risk Factors Surveillance System, the CDC (2015) estimates that 38.2% of rural LGBT people experience depression, compared with 18.9% of rural heterosexual/cisgender people. This, combined with less access to health care providers trained to provide competent services to SM/GD people, shows that living in rural areas may pose additional risk for elders. Medical and mental health professionals who have been trained to work with SM/GD persons and who possess the requisite cultural knowledge to work with this population are in very short supply in rural and impoverished areas.

Socioeconomic Status

For some SM/GD individuals, SES may be the primary determinant in terms of who has access to competent care and who does not. Compared to the general population, sexual and gender minorities are disproportionately poorer overall, but there is variation between subgroups. A recent Pew Research poll (2013) of LGBT individuals found that about 4 in 10 earned $30,000 or less per year, compared to 28% of the U.S. population overall. Poverty rates on average are higher among lesbian and bisexual women, young people, and African Americans.

According to an analysis of the 2006–2010 National Survey of Family Growth, more than one quarter (28%) of lesbian and bisexual women are poor, compared with 21% of heterosexual women. Just over one in five gay and bisexual men (23%) are poor, compared to 15% of heterosexual men. However, when comparing couples, lesbian couples have the highest poverty rates, followed by heterosexual couples and male same-sex couples (who may have the least concerns in this regard, owing to the additive effect of two men with the presumed financial stability that male earning power offers in many cases). Further, a recent survey of more than 6,400 transgender people from across the United States found that the transgender population is approximately four times as likely as the non-transgender population to have an annual income of less than $10,000 (Kates et al., 2016).

Disability

Disability and sexual orientation/gender identity stand at the intersection of the most overlooked populations from a health research standpoint, according to the CDC (Fredriksen-Goldsen, Kim, & Barkan, 2012). A population-based study conducted by the CDC, the Washington State Behavioral Risk Factor Surveillance System, shows that all subgroups within the SM/GD domain report life-altering disability status at a significantly greater rate than heterosexual/cisgender persons. It should be cautioned that SM/GD people with disabilities represent the most under-researched of subgroups in these communities. Nevertheless, given the challenges already noted for able-bodied SM/GD people navigating the health care system, we can only assume, until additional research is available, that the obstacles faced by SM/GD people with disabilities are significant.

We now turn our attention to recommendations that will ameliorate the systemic challenges faced by SM/GD people and increase the availability of competent care.

Creating Cultural Competency

What is required to provide appropriate care to SM/GD persons? Balcazar, Suarez-Balcazar, and Taylor-Ritzler (2009) identify four factors essential to provision of competent care to marginalized groups: *critical examination, cultural knowledge, effective communication*, and *practice*. This will be the framework through which we examine best practices with SM/GD patients, using the guidance provided to psychologists and other mental health professionals through the American Psychological Association (APA)'s *Guidelines for Psychological Practice with Lesbian, Gay and Bisexual Clients* (APA, 2012) and *Guidelines for Psychological Practice with Transgender and Gender Non-Conforming People* (APA, 2015).

Critical Examination

The first step in this model calls upon health care providers to engage in thoughtful and deep introspection regarding their attitudes and beliefs about SM/GD people. Given that all of us grow up an a heterocentric society, it is reasonable to assume that there are, or have been, questions or even negative attitudes about SM/GD people. How does the provider actually feel about SM/GD persons? What exposure has the provider had to individuals with different sexual orientations or gender identities? More importantly, perhaps, is one's process regarding one's own sexuality/gender identity. If it seems puzzling, for instance, that some virulently anti-gay politicians themselves become exposed as engaging in same-sex behavior, we need look no further than studies indicating that those most uncomfortable with same-sex–attracted people are themselves most conflicted about their own sexual orientation (Weinstein et al., 2012). Clinicians are not exempt from this or other potential biases, which in turn affect their ability to provide competent care to SM/GD people. In some cases, religious beliefs may play a role in the provider's attitude. For many, examination of sex and sexuality is uncomfortable. Regardless, it is the responsibility of providers to address their own inner workings and not oblige the patient to suffer the fallout of their unprocessed attitudes about sexuality.

Ultimately, the question is this: Can providers address and overcome any prejudices that may affect their care of SM/GD patients? In most psychology training programs, there is at least passing reference to the needs of SM/GD people. Therapists should ask themselves if they have examined their personal biases sufficiently to work with this population. A psychotherapist's negative attitudes and beliefs about SM/GD people, even if concealed, can do damage to a patient. Before working with SM/GD individuals, both sets of guidelines recommend that therapists conduct a thorough examination of their personal attitudes and beliefs about SM/GD people.

Cultural Knowledge

It is impossible for anyone to be steeped in the norms of all cultural groups, but the APA guidelines provide helpful direction in this regard. Most critical in this area is the ability of the therapist to recognize SM/GD people as a culturally stigmatized group and, as such, to inquire thoughtfully about past experiences of trauma and discrimination. Even the most privileged among SM/GD persons will have experienced some form of rejection, harassment, bullying, discrimination, or even violence as the result of their actual or perceived sexual orientation or gender identity. Even if the patient does not bring these up, the therapist must inquire, given the impact that traumatic events can have on the individual. It also signals to the patient that the therapist is well aware of the added stressors involved with being a sexual minority or gender nonconforming person in this society, which adds to the patient's level of trust.

A second area to consider in this domain concerns the norms associated with the culture(s) of SM/GD people. Again, it is impossible to gain other than a passing familiarity with such norms if the therapist is unacquainted with the communities of SM/GD people; nevertheless, some knowledge in this area is helpful for solidifying the therapeutic relationship. Therapists must also gain a minimal understanding of the differential patterns of relating and social presentation among SM/GD persons so that there is no expectation that the patient will educate the therapist. Additionally, in conjunction with the personal self-examination in which the therapist has engaged, some knowledge of SM/GD culture(s) will inhibit any judgment, even a subliminal one, that could be rendered about the patient's values or behavior.

One important example of SM/GD cultural norms with which the psychotherapist should become familiar has to do with relationship structure. While many SM/GD persons strive to preserve a heteronormative monogamous pair bond as a structure for primary relationships, many do not. Non-monogamy is very common among gay men, as is casual sexual behavior. Alternative relationship structures that involve three or more people are becoming more visible (polyamory). Furthermore, psychotherapists working with SM/GD persons need to have some familiarity with alternative or "kink" sexual practices—at least to the point that they are able to discuss these with a patient without rendering negative judgment. Finally, it is important to recognize that the family systems of many SM/GD persons are chosen and often include persons who are not legally or biologically related.

Another complex but useful area for consideration has to do with the experience and expression of gender. The world is no longer binary (male/female), especially among SM/GD persons. Regardless of a person's outward presentation, it is always respectful to inquire as to how (or if) they identify in gender terms, and what pronouns they use.

Cultural knowledge also requires some understanding of resources for SM/GD persons, either in the local area or on the internet. Organizations and groups that serve the SM/GD communities are readily identified on the internet, and all it takes to discover them is a quick visit to Google. Even some small towns now offer groups and activities, as well as other health care resources, that are appropriate for SM/GD individuals. In remote areas, or even in urban areas, online resources may be accessed.

Effective Communication

Ineffective communication has long been identified as one of the most prominent factors implicated in SM/GD persons' dissatisfaction with psychotherapists. This is an area where medical providers are often less skilled than mental health professionals; nevertheless, it bears saying that inclusive, non-gender-specific language is always the "default setting" in communicating with SM/GD patients. Many providers still engage in heteronormative thinking, and it comes out in the language they use. Heteronormative language superimposes heterocentric cultural norms on SM/GD persons (questions/statements that assume heterosexual orientation or a hetero-monogamous relationship structure). Failing to use pronouns as requested by the patient and expressing confusion or—worse—disapproval at material presented by the patient foreclose one's ability to work with SM/GD persons. Nothing will drive SM/GD patients away faster than a therapist who uses heteronormative language or who assumes a gender binary perspective in dealing with gender-nonconforming patients.

Certainly, communication can be a challenge with SM/GD patients owing to the diversity in these communities that has been noted previously. Differences in gender, age, race/ethnicity, SES status, ability status, and so on influence the ways in which patients see their world—and the language that therapists should strive to employ. For example, in an effort to be helpful with a young person struggling with coming out to their family, it may be tempting for the therapist to provide encouragement—either directly or indirectly—for the person to come out and relieve themselves of the stressful secret. There is, after all, literature to suggest that coming out is a sign of self-efficacy and better mental health for sexual minority persons (Ryan, 2009), enabling SM/GD persons to access greater social support. This may indeed be a helpful therapeutic strategy with many dominant-culture individuals; however, when dealing with clients from different ethnic/racial groups, caution should be exercised. In many cultures, such a disclosure could have a profoundly adverse impact on the person's relationship with their family. Some knowledge of how SM/GD people are viewed in various cultural groups is essential for therapists working with this population.

We have seen that part of what makes clinical work with SM/GD individuals challenging is the diversity within their communities. Sexual orientation and gender identity include not only other identity variables (race, gender, age, SES, ability status, etc.) but also generational differences that inform the use of language. For example, the term "queer" has been used as shorthand for years to include lesbian, gay, bisexual, and asexual persons, and may be used by many—especially younger SM/GD individuals. However, for older SM/GD people, the term "queer" still carries a negative, stigmatizing meaning as an epithet historically used to insult sexually and gender diverse people. Similarly, the identity terms "gay" and "lesbian," favored by older generations, may have less salience for younger people—especially those who do not subscribe to a concept of gender as binary.

Increasingly, we see younger SM/GD individuals eschewing binary-associated identifiers in favor of self-defining as "genderqueer," or rejecting a term altogether. The point is that clinicians need to be flexible in their use of terms and follow the lead of the client. The various permutations of sexual orientation and gender identity, when considered with other identity variables, create a matrix so potentially complex that it behooves the clinician to inquire as to what terms are used (not "preferred") rather than making assumptions. These terms may also change over time for people whose experience of sexual orientation and gender identity is fluid.

Practice

Balcazar et al. (2009) encourage practice as the last key to cultural competency. But how do psychotherapists acquire opportunities to do this as they prepare to enhance their skills in working with SM/GD patients? In the past decade, attention to all diversity variables, including sexual orientation and gender identity, has expanded in education and training for professional psychology. Once a stand-alone topic, diversity is interwoven into the fabric of many graduate training programs. Educational videos for psychologists working in this area are available from a number of sources. Grants that specifically target SM/GD mental health researchers are offered by a number of organizations, including the American Psychological Foundation. Once limited to researchers from the SM/GD communities, study of these groups is now widespread. But is it enough?

Many researchers say no. Despite the increase in opportunities for education, training, and research, most health care professionals are still inadequately trained to provide competent care for the millions of SM/GD people living in the United States (Makadon, 2006; Mayer et al., 2008). Training for health care professionals on SM/GD issues is often delivered as a "one-shot" effort. Students, interns, and professionals alike are frequently offered one seminar or even just one lecture on SM/GD issues. Continuing education for psychologists that focuses exclusively on the SM/GD communities is in short supply. As we have seen, these groups have unique health care concerns and are diverse enough to require an ongoing, integrated approach to clinical training and continuing education.

Effective Strategies and Empirically-Supported Treatments

The declassification of homosexuality as a mental illness was an important first step in moving toward appropriate treatment of SM/GD people—a process that is still ongoing nearly 50 years later. Initially, treatment recommendations for this population were based more on what *not* to do: Emerging from an ignominious history of pathologization and oppression, the nascent gay rights movement in psychology focused on mitigating the damage of the previous era. With the publication of APA's first guidelines for psychotherapy with LGB persons, the profession turned toward affirmative practice. "Gay-affirmative" or "sexual and gender minority (SGM)–affirmative" psychotherapy is often characterized as the antidote to a variety of sociocultural forces that assail SM/GD persons and undermine their health and well-being (e.g., minority stress, systemic oppression and discrimination, conversion therapy).

SGM-affirmative psychotherapy, as defined by Pachankis (2018), "recognizes that SGM individuals possess distinct, and diverse, life experiences not experienced by heterosexual or cisgender individuals that can influence mental health" (p. 1209). He goes on to articulate several principles of SGM-affirmative therapy, including "helping SGM individuals develop insight into the ways in which stigma generates excess stress to compromise mental health; desensitizing SGM individuals to certain negative feelings, such as shame and guilt . . . promoting resilience and community-building, and acting as advocates against societal injustice" (p. 1209). Current practice guidelines support these concepts, but as Pachankis notes, they are based on theory and research on SGM mental health, not on empirical study of the efficacy of SGM-affirmative practice.

Pachankis goes on to observe that, despite the clear evidence that SM/GD persons are at greater risk for stigma-related stress and concomitant negative impact on mental health, only recently has research identified "probable mechanisms shown to underlie the association between stigma-related stress exposure and stress-sensitive mental health outcomes" (Pachankis, 2018, p. 1209). Hatzenbuehler (2009) found that some of these mechanisms, such as emotion-regulation deficits, rumination, social isolation, and depressogenic cognitive biases, are significantly elevated among SM/GD persons in comparison with heterosexuals. Of interest is a recent study that identifies processes specific to SM individuals regarding stigma exposure and internalization of mental health problems (Pachankis, 2015).

A number of studies have described SM/GD-specific adaptations for cognitive behavioral therapy (CBT) (Balsam, Martell, & Safren, 2006)—a logical theoretical choice, given what Pachankis (2018) refers to as CBT's potential for "empowering clients to cope with adverse environmental circumstances, and promoting the replacement of maladaptive cognitive, affective and behavioral stress responses, such as those emerging from stigma exposure" (p. 1210). The advent of population-based studies has created a robust dataset from which further SM/GD-specific adaptations have been and are being created, such as dialectic behavior therapy, mindfulness and acceptance-based approaches, and attachment-based family therapy.

Regardless, stigma itself stands in the way of accurate data collection in the service of developing appropriate treatments for SM/GD persons. It is what limits the inclusion of sexual orientation and gender identity in studies of evidence-based practice in the general population. It is also what dissuades many SM/GD persons from responding honestly to researchers' questions. Nonetheless, it is ultimately research that will provide guidance to the profession as to whether SM/GD-specific treatments are effective, and if so, with whom and under what conditions.

Health Care Policy

Cultural competence requires education and training of health care professionals and research on SM/GD-specific modes of intervention that are seen as effective. However, all the cultural competence in the world does little good if the public has restricted access to health care. It is only through access to appropriate and competent care that health disparities for SM/GD persons can be reduced. Health care policy stands as a formidable gatekeeper, permitting the generating and disseminating of knowledge about the unique health risks faced by SM/GD people, as well as the all-important issue of how it facilitates—or restricts—access to care. Research would suggest that we still have a long way to go in order to adequately resolve health care disparities for this vulnerable population.

A recent survey commissioned by the Center for American Progress found that up to 10% of LGB and 29% of transgender people reported a variety of stigmatizing and discriminatory behaviors on the part of their providers, some of whom expressed justification for such behaviors based on the religious freedom laws being considered in eight jurisdictions (Mizra & Rooney, 2018). Religious freedom laws essentially exempt any health care provider or facility from providing competent treatment to anyone when so doing would contravene the provider's personal religious beliefs. The implications for this are dire and have already been enacted as the U.S. Supreme Court upheld a lower-court ruling that supported the right of a baker to refuse to make a wedding cake for a gay couple. The SM/GD community is holding its collective breath, waiting to see if religious freedom laws will permit medical care providers and health care facilities the right to refuse treatment to SM/GD people.

As stunning an assault on the Hippocratic oath as that may be, to say nothing of the incursion of religious dogma into public policy that it represents, it is part of a cultural backlash that the entire SM/GD community currently faces. Little wonder, then, that a recent study found a significant majority of SM/GD people felt mistrust of health care providers (Veltman & Chaimowitz, 2014). SM/GD patients in this study reported that their providers frequently confused sexual orientation and gender identity, used incorrect pronouns, and were untrained in managing sexual orientation–specific mental health issues resulting from discrimination and trauma; some were openly hostile or dismissive of patient concerns. This explains the chronic mistrust and avoidance of health care on the part of SM/GD people, particularly elders.

The first step in improving health care for underserved SM/GD people lies in addressing inequities in health care policy. In turn, changes in policy require improvements in data collection. Historically, large national population-based studies of health did not include questions about sexual orientation or gender identity. Health disparities for SM/GD people were typically reported anecdotally, as institutional health policy tended to ignore them. Consider, for example, how many years it took before the AIDS crisis was even acknowledged by the federal government. Long after the demise of the "pathology" model of same-sex attraction and behavior was relegated to a shameful entry in the history books, negative attitudes about SM/GD people—ranging from indifference at best to outright hostility at worst—have prevailed, and are actually experiencing a renaissance of sorts at present. Critical efforts to include same-sex couples in the U.S. Census have consistently met with resistance. Yet these data would be enormously helpful in designating SM/GD individuals as an MUP. This would expand resources available for training and education of health care professionals, as well as improving direct service to SM/GD people.

Concurrently, since the available data suggest that SM/GD people living in rural or underserved areas are particularly vulnerable to substandard care, their presence in HPSAs must be documented. HPSAs are determined by geographic area, number and type of health care facilities and providers, and age of inhabitants. Increased resources to incentivize and train providers in offering competent care for SM/GD persons are necessary to improve inequities in care, and the MUP and HPSA designations would be helpful in this regard. However, this cannot happen—especially in the current political environment—without accurate data.

There is reason for cautious optimism in this regard, however. As of this writing, data on sexual orientation and gender identity are collected in the following national surveys:

- Behavioral Risk Factor Surveillance Survey (BRFSS)
- National Health and Nutrition and Examination Survey (NHANES)
- National Survey of Family Growth (NSFG)
- Youth Risk Behavior Survey (YRBS)
- National Crime Victimization Survey (NCVS)
- American Community Survey (ACS)
- National Health Interview Survey (NHIS)
- National Survey of Drug Use and Health (NSDUH)

Of particular importance is the collection of information about a patient's sexual orientation and gender identity in electronic health records, a requirement set forth by the Center for Medicare Services (CMS) and the National Coordinator for Health Information Technology (NCHIT). This practice enables SM/GD people to be included in the agencies' meaningful use guidelines, which is another key to improving health disparities for this population (Cahill, Baker, & Deutsch, 2015). At present, however, due to the precarious nature of political environments, these progressive changes can be in jeopardy. Federal health care policy must acknowledge the existence of SM/GD individuals as a unique group that is disproportionately affected by physical and mental health concerns, and work toward addressing this disparity—not ignore it.

Future Steps

The competent care of the underserved SM/GD populations is grounded in a complex interplay among a variety of personal, institutional, and systemic variables. As such, there is no "one size fits all" approach to working with SM/GD people; rather, flexibility is needed that takes into account the various internal and ecological forces that affect each individual's health and well-being. In summary, we reiterate the salient points of this discussion:

- **Data collection is essential.** We have made significant strides in this area, but much more remains to be done. After all, we still do not have a clear picture of how many SM/GD people inhabit the United States. Data on this population and its health concerns are essential for visibility, development of programs, and access to resources in the service of resolving health disparities.

- **SM/GD people should be specified and included in health care policy.** Such inclusion is the gateway to improved access to care and more competent education and training for care providers.
- **Standardize training for health care professionals.** Seeking a competent care provider can be a gamble for many SM/GD people. Some have a modicum of training in this area, but others—particularly those most likely to be available in rural and/or low-SES areas—have none at all. Coordination of efforts between graduate training programs, as well as the professional organizations that sponsor continuing education, is necessary if mental health practitioners are to be trained to work successfully with SM/GD persons. Understanding basic competencies associated with clinical work with SM/GD individuals is an ethical imperative. According to the APA's Code of Ethics (APA, 2017), gender identity and sexual orientation are included as aspects of diversity in Principle E and Standard 2.01 (b), thereby creating an ethical mandate for possession of basic competencies with these populations.
- **Support research.** Much is still unknown about what specific practices are recommended for clinical work with SM/GD people. So-called conversion therapy and any other related efforts to pathologize or demean same-sex attraction are discredited. Further, APA's comprehensive report on "Appropriate Therapeutic Responses to Sexual Orientation" (APA, 2009) suggests that any number of theoretical approaches and methodologies can be successful in working with LGB clients, given the therapist's open and nonjudgmental stance. However, we know little about what specific strategies might be recommended with the wide range of SM/GD people and the issues they present. Best practices can only be developed and refined through further research.
- **Systemic interventions.** Although the mental health concerns of SM/GD people are experienced personally, they occur in the context of a larger ecological reality. Health care policy and delivery systems, and the access thereto, can make the difference between good and poor health outcomes for SM/GD people. In addition to health care itself, interventions on an institutional level are critical. Anti-bullying programs in schools, for instance, are essential for the protection of SM/GD youth—particularly transgender and gender fluid/questioning teens, whose high suicide rate has been previously mentioned.
- **Focus on prevention.** With the continued increase in new HIV infections among young gay men, especially young gay men of color (CDC, 2012), programs to promote prevention efforts are critical. Further, it has been noted that several health-related issues (STDs, obesity, prostate and cervical cancer, smoking/substance use disorders) among lesbians and gay men are

behaviorally based. This is a point of intervention for clinicians as well as agencies and policymakers.

- **Organizations working together.** As the number of organizations and groups addressing issues related to SM/GD people has proliferated, there is a potential for duplication of efforts and less cohesion between organizations. A central clearinghouse that integrates the work of health care organizations, training programs, and governmental agencies would be a helpful step toward making progress in care for SM/GD people.

We are at a crossroads that was not imagined 40 years ago at the dawn of the modern "gay rights" movement. SM/GD people have unprecedented visibility in American society, and public opinion has shifted markedly toward tolerance. Yet it is perhaps this very progress that has exposed some of the deficiencies in care for underserved SM/GD people, against the current backdrop of uncertain political times. Anti-discrimination protections for SM/GD individuals are under threat in numerous jurisdictions and backlash protests threaten the social progress of the past several decades. SM/GD people everywhere are anxious. Regardless, as we have learned so many times in the past, SM/GD people are nothing if not resilient. Despite years of oppression, the health crisis, and the current specter of sociopolitical backlash, SM/GD individuals are still standing, and more visible than ever. All oppressed groups understand from experience that the arc of justice is not a straight line, but a series of ups and downs, with the overall trajectory toward progress.

References

American Psychological Association. (2009). Report of the APA task force on appropriate therapeutic responses to sexual orientation. Retrieved from https://www.apa.org/pi/lgbt/resources/sexual-orientation.aspx

American Psychological Association. (2012) Guidelines for psychological practice with lesbian, gay and bisexual clients. *American Psychologist*, *67*(1), 10–42.

American Psychological Association. (2015). Guidelines for psychological practice with transgender and gender non-conforming people. *American Psychologist*, *70*(9), 832–864.

American Psychological Association. (2017). Ethical principles of psychologists and code of conduct (2002, amended June 1, 2010, and January 1, 2017). Retrieved from http://www.apa.org/ethics/code/index.aspx

Balcazar, F., Suarez-Balcazar, Y., & Taylor-Ritzler, T. (2009) Cultural competence: Development of a conceptual framework. *Disability and Rehabilitation*, *31*, 14, 1153–1160.

Balsam, K., Martell, C., & Safren, S. (2006). Affirmative cognitive-behavioral therapy with lesbian, gay and bisexual people. In P. A. Hays & G. Y. Iwamasa (Eds.), *Culturally responsive cognitive-behavioral therapy: Assessment, supervision, and practice* (pp. 223–243). Washington, DC: American Psychological Association.

Balsam, K., Rothblum, E., & Beauchaine, T. (2005). Victimization over the lifespan: A comparison of lesbian, gay, bisexual and heterosexual siblings. *Journal of Consulting and Clinical Psychology, 73*(3), 477–487.Brotman, S., Ryan, B., & Cormier, R. (2003). Health and social service needs of gay and lesbian elders and their families in Canada. *The Gerontologist, 43*(2), 192–202.

Cahill, S. R., Baker, K., & Deutsch, M. B. (2015). Inclusion of sexual orientation and gender identity in stage 3 meaningful use guidelines: A huge step forward for LGBT health. *LGBT Health, 3*(2), 1–3.

Centers for Disease Control and Prevention. (2012). HIV surveillance report 24. Retrieved from http://www.cdc.gov/hiv/library

Centers for Disease Control and Prevention. (2015). Behavioral risk factor surveillance system. Retrieved from https://www.cdc.gov/brfss/annual_data/annual_2015.html

Choi, S., & Meyer, I. (2016). *LGBT aging: A review of research findings, needs and policy implications*. Los Angeles: Williams Institute. Retrieved from https://williamsinstitute.law.ucla.edu/wp-content/uploads/LGBT-Aging-A-Review.pdf

de Vries, B. (2014). LGBT persons in the second half of life: The intersections of stigma and cohort. *LGBT Health, 1*(1), 18–23.

Fenway Institute. (2014). The case for designating LGBT people as a medically underserved population and a health professional shortage area population group. Retrieved from https://fenwayhealth.org/wp-content/uploads

Fredriksen-Goldsen, K., Kim, H. J., & Barkan, S. E. (2012). Disability among lesbian, gay and bisexual adults: Disparities in prevalence and risk. *American Journal of Public Health, 102*(1), 16–21.

Fredriksen-Goldsen, K. I., Kim, H. J., Barkan, S. E., Balsam, K. F., & Mincer, S. L. (2010). Disparities in health-related quality of life: A comparison of lesbians and bisexual women. *American Journal of Public Health, 100*(11), 2255–2261.

Gilman, S., Cochran, S., & Mays, V. (2001). Risk of psychiatric disorders among individuals reporting same-gender sexual partners in the National Comorbidity Survey. *American Journal of Public Health, 91*, 933–939.

Grant, J. M., Mottet, L. A., & Tanis, J. (2011). *Injustice at every turn: A report of the National Transgender Discrimination Survey*. Washington, DC: National Center for Transgender Equality and National Gay and Lesbian Task Force. Retrieved from http://endtransdiscrimination.org/PDFs/NTDS_Report.pdf

Hafeetz, H., Zeshan, M., Tahir, M., Jahan, N., & Naveed, S. (2017). Health care disparities among lesbian, gay, bisexual and transgender youth: A literature review. *Cureus, 9*(4), 1184.

Haldeman, D., & Hancock, K. (2017). Lesbian, gay and bisexual health issues: Policy and practice. In K. DeBord, A. Fischer, K. Bieschke, & R. Perez (Eds.), *Handbook of sexual orientation and gender diversity in counseling and psychotherapy*. Washington, DC: APA Books.

Halkitis, P. (2013). *The AIDS generation: Stories of resilience and survival*. New York, NY: Oxford University Press.

Hatzenbuehler, M. (2009). How does sexual minority stigma "get under the skin"? A psychological mediation framework. *Psychological Bulletin, 135*, 707–730.

Hatzenbuehler, M., McLaughlin, K., Keyes, K., & Hasin, D. (2010). The impact of institutional discrimination on psychiatric disorders in lesbian, gay and bisexual populations: A prospective study. *American Journal of Public Health, 100*(3), 452–459.

Hatzenbuehler, M., O'Cleirigh, C., Grasso, C., Meyer, K., Safren, S., & Bradford, J. (2012). Effect of same-sex marriage laws on health care use and expenditures in sexual minority men: A quasi-natural experiment. *American Journal of Public Health, 102*(2), 285–291.

Hooker, E. (1957). The adjustment of the male overt homosexual. *Journal of Projective Techniques, 21*(1), 18–31.

Huygen, C. (2006). Understanding the needs of LGBT people living with mental illness. *Medscape General Medicine, 8*(2), 29.

Institute of Medicine. (2011). *The health of lesbian, gay, bisexual and transgender people: Building a foundation for better understanding.* Washington, DC: National Academies Press.

Kates, J., Ranji, U., Beamesderfer, A., Salganicoff, A., & Dawson, L. (2016). *Health and access to care and coverage for lesbian, gay, bisexual and transgender individuals in the U.S.* Menlo Park, CA: Henry J. Kaiser Family Foundation. Retrieved from http://files.kff.org/attachment/Health-and-Access-to-Care-and-Coverage-for-LGBT-Individuals-in-the-US

Klein, E. (2017). Community mental health disparities facing the LGBT community. In S. Rosenberg & J. Rosenberg (Eds.), *Community mental health: Challenges for the 21st century* (pp. 205–215). New York, NY: Routledge.

Makadon, H. J. (2006). Improving health care for the lesbian and gay communities. *New England Journal of Medicine, 354*, 895–897.

Mayer, K., Bradford, J., Makadon, H., Stall, R., Goldhammer, H., & Landers, S. (2008). Sexual and gender minority health: What we know and what needs to be done. *American Journal of Public Health, 98*(6), 989–995.

Mental Health Net. (2018). Mental health in the LGBT community. Retrieved from https://www.mentalhelp.net/mental-health-in-the-lgbt-community/

Mizra, S., & Rooney, C. (2018). Discrimination prevents LGBTQ people from accessing health care. Washington, DC: Center for American Progress. Retrieved from https://www.americanprogress.org/issues/lgbt/news/2018/01/18/445130/discrimination-prevents-lgbtq-people-accessing-health-care/

National Alliance on Mental Illness. (2018). Mental health of LGBTQ populations. Retrieved from https://www.nami.org/Find-Support/LGBTQ

Office of Disease Prevention and Health Promotion. (2016). Lesbian, gay, bisexual, and transgender health. Retrieved from https://www.healthypeople.gov/2020/topics-objectives/topic/lesbian-gay-bisexual-and-transgender-health

Pachankis, J. E. (2015). A transdiagnostic minority stress treatment approach for gay and bisexual men's syndemic health conditions. *Archives of Sexual Behavior, 44*, 1843–1860.

Pachankis, J. E. (2018). The scientific pursuit of sexual and gender minority mental health treatments: Toward evidence-based affirmative practice. *American Psychologist, 73*(9), 1207–1219.

Pew Center for Research. (2013). Facttank. Retrieved from http://www.pewresearch.org/fact-tank/2013/11/04/as-congress-considers-action-again-21-of-lgbt-adults-say-they-faced-workplace-discrimination/

Ryan, C. (2009). *Helping families support their lesbian, gay, bisexual, and transgender (LGBT) children.* Washington, DC: National Center for Cultural Competence, Georgetown University Center for Child and Human Development.

Ryan, C., Russell, S., & Heubner, D. (2010). Family acceptance in adolescence and the health of young LGBT adults. *Journal of Child and Adolescent Nursing, 23*(4), 205–213.

Ryan, C., Toomey, R., Diaz, R. & Russell, T. (2018). Parent-initiated sexual orientation change efforts with LGBT adolescents: Implications for young adult mental health and adjustment. *Journal of Homosexuality* [Epub before print; doi:10.1080/00918369.2018.1538407].

Suicide Prevention Resource Center. (2015). Comparison of suicide attempts among LGBT and heterosexual teenagers. Retrieved from https://www.google.com/imgres?imgurl=https://annemoss.com/wp-content/uploads/2017/08/29.png&imgrefurl=https://annemoss.com/tag/suicide-rates-higher-with-lgbt-youth

Veltman, L., & Chaimowitz, R. (2014). Mental health care for those who identify as LGBT and (or) queer. *Canadian Journal of Psychiatry, 59*(11), 1–8.

Ward, B. W., Dahlhamer, J. M., Galinsky, A. M., & Joestl, S. S. (2014). Sexual orientation and health among U.S. adults: National health interview survey, 2013. *National Health Statistics Report, 77.* Retrieved from http://www.cdc.gov/nchs/data/nhsr/nhsr077.pdf

Weinstein, N., Ryan, W. S., DeHaan, C. R., Przybylski, A. K., Legate, N., & Ryan, R. M. (2012). Parental autonomy support and discrepancies between implicit and explicit sexual identities: Dynamics of self-acceptance and defense. *Journal of Personality and Social Psychology, 102*(4), 815–832.

Williamson, O. E. (2000). The new institutional economics: Taking stock, looking ahead. *Journal of Economic Literature, 38*(3), 595–613. doi:10.1257/jel.38.3.595

7

Delivering Psychological Services to Religious and Spiritual Clients

Gina Magyar-Russell

Religion and spirituality have historically been, and remain more so than ever, an incredibly powerful force in the world. Religion's far-reaching influence ranges from national and global affairs to intimate matters in the daily lives of individuals. Even as formal religious affiliation is declining in the United States, with 23% of all Americans and 35% of millennials identifying as "nones"—a highly diverse and complex category ranging from atheists and agnostics to unaffiliated believers—61% of nones believe in God or a universal spirit and 37% consider themselves spiritual but not religious (García & Blankholm, 2016; Pew Research Center, 2015). Thus, religion and spirituality remain alive and relevant in the lives of our clients. Moreover, there is increasing consensus among mental health professionals that religion and spirituality represent important cultural and clinical dimensions (American Psychological Association, 2007) associated with treatment outcomes (Koenig, King, & Carson, 2012), and as such, should be attended to when individuals seek psychotherapy.

There have been numerous definitions of religion and spiritualty throughout the history of modern social science. Recent conceptualizations consider religion "a fixed system of ideas or ideological commitments" often expressed via formal, institutional and an doctrinal beliefs and practices (Hill & Pargament, 2008, p. 3). Spirituality "is increasingly used to refer to the personal, subjective side of religious experience" reflected in individuals' emotional and internal perceptions and self-styled expressions (Hill & Pargament, 2008, p. 4). Religious and spiritual clients are underserved in multiple ways for a variety of different reasons. Accordingly, the scope of the problem for both clients and mental health professionals is undeniably large. Even so, an examination of the psychology of religion and spirituality literature reveals that the obstacles are not so big that they cannot be overcome with continued effort by the field. In fact, great strides have been made since the turn of the millennium (Paloutzian, 2017). Within the last decade, the American Psychological Association (APA) has devoted two new journals to the psychological study of religion and spirituality. Annually dozens of empirical studies fill the pages of *Psychology of Religion and Spirituality*, established in 2009, and *Spirituality in Clinical Practice*, established in 2014. *The Journal of Religion and Spiritually in Social Work* was established in 2004. These scientific outlets reflect a noticeable increase in research, openness, and knowledge about the role of religion in psychological processes and its application in clinical settings.

The Scope and Description of the Problem

Sociobiology

If we begin from a sociobiological perspective, which posits that *Homo sapiens*' "capabilities for banding together in intelligently organized social groups for the common good" originated through processes of biological evolution (Griffith, 2010, p. 16), religious prejudice can be found throughout human history. As Griffith (2010) described in his book *Religion That Heals, Religion That Harms*, human sociobiology utilizes religious beliefs and practices to build strong, well-organized groups. Compassion for individuals, however, did not develop as part of effective sociobiological behavior. Thus, religious life organized by sociobiological systems can produce harm to persons outside (out-group), and sometimes inside (in-group), the religious group (Griffith & Magyar-Russell, 2018). Religion, or an anti-religious stance, then becomes a marker of identity rather than a source of concern and compassion for the other. Sociobiological and social neuroscience researchers have provided the most intelligible explanations for religious prejudice (Griffith, 2010). Being cautious or fearful of others different from ourselves is consistent with the "in-group, out-group" dynamics of our sociobiology as humans.

Mental Health Professionals Tend to Be Less Religious Than the General Population

Because mental health professionals tend to be less religious than the general population (Shafranske & Cummings, 2013), being religious in and of itself can be a barrier to treatment for religious clients. In other words, religious clients are often in the "out-group" in mental health treatment settings due to the "in-group" with which many clinicians identify. Shafranske and Cummings (2013) note that 56% of a national general population sample endorsed religion as "very important" while 17% rated religion as "not very important" (Newport, 2007). In comparison, only 21% of a sample of clinical and counseling psychologists rated religion as "very important," while 48% rated religion as "not very important" ($n = 258$; Delaney, Miller, & Bisono, 2007). When interpreting these statistics it is important to keep in mind Principle E of the APA's *Ethical Principles of Psychologists and Code of Conduct* (APA, 2017a), which explicitly states that:

> psychologists are aware of and respect cultural, individual, and role differences, including those based on age, gender, gender identity, race, ethnicity, culture, national origin, religion, sexual orientation, disability, language, and socioeconomic status, and consider these factors when working with members of such groups. Psychologists try to eliminate the effect on their work of biases based on those factors, and they do not knowingly participate in or condone activities of others based upon such prejudices. (p. 4)

The American Counseling Association (ACA, 2014) and the National Association of Social Workers (NASW, 2017) have similar guidelines in their codes of ethical conduct. Even though mental health professionals are required to work toward identifying and reducing the effects of inherent bias, it is important to acknowledge that the human brain is hardwired with sociobiological predispositions to which we must remain vigilant.

Psychology's Strained Past with Religion

Psychology has long had a tenuous relationship with religion (Paloutzian, 2017). Although psychologists of religion have been present since the beginnings of psychology (as evidenced by classic writings such as *The Varieties of Religious Experience* by William James in 1902), the field strived to distinguish itself as an independent science in the mid-20th century. Psychology desired to distance itself from less scientific fields such as philosophy and theology. Occurring roughly during this same period was (a) the creation versus evolution debate, in which many felt religion and science were mutually exclusive, (b) Freud's publication of *The Future of an Illusion* (1927), which argued that religion was a sign of insecurity and neurosis, (c) the advent of behaviorism (Watson, 1925), which viewed behavior as the result of conditioning, leaving social scientists generally uninterested in researching religious and spiritual phenomena, and (d) competition for clients between secular clinicians proclaiming a "new gospel" of human behavior and religious professionals who had devoted their lives to caring for those suffering with mental illness (Paloutzian, 2017). All these circumstances contributed to antagonism between psychology and religion. Not only did psychology distance itself from religion, religious people and institutions considered psychology as contrary to religious teaching. This left psychology and religion with little interface for roughly 40 years (~1927 to 1967; see Paloutzian, 2017, p. 47).

Client Preferences and Clinician Training

The United States is one of the most religious Western nations in the world, with roughly 89% of people believing in God, even if unaffiliated (Newport, 2016), and a majority of adults identifying with some sect of Christianity, even if not currently practicing their faith (Ellison & McFarland, 2013). Accordingly, religion and spirituality are important in the lives of many of our clients. A recent review of 64 peer-reviewed journal articles including over 4,600 clients concludes that many clients prefer to talk about religious and spiritual issues in counseling and believe that it is helpful in resolving their problems (Harris, Randolph, & Gordon, 2016). Additionally, several studies reviewed found that Christian participants preferred a Christian psychotherapist over a secular counselor (Harris et al., 2016). In a study of clients in group therapy, 85% of participants at a university counseling center ($n = 68$) felt religious concerns were an appropriate topic for group therapy and 47% indicated they would like to discuss spiritual or religious topics in psychotherapy (Post, Wade, & Cornish, 2016).

Unfortunately, there is also evidence that, often, religious and spiritual issues are not discussed in psychotherapy, and they are not routinely included in assessment and treatment planning (Hathaway, Scott, & Garver, 2004). Shafranske and Cummings' (2013) review of the literature found that only a small minority of psychology graduate programs offer specific courses in the applied psychology of religion and spirituality and that over 50% of psychology interns reported that religious and spiritual issues were either rarely or never taught or discussed in their academic training (Francis, 2011). Thus, in addition to mental health professionals being less religious and spiritual than the clients they serve, clinicians are also not typically well trained in religious and spiritual assessment and intervention.

Lack of training and comfort with religious and spiritual issues can inhibit the integration of religion and spirituality in a multitude of ways within mental health care. For instance, research that inquires about clients' use of their spiritual and religious beliefs and practices (SRBPs) to manage the problem(s) for which they are seeking treatment may not be carried out due to concerns that clinicians will not know how to address religion and spirituality in session should clients raise them after participating in research on the topic. When these types of situations are recognized, a first step toward increasing clinician familiarity and comfort level is to engage in training in assessment and integration of

SRBPs in psychotherapy. Although training and continuing education are becoming more common, the fact remains that many mental health professionals are not well trained in the assessment and integration of religion and spirituality in psychotherapy.

Client Perspectives of Mental Health Care

Another reason why religious and spiritual clients may be underserved is due to beliefs or interpretations about the appropriateness of talking about personal problems with someone outside of their religious or spiritual tradition, including, and sometimes specifically, mental health professionals (another example of in-group, out-group dynamics). This view may be held by individuals, or the message may come from clergy, leaders, or other church members within a faith tradition. One result of this perspective is that religious individuals may be willing to seek out mental health services only from professionals who they perceive share or will understand and respect their faith tradition. This preference may limit options for efficacious care, and religious individuals may not get the mental health services they need, particularly when they are a member of a minority faith tradition or in areas of the country where there are few mental health professionals.

Misdiagnosis and Missed Opportunities

One of the many consequences of the divide between psychology and religion is that religious and spiritual clients may be misunderstood and misdiagnosed (Vieten & Schammell, 2015). There is even evidence that mental health professionals may appraise religious clients from less mainstream religions as more mentally ill or as having a worse prognosis in comparison to non-religious clients (O'Conner & Vandenberg, 2005; Ruff, 2008). Differential diagnosis between psychosis and religious and spiritual experiences and problems can be difficult to determine. Religious and spiritual content is a common theme for delusions and hallucinations for some individuals. Conversely, religious and spiritual experiences can at times look like psychiatric symptoms but are instead an accepted aspect of a religious or spiritual tradition. For instance, speaking in tongues in the Pentecostal tradition might be misconstrued as psychotic when taken out of context, or consistently speaking to and offering gifts to the dead or benevolent spirts in Native American culture might be viewed as delusional in Western culture. Thus, cultural context is essential for understanding the individual client and making accurate diagnostic assessments.

Vieten and Scammell (2015) suggest that to best serve religious clients when making differential diagnosis decisions clinicians should evaluate whether the information the client is presenting (a) is unfamiliar to you but in line with the client's religious or spiritual tradition, (b) is consistent with the client's religious or spiritual beliefs and practices but also causes significant psychological and emotional distress, or (c) contains religious or spiritual content and is maladaptive or symptomatic of psychopathology. Appropriately evaluating these often complex clinical presentations involves comprehensive assessment, including in-depth conversations with clients about their faith tradition and idiosyncratic beliefs and practices. Several practical sources (Milstein, Manierre, & Yali, 2010; Pargament, 2007, 2013; Vieten & Scammell, 2015) described later in this chapter offer detailed approaches for the assessment of SRBPs.

In addition to misdiagnosis, missed opportunities for accessing resources that could facilitate therapeutic outcomes is another way in which religious and spiritual clients may be underserved. A great deal of empirical evidence exists that SRBPs offer meaning and support in times of stress (Pargament, 2007; Park & Hale, 2014); are associated with an increased sense of purpose, resilience, and well-being (Frederickson, 2002; Fry, 2000; Pargament & Cummings, 2010); and are linked to various dimensions of psychological and physical health (Koenig et al., 2012; Pargament, 2013). Thus, not tapping into a client's religious and spiritual resources may inhibit therapeutic progress and success. Pargament (2007) emphasizes the importance of tailoring religious and spiritual resources "to both the particular case and the particular problem" (p. 243). In other words, rituals or practices that one client may find helpful for dealing with anxiety may in fact exacerbate symptoms of anxiety for another client from the same faith tradition. One of the challenges then for clinicians is to help clients identify the aspects of their faith that are best suited to help them deal with, or even address, their psychological and emotional problems.

For example, clients with obsessive-compulsive disorder (OCD) who suffer from religious obsessions and compulsions (see Griffith & Magyar-Russell, 2018 for an extensive case study) may struggle to engage in some of the practices of their faith tradition because they trigger religious obsessions. To complicate matters, rituals within a tradition may serve as compulsions and temporarily relieve anxiety yet maintain the destructive cycle of OCD. Clinicians must work collaboratively with their clients, and consult clergy as needed, to be creative about what aspects of faith may be problematic for the client, while utilizing other religious resources to further treatment. For instance, attending Bible study and other social events at church might be a better source of spiritual sustenance for individuals with OCD than engaging in religious rituals or solitary activities. Pargament (2007) provides useful guidelines for helping clients draw on their spiritual knowledge, strivings, and experience (see pp. 242–259) as resources in psychotherapy.

Barriers to Service Delivery

A significant barrier to service delivery for religious and spiritual clients is simply that many mental health professionals do not feel comfortable addressing religion or spirituality in psychotherapy (Gladding & Crockett, 2018). Saunders, Miller, and Bright (2010) describe "spiritually avoidant care" (p. 357) in which clinicians are hesitant to discuss, or even avoid discussing, religious, spiritual, existential or an mystical experiences in the lives of their clients. Some clinicians report concerns such as overstepping boundaries (Koenig et al., 2012) or their ability to address religious and spiritual issues without feeling emotionally triggered, misguiding clients, making embarrassing mistakes, or imposing values (Gladding & Crockett, 2018). Still other practitioners may be overwhelmed by the challenge of learning what is normative for various religions and cultures in order to interpret whether their clients' beliefs and practices are consistent with the norms of their faith tradition (Saunders et al., 2010). Moreover, norms can vary both within and across faith traditions depending on many factors, such as region, culture, and gender (McMinn, Snow, & Orton, 2012).

A few common areas of uncertainty for psychotherapists include the appropriateness of dress, behaviors, and discussion of topics that may not be permitted in some faith traditions, particularly when the client and clinician are members of the opposite sex. For example, a female clinician might unintentionally insult an Orthodox Jewish male client if she reaches to shake hands, and a male clinician might inadvertently offend a Muslim female client if he attempts to make direct eye contact. It is impossible to know everything about each faith tradition and its cultural variations; thus, there are inevitably going to be some awkward moments and "mistakes" (however, this happens when discussing many topics in psychotherapy, not just when addressing religious and spiritual issues). Clinicians may feel discouraged and overwhelmed when trying to learn the norms of different faith traditions and cultures. There are many approaches for gaining knowledge about different faiths (see Vieten & Scammell, 2015, pp. 45–50). One of the most helpful and practical strategies is to learn from each client. In other words, once you glean the faith tradition of your client at intake, begin researching and reading about that tradition, and even visit a place of worship or contact a clergy member for a consultation in that tradition. Learning from clients by first asking permission to discuss their faith and then asking open-ended questions about their tradition and personal beliefs and practices (e.g., "What does it mean to you to be Buddhist/Christian/Muslim/etc.?," "Please tell me more about your faith community") is essential for overcoming barriers in psychotherapy. Although it is important for clinicians to educate themselves about RSBPs outside of sessions, it is also necessary to ask clients for further information and personal preferences to gain greater understanding of their particular faith community and traditions, and to attempt to avoid misinterpretations or misunderstandings. After a few years of clinical work, the average clinician working in a metropolitan area is likely to have learned a great deal about multiple faith traditions.

Gladding and Crockett (2018) also note that some psychotherapists do not think they have time to delve into religious and spiritual issues if they are limited by number of sessions or are compensated based on the number of clients they see. Additionally, psychotherapists may be reluctant to discuss religious and spiritual issues with clients for fear that clients will be dogmatic or inflexible, will proselytize to the psychotherapist, or will engage in strategies such as spiritual bypass (the use of spirituality to avoid dealing with difficult issues; Welwood, 2000) that can undermine treatment. Another barrier to service delivery can occur when psychotherapists find it difficult to know whether to treat or refer a client to a clinician with greater experience working with clients from a particular religious or spiritual tradition, or working with religious and spiritual issues in general. Magyar-Russell and Griffith (2016) suggest that the option of transferring clients to a different clinician should be used as a last recourse because it can discourage clients and inhibit their therapeutic process. It also limits the clinician's ability to work with clients from diverse backgrounds.

A final barrier to services for religious and spiritual clients is lack of proper training for both mental health professionals and clergy. Although training was previously discussed as part of the "problem," it is also a substantial barrier to getting the most efficacious mental health treatment for religious and spiritual individuals. There simply are not enough clinicians well trained in ethically, sensitively, and effectively assessing and addressing SRBPs in the context of psychotherapy. Thus, these issues are often not adequately attended to in treatment (Hathaway, Scott, & Garver, 2004; Shafranske, 2014). Moreover, Gross and Simmons (2007) found that psychology professors are among the least religious in academia; therefore, those responsible for training mental health professionals may have a "blind spot" when it comes to providing knowledge and training in the integration of religion and spirituality in psychotherapy.

On the other hand, most clergy members are not dually trained as both spiritual leaders in their faith tradition and in mental health treatment. In a nationally representative general population survey of over 8,000 respondents ages 15 to 54, Wang, Berglund, and Kessler (2003) found that one fourth of individuals who sought treatment for mental disorders did so from a clergy member, and that most of these individuals were seen solely by clergy (i.e., not by a mental health professional or physician). This statistic represents a very serious, and even dangerous, barrier to adequate mental health care for religious and spiritual clients. Since clergy continue to play a critical role in mental health care delivery in this country, sufficient training is needed in seminary, and after ordination, to ensure that clergy recognize the presence and severity of mental disorders, collaborate with health care professionals, and refer parishioners to mental health practitioners when needed.

Creating Cultural Competency

Even though there are numerous barriers to providing religious and spiritual clients with spiritually sensitive, ethical, and effective mental health care, efforts to overcome these obstacles are underway. Within the last decade, competencies for working with religious and spiritual issues in psychotherapy, supervision, and graduate training have been developed (Hathaway, 2013; Saunders et al., 2010; Shafranske, 2014; Vieten & Scammell, 2015). In the updated 2017 *Multicultural Guidelines: An Ecological Approach to Context, Identity, and Intersectionality*, the APA defines culture as "the embodiment of a worldview through learned and transmitted beliefs, values, and practices, including religious and spiritual traditions" (APA, 2017b, p. 165). This definition, in combination with Principle E of the APA's *Ethical Principles of Psychologists and Code of Conduct* (2017a; quoted earlier), suggests that taking into consideration the SRBPs of clients is not only clinically useful, it is an ethical requirement.

In one of the early efforts to set forth religious and spiritual clinical competencies, Saunders et al. (2010) suggest that the minimum standard practice with all clients should be "spiritually conscious care" (p. 355). Spiritually conscious care requires the assessment of SRBPs in a respectful manner to determine their relevance to the client's presenting problems, psychological health, and salience in daily life. Saunders et al. (2010) provide a helpful continuum of spiritual care in psychotherapy ranging from "spiritually avoidant care" (p. 357; avoiding conversation about clients' SRBPs) through "spiritually directive care" (p. 356; SRBPs are the focus of clinical attention). The authors note that as clinicians move up the continuum of spiritual care in psychotherapy, a greater level of training is required.

Similarly, the most comprehensive set of spiritual and religious standards for mental health professionals published to date (Vieten & Scammell, 2015) makes explicit the distinction between competence, "the basic attitudes, knowledge, and skills clinicians should possess to conduct effective therapy" (p. xiii), and proficiency, "a high degree of expertise or skill" (p. xiii). In their book *Spiritual & Religious Competencies in Clinical Practice*, Vieten and Scammell (2015) apply the general multicultural competence strategies of attitudes, knowledge, and skills to the spiritual and religious domain of clinical practice. More specifically, attitudes refer to engaging in a process of consciously examining the assumptions, bias, values, perceptions, and personal limitations the clinician currently holds about religious and spiritual issues; knowledge is the effort to learn about and understand the worldview of religiously and spiritually diverse clients without judgment; and skills include the ability to implement ethical, religiously and spiritually sensitive assessment, diagnosis, and therapeutic strategies in the context of psychotherapy (Vieten & Scammell, 2015).

Within this cultural competency framework, the authors describe in detail 16 research-based spiritual and religious competencies for mental health professionals, along with case examples and strategies for working toward each standard. The 16 competencies were based on a comprehensive review of the literature, focus groups with clinicians and scholars, and an online survey of clinicians and scholars (n = 184) experienced in the integration of SRBP within psychology and psychotherapy (Vieten et al., 2013). Since the publication of the competencies, Vieten et al. (2016) conducted a survey of a broad group of practicing psychologists. Although 73% to 94% of respondents agreed that psychologists should receive training and obtain competency in the 16 areas, the majority (~52% to 81%) reported they had received little or no training in these areas. *Spiritual & Religious Competencies in Clinical Practice* also contains a "resources" section that lists articles, books, videos, and websites to facilitate achieving each competency. Clearly, Vieten and Scummell's (2015) book is a key resource for clinicians working toward cultural competence in clinical practice.

Shafranske (2014) provides another useful resource for developing culturally sensitive integration of religion and spirituality into psychotherapy. He outlines a competency-based clinical supervision model (Falender & Shafranske, 2004) that provides supervisors with detailed and practical recommendations for implementing supervisory practices that enhance supervisee development in religious and spiritual competencies. This model also uses the attitudes, knowledge, and skills framework to guide supervision.

As noted earlier, a critical place for facilitating culturally competent religious and spiritual care is in graduate education and training. Hathaway (2013) identified graduate programs and training sites that currently offer a formal structure for instilling the attitudes, knowledge, and skills necessary for religious and spiritual competency, and in some cases proficiency. The curriculum objectives for religious and spiritual competency in psychology training can be found in Hathaway (2013) and closely resemble the competencies detailed by Veiten and Scummell (2015).

Another useful tool for clinicians is applying an ethical decision-making process to an evaluation of religious and spiritual issues in psychotherapy. Barnett and Johnson (2011) suggest implementing the nine non-sequential stages of their model to assist "in determining whether a client's religious or spiritual beliefs may be clinically salient, and if so, how a psychotherapist might consider ethical principles and standards in determining how to proceed" (p. 158).

Finally, Oxhandler and Pargament (2018) provide a summary of measures that have been used across helping professions to measure providers' religious and spiritual competencies. Although the authors conclude that there is much work to be done in this area of assessment, they highlight scales that practitioners and supervisors can use to measure progress in ethically attending to issues of religious and spiritual diversity in sessions. For instance, the Religious/Spiritually Integrated Practice Assessment Scale (RSIPAS; Oxhandler & Parrish, 2016) measures "practitioners' overall orientation to integrating clients' religion and spirituality [RS] in practice, including their attitudes, self-efficacy, perceived feasibility, and behaviors related to integrating clients' RS in practice" (Oxhandler & Pargament, 2016, p. 125).

Effective Strategies and Empirically-Supported Treatments

One of the most widely used models for integrating culturally sensitive, compassionate, and effective integration of religion and spirituality into clinical practice is found in Pargament's (2007) seminal book, *Spiritually Integrated Psychotherapy: Understanding and Addressing the Sacred.* Pargament's (2007) model begins by "setting the stage for spiritual dialogue" (p. 202) in psychotherapy and guides the clinician through a multifaceted and dynamic assessment process that develops in depth over time with the client. More specifically, the first half of the book describes (a) *initial spiritual assessment,* which focuses on four areas of clinical relevance: (i) salience of spirituality to the client, (ii) importance of religious affiliation or community, (iii) prominence of spirituality as part of the problem, and (iv) the degree to which spirituality might be part of the solution (see Pargament, 2007, pp. 211–216); (b) *implicit spiritual assessment,* which takes "a more covert approach that does not initiate the discussion of religious or spiritual issues and does not openly, directly, or systematically use spiritual resources" (Tan, 1996, p. 368; see Pargament, 2007, pp. 216–220); and (c) *explicit spiritual assessment,* which involves a direct and intentional focus on the role of religion and spirituality within the context of the client's life (see Pargament, 2007, pp. 221–241).

The second half of the book provides clinicians with strategies for helping clients draw on their spiritual and religious beliefs and practices, relationships, and coping methods. Several chapters are devoted to teaching clinicians how to address different types of religious and spiritual issues that may arise and can adversely impact the client's presenting problem(s). Finally, Pargament provides a summary of manualized spiritually integrated therapies that offers the reader a sense of the session-by-session content and goals of various religious and spiritual interventions. Pargament's (2007) work provides an excellent and accessible approach for integrating religion and spirituality into the practice of psychotherapy.

Another invaluable resource for developing competence is the *APA Handbook of Psychology, Religion, and Spirituality* (Pargament, 2013; Volumes 1 and 2). Volume 1 is focused on theory, research, and context and devotes 15 chapters, written by experts in each area, to understanding religion and spirituality among different populations, such as adolescents, older adults, African Americans, Buddhists, gay and lesbian persons of faith, atheists, and Hindus. Volume 2 focuses on an applied psychology of religion and spirituality. In this volume's 34 chapters the practitioner will find detailed information about how to carry out thorough religious and spiritual assessment strategies (Hodge, 2013) and address religion and spirituality within different therapeutic frameworks (e.g., psychodynamic, cognitive behavioral, family systems) and among different client populations (e.g., trauma, acute and chronic illness, military personnel, couples, eating disorders). The sheer size of these volumes is testament to all the work that is being carried out in the psychology of religion and spirituality and the abundance of quality resources available to clinicians.

Milstein et al. (2010) offer mental health professionals a model of mental health care for persons of diverse religions. At the heart of this model are strategies to break down some of the barriers to obtaining efficacious treatment for religious and spiritual clients. The Clergy Outreach and Professional Engagement (COPE) model "delineates boundaries between clinical care provided by mental health professionals and religious care provided by clergy, as well as describes pathways of collaboration across these boundaries" (p. 371). Developed in an effort to help clinicians uphold the APA's 2008 Resolution on Religious, Religion-Based and/or Religion-Derived Prejudice, the COPE model is comprised of four parts: (a) recognition of the positive psychological and behavioral influences that congregational communities can have on their members, (b) description of the support, both spiritual and social, that congregations can provide when members are stressed, (c) promotion of (i.e., referral to) professional assessment and treatment when serious emotional problems or mental disorders are evident, and (d) supportive of the recovery process of individuals with chronic mental health problems via ongoing and collaborative care among individuals, their mental health provider(s), and their religious communities. The authors emphasize that the ever-changing elements of collaboration among the four parts of the continuum aid clinicians' ability to assess, comprehend, and engage the religious values and resources of their clients while simultaneously offering congregations and clergy trusted relationships with mental health professionals when it is necessary to refer. Milstein et al. (2010) provide useful websites and practical resources to help clinicians execute the COPE model.

There have been dozens of interventions developed and tested, the majority within the past 25 years, that either (a) assimilate religious and spiritual strategies within the context of an established treatment (*assimilative approach*); (b) are purposefully "altered to incorporate a particular religious or spiritual approach" (McMinn et al., 2012, p. 262; *accommodative approach*); or (c) involve the collaboration of mental health professionals and religious leaders (*collaborative approach*). A recent example of using the accommodative approach to create religious interventions is Koenig et al.'s (2015) development of Christian, Jewish, Buddhist, Hindu, and Muslim versions of Religious Cognitive Behavioral Therapy (RCBT) for major depression in persons with chronic medical illness. The Duke Center for Spirituality, Theology, and Health website provides all six treatment manuals and workbooks (RCBTS and conventional CBT), a training video, and detailed information about the study design, protocol, and research findings when compared to conventional CBT (https://spiritualityandhealth.duke.edu/index.php).

Although most religious and spiritual interventions have been examined for their effectiveness on specific outcomes, a relatively small number have been tested in randomized clinical trials (RCTs). Hook et al. (2010) applied rigorous evaluation criteria to assess the efficacy of religious and spiritual treatments for a variety of mental health problems. In addition to the five studies that utilized a general spiritual strategy, religions represented in the 24 RCTs were Christianity (10 studies), Islam (seven studies), Taoism (one study), and Buddhism (one study). Only two religious and spiritual treatments met criteria for *efficacious* (Christian accommodative cognitive therapy for depression and 12-step facilitation for alcoholism), two more met criteria for *efficacious when used in the context of medication* (Muslim psychotherapy for depression and Muslim psychotherapy for anxiety), and the remaining treatments were deemed *efficacious when combined with existing inpatient treatment* and *possibly efficacious treatments* (see Hook et al., 2010, for detailed information on each RCT). The authors surmise that most of the religious and spiritual treatments evaluated were helpful for clients with various types of psychological problems but did not meet criteria as *efficacious* treatment due to the small number of high-quality, replicated, and controlled outcome studies. Additionally, most of the RCTs found that religiously and spiritually integrated treatments are at least as efficacious as existing secular treatments; however, there is currently insufficient evidence to suggest that religious and spiritual treatments perform *better* than established secular treatments (Hook et al., 2010; Pargament, 2007). Hook et al. (2010) conclude that practitioners who would like to use existing religious and spiritual interventions can be assured that evidence-based research generally supports their use.

Future Steps

This chapter highlighted some of the central problems and barriers to providing culturally competent and compassionate mental health care to religious and spiritual clients. Hopefully it has also demonstrated the great progress that has been made toward better serving the psychological needs of religious and spiritual clients, especially in the last few decades. Nevertheless, there remains room for improvement, particularly in dissemination and evaluation of culturally competent training and advancement of treatment outcomes research.

A critical step forward is the dissemination and implementation of the recently developed spiritual and religious competencies in graduate programs, internship sites, postdoctoral fellowships, and in continuing education formats for practicing mental health professionals. Development of standardized training programs and measures to evaluate religious and spiritual competencies could also facilitate fidelity to best practices and service delivery among clinicians (Oxhandler & Pargament, 2018). Mental health professionals with specialized training in the integration of religion and spirituality in psychotherapy should seek out opportunities to share their knowledge and experience via teaching formal courses, clinical supervision, or presenting continuing education workshops.

Leaders in the field suggest both formal and informal training efforts (Hathaway, 2013; Pargament, 2007; Shafranske, 2014; Veiten & Scummell, 2015). Formal training in graduate education might include a seminar in the psychology of religion and spirituality, a class in comparative religions, and a course in spiritually integrated psychotherapy. This combination of coursework would offer students information in theory, research, practice, and the diversity of RSBPs. In addition, integration of religious and spiritual issues in other courses, such as assessment and psychopathology, would help students make practical connections. Formal training for both graduate students and established professionals should include culturally competent religious and spiritual supervision of clinical cases (Shafranske, 2014) and continuing education seminars and workshops. Because there is always more to learn about RSBPs and their ethical integration in psychotherapy, mental health professionals should consider a lifelong learning approach by seeking opportunities to gain information and greater understanding from multiple sources and experiences. Informal training may take several forms, such as visiting places of worship, reading about faith traditions, consulting with clergy members and religious leaders, talking with friends whose beliefs are different from your own, and engaging in reflection about your own spiritual self-awareness, such as writing your own "spiritual autobiography" (see Pargament, 2007, pp. 334–336).

Dissemination of information to clergy and religious leaders about culturally competent psychotherapies available for religious and spiritual individuals is also a vital step in moving forward. Mental health professionals must strive to reduce the barriers for religious and spiritual individuals who might benefit from working with appropriately trained clinicians but who may not seek out mental health treatment due to misinformation or misunderstanding. The COPE model (Milstein et al., 2010, described earlier in the chapter) represents a collaborative strategy in which mental health professionals and clergy work in tandem, utilizing their unique knowledge and skill sets, to educate one another for the benefit of religious and spiritual individuals in need of holistic mental health and spiritual care. Given the large number of individuals in the United States who seek treatment for mental disorders from clergy (Wang et al., 2003), propagation of and engagement in the COPE model, similar collaborative approaches, or workshops for educating clergy are imperative for helping religious and spiritual individuals obtain effective mental health care.

Another necessary step toward better serving religious and spiritual clients is advancing treatment outcomes research, with specific emphasis on developing empirically supported treatments. Due to the relatively recent resurgence of interest in and acceptance of the integration of religion and spirituality in psychotherapy, psychologists and other social scientists of religion must engage in an aggressive clinical research agenda to "catch up" with established secular treatments and culturally competent therapies in other areas of diversity. Specifically, an increase in the sheer number of treatment studies, larger sample sizes, replication of findings, and more well-controlled RCTs are needed (Hook et al., 2010). Finally, researchers should start asking more nuanced questions, such as "To what extent do the therapist and client need to share a similar faith perspective when an accommodative intervention is used?" and "Which therapies are useful for which individuals holding which religious and spiritual beliefs?" (McMinn et al., 2012, p. 267). As knowledge from religious and spiritual treatment outcomes research continues to grow and mental health professionals move closer to reaching the standards of culturally competent practice, the gaps in service delivery will narrow for religious and spiritual clients seeking psychotherapy.

References

American Counseling Association. (2014). *ACA code of ethics*. Alexandria, VA: Author.

American Psychological Association. (2007). *Resolution on religious, religion-based and/or religion-derived prejudice*. Washington, DC: Author. Retrieved from https://www.apa.org/about/policy/religious-discrimination.pdf

American Psychological Association. (2017a). *Ethical principles of psychologists and code of conduct* (adopted June 1, 2003; amended June 1, 2010, and January 17, 2017). Retrieved from http://www.apa.org/ethics/code/index.aspx

American Psychological Association. (2017b). *Multicultural guidelines: An ecological approach to context, identity, and intersectionality*. Retrieved from http://www.apa.org/about/policy/multicultural-guidelines.pdf

Barnett, J. E., & Johnson, W. B. (2011). Integrating spirituality and religion into psychotherapy: Persistent dilemmas, ethical issues, and a proposed decision-making process. *Ethics and Behavior*, *21*(2), 147–164.

Delaney, H. D., Miller, W. R., & Bisono, A. M. (2007). Religiosity and spirituality among psychologists: A survey of clinical members of the American Psychological Association. *Professional Psychology: Research and Practice*, *38*, 538–546.

Ellison, C. G., & McFarland, M. J. (2013). The social context of religion and spirituality in the United States. In K. I. Pargament, J. J. Exline, & J. W. Jones (Eds.), *APA handbook of psychology, religion, and spirituality: Vol. 1, Context, theory, and research* (pp. 21–51). Washington, DC: American Psychological Association.

Falender, C. A., & Shafranske, E. P. (2004). *Clinical supervision: A competency-based approach*. Washington, DC: American Psychological Association.

Francis, J. (2011). Religious and spiritual beliefs, practices, professional attitudes, and behaviors of clinical and counseling psychology interns. *Dissertation Abstracts International: Section B: The Sciences and Engineering*, *72*(10-B), 6383.

Fredrickson, B. L. (2002). How does religion benefit health and well-being? Are positive emotions active ingredients? *Psychological Inquiry*, *13*(3), 209–213.

Freud, S. (1961). *The future of an illusion* (J. Strachey, Ed. & Trans.). New York, NY: Norton. (Original work published in 1927.)

Fry, P. S. (2000). Religious involvement, spirituality, and personal meaning for life: Existential predicators of psychological well-being in community-residing and institutional care elders. *Aging and Mental Health*, *4*(4), 375–387.

García, A., & Blankhom, J. (2016). The social content of organized nonbelief: County-level predictors of nonbeliever organizations in the United States. *Journal for the Scientific Study of Religion*, *55*(1), 70–90.

Gladding, S. T., & Crockett, J. E. (2018). Religious and spiritual issues in counseling and therapy: Overcoming clinical barriers. *Journal of Spirituality in Mental Health*. Retrieved from https://doi.org/10.1080/19349637.2018.1476947

Griffith, J. (2010). *Religion that heals, religion that harms*. New York, NY: Guilford Press.

Griffith, J. L., & Magyar-Russell, G. (2018). Unhealthy and potentially harmful uses of religion. In J. Peteet & A. Fung (Eds.), *Ethical considerations at the intersection of psychiatry and religion* (pp. 43–59). New York, NY: Oxford University Press.

Gross, N., & Simmons, S. (2007, February 6). *How religious are America's college and university professors?* Social Science Research Council. Retrieved from http://religion.ssrc.org/reforum/Gross_Simmons.pdf

Harris, K. A., Randolph, B. E., & Gordon, T. D. (2016). What do clients want? Assessing spiritual needs in counseling: A literature review. *Spirituality in Clinical Practice*, *3*(4), 250–275.

Hathaway, W. L. (2013). Pathways toward graduate training in the clinical psychology of religion and spirituality: A spiritual competencies model. In K. I. Pargament, A. Mahoney, & E. P. Shafranske (Eds.), *APA handbook of psychology, religion, and spirituality: Vol. 2, An applied psychology of religions and spirituality* (pp. 635–649). Washington, DC: American Psychological Association.

Hathaway, W. L., Scott, S. Y., & Garver, S. A. (2004). Assessing religious/spiritual functioning: A neglected domain in clinical practice? *Professional Psychology: Research and Practice, 35*(1), 97–104.

Hill, P. C., & Pargament, K. I. (2008). Advances in the conceptualization and measurement of religion and spirituality: Implications for physical and mental health research. *Psychology of Religions and Spirituality, S*(1) 3–17.

Hook, J. N., Worthington, E. L. Jr., Davis, D. E., Jennings, D. J., Gartner, A. L., & Hook, J. P. (2010). Empirically supported religious and spiritual therapies. *Journal of Clinical Psychology, 66*(1), 46–72.

James, W. (1991). *Varieties of religious experience*. New York, NY: Triumph Books. (Original work published in 1902.)

Koenig, H. G., King, D., & Carson, V. B. (2012). *Handbook of religion and health* (2nd ed.). New York, NY: Oxford University Press.

Koenig, H. G., Pearce, M. J., Nelson, B., Shaw, S. F., Robins, C. J., Daher, N. S., . . . King, M. B. (2015). Religious vs. conventional cognitive behavioral therapy for major depression in persons with chronic medical illness: A pilot randomized trial. *Journal of Nervous and Mental Disease, 203*, 243–251.

Magyar-Russell, G., & Griffith, J. L. (2016). Addressing unhealthy and potentially harmful expressions of religiousness and spirituality in clinical practice. *Spirituality in Clinical Practice, 3*(3), 159–162.

McMinn, M. R, Snow, K. N., & Orton, J. J. (2012). Counseling and psychotherapy within and across faith traditions. In L. J. Miller (Ed.), *The Oxford handbook of psychology and spirituality* (pp. 255–270). New York, NY: Oxford University Press

Milstein, G., Manierre, A., & Yali, A.M. (2010). Psychological care for persons of diverse religions: A collaborative continuum. *Professional Psychology: Research and Practice, 41*(5), 371–381.

National Association of Social Workers. (2017). *NASW code of ethics* (adopted 1996; revised 2017). Retrieved from https://www.socialworkers.org/About/Ethics/Code-of-Ethics/Code-of-Ethics-English

Newport, F. (2007, December 24). Questions and answers about Americans' religion. Retrieved from https://news.gallup.com/poll/103459/questions-answers-about-americans-religion.aspx

Newport, F. (2016, June 29). Most Americans still believe in God. Retrieved from https://news.gallup.com/poll/193271/americans-believe-god.aspx?version=print

O'Conner, S., & Vandenberg, B. (2005). Psychosis or faith? Clinicians' assessment of religious beliefs. *Journal of Consulting and Clinical Psychology, 73*(4), 610–616.

Oxhandler, H. K., & Pargament, K. I. (2018). Measuring religious and spiritual competence across helping professions: Previous efforts and future directions. *Spirituality in Clinical Practice, 5*(2), 120–132.

Oxhandler, H. K., & Parrish, D. E. (2016). The development and validation of the Religious/Spiritually Integrated Practice Assessment Scale. *Research on Social Work Practice, 26*, 295–307.

Paloutzian, R. F. (2017). *Invitation to the psychology of religion* (3rd ed.). New York, NY: Guilford Press.

Pargament, K. I. (2007). *Spiritually integrated psychotherapy: Understanding and addressing the sacred*. New York, NY: Guilford Press.

Pargament, K. I. (Ed.). (2013). *APA handbook of psychology, religion, and spirituality. Vols. 1 & 2.* Washington, DC: American Psychological Association.

Pargament, K. I., & Cummings, J. (2010). Anchored by faith: Religion as a resilience factor. In J. W. Reich, A. J. Zautra, & J. S. Hall (Eds.), *Handbook of adult resilience* (pp. 193–210). New York, NY: Guilford Press.

Park, C. L., & Hale, A. (2014). Religious/spiritual meaning systems: Multiple pathways to well-being. In K. P. Chu (Ed.), *Religion and spiritualty across cultures* (pp. 177–201). New York, NY: Springer.

Pew Research Center. (2015). *Religious nones are not only growing they're becoming more secular.* Retrieved from http://www.pewresearch.org/fact-tank/2015/11/11/religious-nones-are-not-only-growing-theyre-becoming-more-secular/

Post, B. C., Wade, N. G., & Cornish, M. A. (2016). Religion and spirituality in group counseling: Beliefs and preferences of university counseling center clients. *Group Dynamics: Theory, Research, and Practice, 18*(1), 53–68.

Ruff, J. L. (2008). Clinician religiosity and response to divergent patient religiosity: An investigation into the effects of implicit and explicit stereotyping on empathy and prognosis in initial responding to patients who are religiously diverse from psychologists. *US Dissertation Abstracts International: Section B: The Sciences and Engineering,* 69(4-B), 2639.

Saunders, S. M., Miller, M. L., & Bright, M. M. (2010). Spiritually conscious psychological care. *Professional Psychology: Research and Practice, 41*(5), 355–362.

Shafranske, E. P. (2014). Addressing religiousness and spirituality as clinically relevant cultural features in supervision. In C. A. Falender, E. P. Shafranske, & C. J. Falicov (Eds.), *Multiculturalism and diversity in clinical supervision: A competency-based approach* (pp. 181–207). Washington, DC: American Psychological Association.

Shafranske, E. P., & Cummings, J. P. (2013). Religious and spiritual beliefs, affiliations, and practices of psychologists. In K. I. Pargament, A. Mahoney, & E. P. Shafranske (Eds.), *APA handbook of psychology, religion, and spirituality: Vol. 2, An applied psychology of religion and spirituality* (pp. 23–41). Washington, DC: American Psychological Association.

Tan, S. Y. (1996). Religion in clinical practice: Implicit and explicit integration. In E. P. Shafranske (Ed.), *Religion and the clinical practice of psychology* (pp. 365–387). Washington, DC: American Psychological Association.

Vieten, C., & Scammell, S. (2015). *Spiritual and religious competencies in clinical practice: Guidelines for psychotherapists and mental health professionals.* Oakland, CA: New Harbinger Publications.

Vieten, C., Scammell, S., Pierce, A., Pilato, R., Ammondson, I., & Pargament, K. I. (2016). Competencies for psychologists in the domains of religion and spirituality. *Spirituality in Clinical Practice, 3*(2), 92–114.

Vieten, C., Scammell, S., Pilato, R., Ammonson, I., Pargament, K. I., & Lukoff, D. (2013). Spiritual and religious competencies for psychologists. *Psychology of Religion and Spirituality, 5*(3), 129–144.

Wang, P. S., Berglund, P. A., & Kessler, R. C. (2003). Patterns and correlates of contacting clergy for mental disorders in the United States. *Health Services Research, 38*(2), 647–673.

Watson, J. B. (1925). *Behaviorism.* Chicago, IL: University of Chicago Press.

Welwood, J. (2000). *Toward a psychology of awakening: Buddhism, psychotherapy and the path of personal and spiritual transformation.* Boston, MA: Shambhala Publications.

SECTION 3

PEOPLE IN TRANSITION AND UNDERSERVED LOCATIONS

8

Delivering Psychological Services to Refugees Resettled in the United States

Johanna E. Nilsson, Sally Stratmann, Aurora Molitoris, Marcella A. Beaumont, and Jessica Horine

According to data from the United Nations High Commissioner for Refugees (UNHCR, 2018), over 68 million individuals have been forced to leave their homes due to war, persecution, human right violations, natural disasters, or other threats to life and safety. An estimated 40 million of these individuals are internally displaced, meaning that they are still within their country of origin. About 25 million are considered refugees and about half are believed to be minors. The largest groups of refugees are currently from Syria, Afghanistan, South Sudan, Myanmar, and Somalia (UNHCR, 2018). Most of them reside in developing countries, such as Turkey, Pakistan, Ethiopia, and Lebanon, with a relatively small percentage being resettled in developed countries (Armbrecht, 2015). This chapter will provide information about refugees, including definition and resettlement policies, unique and common pre- and post-migration concerns, barriers to services, cultural competences, and available effective treatments.

Endorsed by 148 nations, the only two legal and globally recognized documents to define and address the rights of refugees are the 1951 Geneva Convention and the later 1967 Protocol of the Convention (UNHCR, 2001). The Geneva Convention Article 1A defines refugees as any persons having

> a well-founded fear of being persecuted for reasons of race, religion, nationality, membership of a particular social group or political opinion, is outside the country of his nationality and is unable or, owing to such fear, is unwilling to avail himself of the protection of that country; or who, not having a nationality and being outside the country of his former habitual residence as a result of such events, is unable or, owing to such fear, is unwilling to return to it. (Convention of 1951, Article 1A (2))

Articles based on the Geneva Convention also outline responsibilities of nations hosting refugees, such as non-refoulement (i.e., refugees cannot be sent back to their country of origin if they will experience threat to their life and freedom there; Article 3, UNHCR, 2001). Other protections that are awarded to refugees include treating them with similar civil, economic, and social rights as the nation's citizens (UNHCR, 2016).

The large number of displaced individuals and refugees has resulted in what has been declared a worldwide refugee crisis (Lennard, 2013), with millions of people seeking resettlement in other countries. Refugee resettlement falls under the auspices of the UNHCR. As of 2016, only 37 of the world's 195 total countries had agreed to formally resettle refugees, with the United States being one of those countries (UNHCR, 2016).

Perhaps owing to the limited number of participating countries, only a small portion of refugees are resettled each year. Resettlement, the opportunity to be permanently relocated in another country, generally takes place in one of two ways. The first method involves refugees waiting for UNHCR to place them in a participating country. UNHCR screens and determines whether a person has a unique need to be resettled. An example of this process would be individuals from Somalia and South Sudan who, after fleeing their countries of origin, have ended up living in UN refugee camps in other African counties. These individuals will remain in these camps indefinitely until their application for resettlement is processed, at which point they will go live in a host country should they qualify for refugee status.

A second possible pathway to obtain refugee status is for individuals to enter the country in which they wish to resettle and seek asylum upon entry in that country. Asylum seeking has been utilized by many Syrian refugees, who fled the war in Syria by traveling to Europe and requesting asylum in countries such as Germany, France, or Sweden. Asylum seekers also include individuals from Central and South America seeking asylum in the United States. In an effort to decrease the number of asylum seekers from this region, the U.S. government, in December 2018, reported a new, rather unprecedented method to process asylum seekers at the Mexican border. Rather than having them reside in the United States while waiting for their asylum request to be determined, they will now have to remain in shelters in Mexico (Burnette, 2018).

Almost 3 million refugees have officially resettled in the United States since the U.S. Congress passed the Refugee Act in 1980. The annual number of refugees admitted to the United States is set by the seated president and has thus experienced significant fluctuation. While yearly admissions in the mid-1900s averaged around 100,000, 2002 (one year after the September 11, 2001, terrorist attacks on the United States) saw a dramatic plunge to 27,000, later rising to 85,000 in 2016, under President Obama's leadership. During President Trump's tenure, the number of refugees has again decreased, and it is expected that only 21,000 refugees will be able to resettle in the United States in 2018 (Ryan, 2018).

The refugees recently resettled in the United States include individuals from Congo, Syria, Burma, Iraq, and Somalia (Igielnik & Krogstad, 2017).

Once refugees arrive in the United States, they are provided with basic services by the U.S. Department of State's Reception and Placement Program, via local resettlement agencies. Upon arrival, refugees are met at the airport by a family member, friend, or resettlement agency staff. They are provided an apartment with some furniture, food and clothing, and access to various services. The Reception and Placement Program financially supports refugees for the first three months, after which they are expected to be self-reliant. However, three months is often not enough time for many refugees to adjust and become financially independent. Fortunately, other federal agencies such as the Department of Health and Human Service's Office of Refugee Resettlement can provide additional support such as English classes and employment services. Refugees can apply for permanent residence after one year in the United States and are eligible for citizenship five years later (U.S. Department of State, 2018).

The Scope and Description of the Problem

While many refugees successfully adjust to life in their host nation after resettlement, others experience significant adversities. Both pre-migration trauma and post-migration challenges contribute to these difficulties. Some of these challenges also act as barriers to psychological services.

Pre-migration Trauma

Many refugees have faced arduous and horrifying experiences in their journey toward safety. Traumatic events may include witnessing or being subjected to torture, forced labor, starvation/deprivation of food or shelter, rape, sexual assault, disease and illness, and loss of family members and friends (Schweitzer, Melville, Steel, & Lacherez, 2006). Such traumatic experiences can have a detrimental impact on the mental and physical well-being of refugees and are associated with post-traumatic stress disorder (PTSD), depression, and anxiety (e.g., Anna et al., 2017; Fazel, Wheeler, & Danesh, 2005; Steel et al., 2009). For example, Fazel et al. (2005) found that among refugees in Western countries, 10% were diagnosed with PTSD, 5% with major depression, and 4% with generalized anxiety disorder. In a more recent study of 385 mostly young male refugees, 50% could be diagnosed with mental health disorders; of these, about 31% met the criteria for PTSD and 20% for depression (Anna et al., 2017). Traumatic experiences in this study were defined as combat and detention experiences, threat of death, and witnessing violence or death. Similarly, in a meta-analysis of over 80,000 refugees and other displaced individuals identified, torture was the strongest predictor of PTSD (Steel et al., 2009).

High incidences of PTSD and depression also exist among refugee children. A relationship between poorer mental health and increased exposure to violence, including war trauma and violent death and/or abuse of a family member, has been reported. Additionally, children migrating without family members report higher rates of PTSD than those who migrate with family (Reavall & Fazil, 2016).

Post-Migration Challenges

While many refugees are excited and deeply grateful for the opportunity to resettle in a new country, resettlement also brings unique challenges. Refugees are faced with beginning the acculturation process while simultaneously grieving the loss of their home country, culture, identity, and often family and friends. Broadly defined, the term "acculturation" describes the ways in which individuals change due to contact with another culture (Graves, 1967).

In a longitudinal study, LeMaster et al. (2018) examined the relationship between acculturation and pre-migration factors (demographics, chronic disease, trauma, social support, and resilience) in a group of recently arrived Iraqi refugees. The findings suggested that pre-migration trauma, medical illness, and more depressive symptoms at baseline had an adverse impact on refugees' acculturation at least through the first year of post-migration. Yet there is evidence to suggest that post-migration stressors, such as socioeconomic disadvantage, lack of social support, and challenges in acculturation, not only add to but can be unique predictors of post-migration mental health problems (Carswell, Blackburn, & Barker, 2009).

Employment and Financial Challenges

An important aspect of acculturation, and often a great stressor, is learning the host country's language (Baranik, Hurst, & Eby, 2018). Learning English is almost impossible for those who are illiterate in their native language. Roughly 20% of Congolese individuals over the age of 18 are illiterate. It is estimated that over half of Congolese refugees resettled in the United States do not speak English, and that even a larger proportion cannot read or write in English, the majority of this group being Congolese women. Language barriers and lack of formal education can make acculturation even more challenging, often impeding the person's ability to learn how to drive and use computers and appliances (Cultural Orientation Resource Center, 2014).

Due to education and language barriers, many refugees struggle to find employment and to become financially stable. Research on employment stressors and barriers among Muslim Arabs at two different refugee resettlement agencies showed that their greatest concern was getting access to and opportunity for employment. Challenges described by the participants included difficulties finding a job, which were exacerbated by a lack of recognition of past education and employment experiences in their native country. Overt and covert discrimination is another stressor that can prevent access to employment (Baranik et al., 2018), as well as housing, health care, and various other basic needs (Chung, Bemak, Ortiz, & Sandoval-Perez, 2008).

Given these difficulties securing employment, financial hardship and poverty are rather common in these populations. Among U.S. immigrant groups, Somalis are among the poorest, with approximately 79% living in low-income households (Capps et al., 2015). Compared to Asian and Pacific Islanders, of whom about 13% live below the poverty line, about 30% of the Burmese population live in poverty (Vang & Trieu, 2014).

Family Dynamics

As family members, individually, adjust and acculturate to their new cultural context, many face changes in family dynamics, gender roles, and responsibilities. Diverging from traditional cultural expectations, women—who may for the first time be working outside the home—may experience an increased sense of independence and self-esteem. For men, resettlement and unemployment may lead to a loss of identity and status. Such role reversals can contribute to marital conflicts and domestic violence (Darvishpour, 2002; Nilsson, Brown, Russell, & Khamphakdy-Brown, 2008).

Similar to adults, refugee children face unique struggles during the post-migration period. While children often acculturate faster than their parents (Deng & Marlowe, 2013), many children and adolescents experience academic difficulties, lack of peer relationships, frequent moves, challenges in managing cultural differences, and potential financial hardships—all of which can result in stress, depression, and other mental health problems (Heptinstall, Sethna, & Taylor, 2004; Sack, 1998). Trauma also manifests developmentally, creating academic and interpersonal difficulties such as disconnection from school and friends or antisocial behavior (Saltzman, Layne, Steinberg, Arslanagic, & Pynoos, 2003). It has also been noted that parental trauma may negatively affect the quality of family functioning and relationships among parents and children (CMAS, 2015).

Barriers to Service Delivery

As has been described, refugees can face a host of difficulties, ranging from significant pre-migration trauma to dealing with language and cultural barriers, financial hardship, discrimination, and family conflict during the resettlement period. Clearly such stressors can lead to psychological symptoms of depression and anxiety, as well as somatic concerns. In addition, many refugees experience grief and loneliness as a result of leaving a familiar culture behind and the loss of family members and support systems. Given all those challenges, it would seem that mental health counseling would be a relevant choice of support for this population; however, due to the more urgent post-migration concerns previously described, seeking help for mental health problems may seem less important or even as a potentially ineffective solution for these concerns (O'Driscoll, Serneels, & Imeraj, 2017). Some groups of refugees also hold strong, often cultural, biases against mental illness (see Marshall, Butler, Roche, Cumming, & Taknint, 2016). Additionally, based on our experience, a lack of access to transportation and childcare services can further prevent individuals from seeking help.

Another barrier to mental health services is that psychotherapy and counseling are a largely Western phenomenon (O'Driscoll et al. 2017). Many refugees are unfamiliar with the context of individual psychotherapy and may feel uncomfortable engaging in intimate conversations with a stranger (Bemak & Chung, 2017). To further complicate this issue, few mental health practitioners are specifically trained to work with refugee populations, and there is a lack of bilingual and bicultural mental health staff. In a large review of studies on mental health practitioners working with ethnic and racial minority clients, Dune, Caputi, and Walker (2018) concluded that low levels of cultural competence and high levels of ethnic and racial blindness on the part of practitioners functioned as a barrier in the development of effective therapeutic alliances.

The current mental health system itself can also serve as a hindrance for services as it is often separated from other services that refugees may need, such as medical, employment, housing, and social services. Mental health professionals and refugees alike have expressed the need for more holistic or multimodal treatment modalities that encompass multiple services to improve refugee mental health and well-being (Elsass & Phuntsok, 2009; Vrana, Campbell, & Clay, 2013). Given the myriad challenges that refugees may have, such as transportation, language, employment, social isolation, social services, and even empowerment, in addition to mental health concerns, their situation could be understood using holistic and humanistic theoretical frameworks, such as Abraham Maslow's (1954) hierarchy of needs (Lonn & Dantzler, 2017). The current lack of multimodal care systems calls for mental health professionals to work outside of their traditional role to provide refugee clients with the services they need.

Creating Cultural Competency

While not many training models or curricula specifically address how to work with a refugee population (Pieterse, Evans, Risner-Butner, Collins, & Mason, 2009), the American Psychological Association (APA) and other mental health organizations have provided general multicultural competencies guidelines. The most recent guidelines, *Multicultural Guidelines: An Ecological Approach to Context, Identity, and Intersectionality* (APA, 2017), were developed to direct clinical practice and give practitioners a model to aspire to in relating to clients of varying cultural backgrounds. The guidelines acknowledge that practice is influenced by globalization and provide a case study that illustrates issues that accompany refugee status. The guidelines address various aspects of cultural competence, such as awareness that the client and clinician each are cultural beings, the role of language, intersectionality, awareness of discrimination, privilege and power, and the need to use culturally adaptive interventions and strengths-based approaches when working with individuals. These tenets are also of value for practitioners working with refugee populations.

The basic pillars of cultural competence when working with refugees, based on available literature and our experiences, can be summarized as follows. Practitioners working with refugees should:

- Understand that refugees come from many regions of the world and represent a wide range of national, cultural, religious, educational and professional backgrounds—as well as that their journeys toward safety and their experiences in the United States can vary greatly
- Know about refugee policies, definitions, and rights
- Be willing to learn about each client's cultural background while keeping in mind that each client is a unique individual within her or his cultural context
- Know about the impact of trauma on functioning
- Understand potential pre- and post-migration experiences that refugees may have
- Be aware of resources and services available for refugees
- Be willing to step outside the traditional role of a mental health professional, and work closely with cultural brokers, interpreters, paraprofessionals, and community agencies
- Be aware of their own culture, biases, and privileges, and how to not project these onto their clients
- Use pertinent, culturally effective interventions based on the context of the unique client's cultural identity.

Due to the ever-changing demographics and composition of the refugee population, practitioners working with refugees must also be open, willing, and flexible to learn about new groups of refugees and develop interventions that meet the needs of a specific group (APA, 2010).

The Empowerment Program

Since 2001, one of us (J.E.N.) has coordinated a mental health program for refugees in Kansas City. The Empowerment Program was created by a small group of women, both U.S. citizens and refugees, to better meet the needs of refugee women. Its mission is to serve refugee women and their families in the areas of adjustment, mental health, and domestic violence via counseling, home visits, community workshops, advocacy/case management, assistance with domestic violence concerns, interpretation, and transportation, without charge. One of its main goals is to eliminate barriers to mental health services. The program has worked toward this goal by working closely with refugee and immigrant communities. The program employs staff who are bilingual and bicultural and who come from refugee and immigrant backgrounds. The staff, titled advocates/case managers, some of whom are paraprofessionals, provide clients with support services, link them with other resources, and function as liaisons between the refugee community and U.S. social and health services. They provide transportation and emotional support and serve as interpreters and cultural mentors, helping to meet the needs of refugees that often remain unmet by other services (APA, 2010). The program serves about 150 refugee women and their families each year from a wide range of national backgrounds, including Somalia, Sudan, Afghanistan, Vietnam, Russia, Iraq, and Mexico (for more information see Khamhakdy-Brown, Jones, Nilsson, Russell, & Klevens, 2006).

One of the main lessons learned from the Empowerment Program is that even after years of working in the community, very few individuals seek traditional mental health services, even if a need for such services exists. This is predominantly due to the barriers previously discussed in this chapter. Other methods had to be developed to meet the psychological needs of this group, and the Empowerment Program worked to build a network of social support via its staff of advocates. Data show that social support and belongingness are two critical components of post-migration success and mental well-being (LeMaster et al., 2018; Schweitzer et al., 2006). Hence, it is not surprising that many refugees settle close to other individuals who share their nationality if possible. Often this community provides considerable support for newly arrived refugees, as well as for individuals who have resided in the country for longer periods.

In addition to the work of the advocates, the community workshops have become the Empowerment Program's most effective service. They provide social support and empowerment, build community, and address various mental health and other physical and social needs. The specific topics of the workshops are based on the communities' input on their specific areas of interest. Over the years a wide range of topics have been addressed, including skills for teenagers and parents, women's health care, acculturation, mental health, self-care, employment, and the school systems; workshop participants have met with the police to develop a better relationship and have visited domestic violence shelters. While the workshops have a psychoeducational focus, they also use a multimodal approach to services to help build community and relationships within and among different refugee communities and to build bridges to U.S. services and agencies (see Khamhakdy-Brown et al., 2006).

Effective Strategies and Empirically-Supported Treatments

Due to the cultural diversity among refugees, treatments found to be efficacious with one group may not be effective for another (Zayfert, 2008). Effective strategies for developing a therapeutic alliance, conducting assessments, and diagnosing will be discussed, followed by a review of both traditional and obscure empirically supported treatments, as well as treatments for adolescents and children.

Therapeutic Alliance

A strong therapeutic alliance, based on trust and security, is the foundation of culturally competent counseling with refugees (Warr, 2010). Refugees may not understand how or why to disclose their turbulent stories, and mental health professionals, who are commonly far removed from these often unimaginable notions of survival and chaos, may have to strive to build a framework of understanding of these experiences (Davidson, Murray, & Schweitzer, 2010). Power dynamics are an important consideration in the alliance, as the refugee inherently has less power than the mental health clinician. Personal disclosure and connection can help the refugee client develop trust (Guregård & Seikkula, 2014).

Educating clients about the context of treatment and confidentiality can aid in building rapport, can help the client to understand the purpose of disclosure, and can prepare the client for what may seem to be an inappropriate focus on the self. The majority of refugees are fleeing nations that ascribe to collectivist values, so the individualism typical of Western counseling must adapted to suit these values by understanding how clients' paradigms are tied to their community (Bemak & Chung, 2017). In the Empowerment Program, students are trained to spend time developing rapport first before obtaining extensive detail about their clients' experiences.

Within the process of psychotherapy itself, common topics may include difficulties pertaining to the loss of the culture of origin and issues with acculturation (Kaczorowski et al., 2011). Showing an understanding of and a desire to address inequities, racism and discrimination, and violations of human rights can also support refugees' mental health and well-being (Bemak & Chung, 2017); in our experience, it can also strengthen rapport.

Assessment and Diagnosis

Mental health professionals should hold the cultural background of the refugee in mind when conducting assessments, diagnostic interviews, and other means of defining mental distress and disorders. Since only a few instruments have demonstrated evidence for reliability and validity in refugee populations, researchers have advocated for using narrative or open-ended formats that allow for flexibility in the expression of mental health status, as opposed to highly structured assessments (Kaczorowski et al., 2011). Before administering measures to or conducting interviews with refugee patients, clinicians must investigate the evidence of validity of the assessment or diagnosis for patients of that nationality, ethnic group, or geographic area. In refugee patients, it is possible that somatic symptoms or beliefs around supernatural phenomena may be more indicative of psychological distress than the diagnostic criteria most Western assessments utilize, making Western assessments less useful (McLellan, 2015; Rohlof, Knipscheer, & Kleber, 2014).

Traditional, Empirically Supported Treatments

While it should not be assumed that all refugees are traumatized, the estimate that slightly under one third of refugees meet diagnostic requirements for PTSD indicates that focusing on effective treatments is vital (Anna et al., 2017). We will address a few therapies with evidence for efficacy in alleviating PTSD symptoms in refugee patients: narrative exposure therapy (NET), eye movement desensitization and reprocessing (EMDR), and cognitive behavioral therapy (CBT). These therapies must be used with some caution, however: Many studies of whether trauma therapies "work" for refugees use small samples, do not contain control groups, and do not assess whether positive outcomes are maintained in the long term (Nickerson, Bryant, Silove, & Steel, 2011).

NET

NET is a standardized short-term approach that involves the construction of a cohesive life story. The goal is to help the patient integrate the fragmented memory of traumatic events into a coherent narrative. By telling a chronological narrative of their life, either to a therapist individually or in a small-group setting, patients are able to develop a story that is less fractured. Both positive and negative experiences of a sensory, emotional, and cognitive nature are integrated, resulting in a more holistic view of one's life and sense of self. Patients recount their life stories with traumatic experiences interwoven, instead of splintered, until symptomology associated with the recollection of those memories dissipates. This new story overcomes the trauma-focused narrative, which was previously at the forefront of the person's self-understanding. At the end of the treatment, the therapist provides the patients with an autobiography of their lives and serves as a witness to their experiences, strength, and human rights (Schauer, Neuner, & Elbert, 2011). NET currently appears to be one of the most efficacious PTSD treatments for refugees (see Nosè et al., 2017; Thompson, Vidgen, & Roberts, 2018).

EMDR

In EMDR, the client processes the difficult traumatic memories for a short period of time while simultaneously attending to an outside stimulus, facilitating the achievement of adaptive paradigms and adaptive functioning in response to trauma-related stimuli (EMDR Institute, Inc., 2018). The patient recounts the traumatic memory in great detail while following some form of stimulation, such as following the movement of a finger back and forth. Recounting the memory, a cognitive and affective process, while attending to a sensory stimulus is thought to help with integrating the traumatic memory (EMDR Institute, Inc., 2018). EMDR, however, is considered a controversial treatment. Despite some evidence for its ability to treat PTSD, some find the sensory stimulation used in EMDR unnecessary, viewing its success as a result of its exposure component (Davidson & Parker, 2001). There is some evidence that EMDR is efficacious with refugee populations (e.g., Schubert, Lee, Araujo, Butler, & Taylor, 2016; Thompson et al., 2018).

CBT

CBT is a brief intervention targeting maladaptive thoughts and behaviors, with the understanding that changing these patterns will lead to positive changes in mood and well-being (Beck Institute for Cognitive Behavior Therapy, 2017).

CBT with traumatized refugees holds promise, as well as derivatives such as culturally adapted CBT (CA-CBT). CA-CBT involves a variety of CBT techniques and protocols modified to suit different populations—for example, using emotional regulation techniques that involve stretching, meditation, and culturally appropriate and applicable imagery to meet the salient somatic needs of many traumatized refugee and ethnic minority populations (Hinton, Rivera, Hoffman, Barlow & Otto, 2012).

Other Treatments

Indigenous Treatments

Mental health professionals may also want to elicit the help of indigenous healers from the refugee's culture of origin in the treatment of the refugee to improve outcomes in psychotherapy. This process should involve healing techniques useful to the therapeutic process and healers that are vetted for authenticity (Bemak & Chung, 2017). Having established relationships with the specific refugee community aids in finding elders and professionals to ask when trying to find authentic and respected healers.

Indigenous treatments for mental health needs have shown success in many of the communities in which they've been studied. For example, participation in religious rituals was found to alleviate symptoms of depression, anxiety, and stress in indigenous refugees in India (Snodgrass, Most, & Upadhyay, 2017). The treatment model developed and employed by the Center for Victims of Torture in Guinea, which incorporates native West African cultural activities such as "traditional stories, drumming, chants, rhythmic clapping, and song" (p. 926), produced reductions in trauma symptomology, elevated levels of social support, and better overall daily functioning in Liberian and Sierra Leonean refugees (Stepakoff et al., 2006).

Collaborative Care

One potential model for meeting refugee needs involves collaborative or integrated care, in which a team of health professionals take a unified and systemic approach to patient care to maximize outcomes by treating multiple presenting concerns simultaneously and in conjunction with one another (Peek & the National Integration Academy Council, 2013). A review by Esala, Vukovich, Hanbury, Kashyap, and Joscelyne (2018) concluded that there is evidence for the usefulness of collaborative care for mental health concerns that commonly affect refugees, such as PTSD, anxiety, depression, severe and persistent mental illness, and certain chronic health conditions. However, similarly to multimodal approaches, there are multiple and sometimes disparate approaches to collaborative care with poor model specification, making the effectiveness of these approaches difficult to assess.

Care for Children and Adolescents

Consistent with the discussion of multimodal approaches, it is important for psychotherapists to serve both the refugee child's mental health needs and environmental needs in a culturally competent manner (Saltzman et al., 2003; Warr, 2010). The lives of these children are often marred by insecurities about basic needs and asylum status. The mental health professionals interviewed by Warr (2010) asserted that feelings of safety in refugee children are necessary for successful therapy. It should be the goal of the psychotherapist to help the refugee child develop a coherent, empowered narrative that includes pre- and post-migration experiences (Davies & Webb, 2000). Developing a cohesive trauma narrative, learning to cope with trauma-related cues in the environment that may trigger intrusive memories, and facilitating an adaptive bereavement process after the prevalent loss of loved ones are crucial discussion points (Davies & Webb, 2000). Grief and loss may be defined, manifested, and dealt with in culturally specific ways, making it vital to understand indigenous bereavement processes and coping mechanisms (Eisenbruch, 1991).

It is also imperative to address the ways, insidious and overt, in which the trauma has seeped into the child's life. The ripple effect of war trauma can create financial difficulties, dramatically alter family dynamics or proximity, and lead to geographic dislocation. Consequently, addressing trauma should involve the internal symptomology and distress, as well as psychosocial and environmental issues. Therapies such as CBT, NET, and EMDR have demonstrated potential for addressing trauma symptoms in children and adolescents (Ehntholt & Yule, 2006). While it is often the notion that psychotherapy with child and adolescent refugees should focus on presenting psychopathology, failing to see a client's abilities may be damaging to children and teens seeking a sense of direction and hope in an unfamiliar nation. Mental health professionals may want to balance their focus on issues of mental health with ways in which to empower these clients and bring their strengths and sense of resilience into the counseling context (Marshall et al., 2016).

In general, flexibility and adaptability in the therapeutic process are crucial when working with child and adolescent refugees. Alternative therapies involving creative expression and social interaction may be useful as they transition into a new school and new society by helping the patient understand emotions and connect with peers (Marshall et al., 2016). For example, reflective writing has been shown to alleviate symptoms of traumatic grief in child and adolescent refugees (Kalantari, Yule, Dyregrov, Neshatdoost, & Ahmadi, 2012). Utilizing online and mobile resources as part of the counseling process may improve access to youth populations (Marshall et al., 2016).

Finally, a quick note on language. Researchers have shown that although teachers and pediatricians may suggest to refugee parents that they only communicate with children via their new host language, it is recommended that communication continues in the heritage language. This retention enables refugee children to maintain close connection with family, elders, and their cultural heritage. Further, a connection to one's heritage language is related to the well-being of children through more positive family relationships. However, the importance for refugee children of mastering their host language has also been noted. This enables them to not only connect to their newfound world, but also helps them to successfully navigate life in a new country, make friends outside of their comfort zone, and succeed in school and eventually a career of their own (Leyendecker et al., 2018).

Future Steps

While we have covered a range of topics in this chapter, it should be known that training in the treatment of refugees is still sparse. To ensure effective care for current and future refugees, we urge training programs at every level to teach skills for working with immigrant populations. We also encourage training programs, organizations, and independent practitioners to develop partnerships with their local resettlement agency and other community agencies that support refugees. As previously mentioned, there is often a wide gap between the refugee community and mental health services. Bridging this gap may involve counseling and workshops for refugees in many specialty areas. It may also involve educating the staff working with refugees on their potential mental health needs and offering consultations. Steps like these create an invaluable level of accessibility and ensure a more positive transition process. Finally, it is also important to be actively involved in refugee communities, to listen and learn from leaders, from elders, and in our experience especially from women, so that we can provide services that will support the health and well-being of the community. Women's voices have guided us to learn not only what they need, but also the needs of their children, parents, and community at large.

While most multimodal approaches seek to remedy gaps in service delivery that are well documented in the current literature and strive to deliver services using evidence-based and culturally competent methodologies (e.g., Bemak & Chung, 2017), data on efficacy are still limited. This is mainly due to the lack of a uniform system in multimodal approaches and the nature of using multiple services to address needs, which may be difficult to empirically test (Nickerson et al., 2011). Outlining and testing these approaches should be considered a vital first step in learning how to best serve refugees.

We hope that this chapter has provided helpful information about the unique experiences and needs of the refugee community. While we have addressed the many challenges refugees may face, it is important to acknowledge that they also demonstrate remarkable resilience and ability to cope with stressors (Schweitzer, Greenslade, & Kagee, 2007). Many refugee children are resilient and successfully employ coping skills to reduce the harmful effects of displacement (Davies & Webb, 2000). Adults even report positive psychological changes and growth as a result of their struggle with highly challenging life circumstances (Hussain & Bhushan, 2013; Maung, 2018).

If we are fortunate enough, we will have the opportunity as mental health professionals to work with refugees, many of whom have traveled far and waited for years to reach a place of safety. Many have experienced more horrific events and losses than most of us can fathom. Some have psychological scars that are almost impossible to overcome, and for others the resettlement is easier. The privilege to work with this culturally rich, resilient, and wise group of individuals is immense. We can sit in our offices and wait for them to seek our help, or we can reach out to offer our services and support their resettlement and healing process.

References

American Psychological Association. (2010). *Resilience and recovery after war: Refugee children and families in the United States*. Retrieved from http://www.apa.org/pubs/info/reports/refugees.aspx

American Psychological Association. (2017). *Multicultural guidelines: An ecological approach to context, identity, and intersectionality*. Retrieved from http://www.apa.org/about/policy/multicultural guidelines.pdf

Anna, C., Rita, F., Reid, A., Van den Boogaard, W., Deiana, P., Quaranta, G., & Di Carlo, S. (2017). Mental health and trauma in asylum seekers landing in Sicily in 2015: A descriptive study of neglected invisible wounds. *Conflict & Health, 11*, 1–11.

Armbrecht, A. (2015). Which country has hosted the most refugees? *World Economic Forum*. Retrieved from https://www.weforum.org/agenda/2015/12/which-country-has-hosted-the-most-refugees-this-century/

Baranik, L. E., Hurst, C. S., & Eby, L. T. (2018). The stigma of being a refugee: A mixed-method study of refugees' experiences of vocational stress. *Journal of Vocational Behavior, 105*, 116–130.

Beck Institute for Cognitive Behavior Therapy. (2017, July 31). What is cognitive behavior therapy (CBT)? Retrieved from https://beckinstitute.org/get-informed/what-is-cognitive-therapy/

Bemak, F., & Chung, R. C. (2017). Refugee trauma: Culturally responsive counseling interventions. *Journal of Counseling & Development, 95*(3), 299–308.

Burnette, J. (2018). Trump administration changes border policy to discourage asylum-seekers. Retrieved from https://www.npr.org/2018/12/21/679057325/trump-administration-changes-border-policy-to-discourage-asylum-seekers

Capps, R., Newland, K., Fratzke, S., Groves, S., Auclair, G., Fix, M., & McHugh, M. (2015). *The integration outcome of U.S. refugees: Successes and challenges.* Washington, DC: Migration Policy Institute.

Carswell, K., Blackburn, P., & Barker, C. (2009). The relationship between trauma, post-migration problems and the psychological well-being of refugees and asylum seekers. *International Journal of Social Psychiatry, 57*(2), 107–119.

Chung, R. C.-Y., Bemak, F., Ortiz, D. P., & Sandoval-Perez, P. A. (2008). Promoting the mental health of migrants: A multicultural–social justice perspective. *Journal of Counseling & Development, 38*, 310–317.

CMAS (Childminding, Monitoring, Advisory and Support) (2015). *Caring for Syrian refugee children: A program guide for welcoming young children and their families.* Retrieved from https://cmascanada.ca//wp-content/uploads/2015/12/Supporting_Refugees/Caring%20for%20Syrian%20Refugee%20Children-final.pdf

Cultural Orientation Resource Center. (2014). Refugees from the Democratic Republic of the Congo. Retrieved from file:///C:/Users/nilssonj/Downloads/CAL+Backgrounder+07+-+Congolese+FINAL.pdf

Darvishpour, M. (2002). Immigrant women challenge the role of men: How the changing power relationship within Iranian families in Sweden intensifies family conflicts after immigration. *Journal of Comparative Family Studies, 33*, 271–296.

Davidson, G. R., Murray, K. E., & Schweitzer, R. D. (2010). Review of refugee mental health assessment: Best practices and recommendations. *Journal of Pacific Rim Psychology, 4*(1), 72–85.

Davidson, P. R., & Parker, K. C. H. (2001). Eye movement desensitization and reprocessing (EMDR): A meta-analysis. *Journal of Consulting and Clinical Psychology, 69*(2), 305–316.

Davies, M. & Webb, E. (2000). Promoting the psychological well-being of refugee children. *Clinical Child Psychology and Psychiatry, 5*, 541–554.

Deng, S. A., & Marlowe, J. M. (2013). Refugee resettlement and parenting in a different context. *Journal of Immigrant & Refugee Studies, 11*, 416–430.

Dune, T., Caputi, P., & Walker, B. (2018). A systematic review of mental health care workers' constructions about culturally and linguistically diverse people. *PLoS One, 13*(7), e0200662.

Ehntholt, K. A., & Yule, W. (2006). Practitioner review: Assessment and treatment of refugee children and adolescents who have experienced war-related trauma. *Journal of Child Psychology and Psychiatry, 47*, 1197–1210.

Eisenbruch, M. (1991). From post-traumatic stress disorder to cultural bereavement: Diagnosis of Southeast Asian refugees. *Social Science and Medicine, 33*, 673–680.

Elsass, P., & Phuntsok, K. (2009). Tibetans' coping mechanism following torture: An interview study of Tibetan torture survivors' use of coping mechanism and how these were supported by Western counseling. *Traumatology, 15*, 3–10.

EMDR Institute, Inc. (2018). What is EMDR? Retrieved from http://www.emdr.com/what-is-emdr/

Esala, J. J., Vukovich, M. M., Hanbury, A., Kashyap, S., & Joscelyne, A. (2018). Collaborative care for refugees and torture survivors: Key findings from the literature. *Traumatology, 24*(3), 168–185.

Fazel, M., Wheeler, J., & Danesh, J. (2005). Prevalence of serious mental disorder in 7000 refugees resettled in western countries: A systematic review. *Lancet, 365*, 1309–1314.

Graves, T. D. (1967). Acculturation, access, and alcohol in a tri-ethnic community. *American Anthropologist, 69*(3-4), 306–321.

Guregård, S., & Seikkula, J. (2014). Establishing therapeutic dialogue with refugee families. *Contemporary Family Therapy: An International Journal, 36*(1), 41–57.

Heptinstall, E., Sethna, V., & Taylor, E. (2004). PTSD and depression in refugee children: Association with pre-migration trauma and post-migration stress. *European Child Adolescent Psychiatry, 13*, 373–380.

Hinton, D. E., Rivera, E. I., Hoffman, S. G., Barlow, D. H., & Otto, M. W. (2012). Adapting CBT for traumatized refugees and ethnic minority patients: Examples from culturally-adapted CBT (CA-CBT). *Transcultural Psychiatry, 49*, 340–365.

Hussain, D., & Bhushan, B. (2013). Posttraumatic growth experiences among Tibetan refugees: A qualitative investigation. *Qualitative Research in Psychology, 10*, 204–216.

Igielnik, R., & Krogstad, J. M. (2017). *Where refugees to the U.S. come from*. Pew Research Center. Retrieved from http://www.pewresearch.org/fact-tank/2017/02/03/where-refugees-to-the-u-s-come-from/

Kaczorowski, J. A., Williams, A. S., Smith, T. F., Fallah, N., Mendez, J. L., & Nelson-Gray, R. (2011). Adapting clinical services to accommodate needs of refugee populations. *Professional Psychology: Research and Practice, 42*, 361–367.

Kalantari, M., Yule, W., Dyregrov, A., Netshatdoost, H., & Ahmadi, S. J. (2012). Efficacy of writing for recovery on traumatic grief symptoms of Afghani refugee bereaved adolescents: A randomized control trial. *Omega: Journal of Death and Dying, 65*, 139–150.

Khamphakdy-Brown, S., Jones, L. N., Nilsson, J. E., Russell, E. B., & Klevens, C. L. (2006). The Empowerment Program: An application of an outreach program for refugee and immigrant women. *Journal of Mental Health Counseling, 28*, 38–47.

LeMaster, J. W., Broadbridge, C. L., Lumley, M. A., Arnetz, J. E., Arfken, C., Fetters, M. D., & Arnetz, B. B. (2018). Acculturation and post-migration psychological symptoms among Iraqi refugees: A path analysis. *American Journal of Orthopsychiatry, 88*, 38–47.

Lennard, N. (2013, June 19). UN: Global refugee crisis worst in decades. *Salon*. Retrieved from http://www.salon.com/2013/06/19/un_global_refugee_crisis_worst_in_decades/

Leyendecker, B., Cabrera, N., Lembcke, H., Willard, J., Kohl, K., & Spiegler, O. (2018). Parenting in a new land: Immigrant parents and the positive development of their children and youth. *European Psychologist, 23*, 57–71.

Lonn, M. R., & Dantzler, J. Z. (2017). A practical approach to counseling refugees: Applying Maslow's hierarchy of needs. *Journal of Counseling Practice, 8*(2), 61–82.

Marshall, A. E., Butler, K., Roche, T., Cumming, J., & Taknint, J. T. (2016). Refugee youth: A review of mental health counseling issues and practices. *Canadian Psychology, 57*, 308–319.

Maslow, A. (1954). *Motivation and personality*. New York, NY: Harper.

Maung, J. C. (2018). *Burmanese refugee women in resettlement: Narratives of strength, resilience and posttraumatic growth*. University of Missouri-Kansas City. Unpublished Dissertation.

McLellan, J. (2015). Religious responses to bereavement, grief, and loss among refugees. *Journal of Loss and Trauma, 20*, 131–138.

Nickerson, A., Bryant, R. A., Silove, D., & Steel, Z. (2011). A critical review of psychological treatments of posttraumatic stress disorder in refugees. *Clinical Psychology Review, 31*, 399–417.

Nilsson, J. E., Brown, C., Russell, E. B., & Khamphakdy-Brown, S. (2008). Acculturation, partner violence, and psychological distress in refugee women from Somalia. *Journal of Interpersonal Violence, 23*, 1654–1663.

Nosè, M., Ballette, F., Bighelli, I., Turrini, G., Purgato, M., Tol, W., . . . Barbui, C. (2017). Psychosocial interventions for post-traumatic stress disorder in refugees and asylum seekers resettled in high-income countries: Systematic review and meta-analysis. *PLoS One, 12*(2), e0171030.

O'Driscoll, J. V., Serneels, G., & Imeraj, L. (2017). A file study of refugee children referred to specialized mental health care: From an individual diagnostic to an ecological perspective. *European Child and Adolescent Psychiatry, 26*, 131–1341.

Peek, C. J., & the National Integration Academy Council. (2013). *Lexicon for behavioral health and primary care integration: Concepts and definitions developed by expert consensus* (AHRQ Publication No. 13- IP001-EF). Rockville, MD: Agency for Healthcare Research and Quality. Retrieved from http://integrationacademy.ahrq.gov/sites/default/files/ Lexicon.pdf

Pieterse, A. L., Evans, S. A., Risner-Butner, A., Collins, N. M., & Mason, L. B. (2009). Multicultural competence and social justice training in counseling psychology and counselor education. *The Counseling Psychologist, 37*(1), 93–115.

Reavell, J., & Fazil, Q. (2016). The epidemiology of PTSD and depression in refugee minors who have resettled in developed countries. *Journal of Mental Health, 26*, 74–83.

Rohlof, H. G., Knipscheer, J. W., & Kleber, R. J. (2014). Somatization in refugees: A review. *Social Psychiatry and Psychiatric Epidemiology, 49*, 1793–1804.

Ryan, K. (2018, March 27). U.S. policy leads to "astounding" drop in number of refugees in KC, pulls families apart. *Kansas City Star*. Retrieved from https://www.kansascity.com/news/politics-government/article206632989.html

Sack, W. H. (1998). Multiple forms of stress in refugee and immigrant children. *Child and Adolescent Psychiatric Clinics of North America, 7*, 153–167.

Saltzman, W. R., Layne, C. M., Steinberg, A. M., Arslanagic, B., & Pynoos, R. S. (2003). Developing a culturally and ecologically sound intervention program for youth exposed to war and terrorism. *Child and Adolescent Psychiatric Clinics of North America, 12*, 319–342.

Schauer, M., Neuner, F., & Elbert, T. (2011). *Narrative exposure therapy: A short-term treatment for traumatic stress disorders* (2nd ed.). Cambridge, MA: Hogrefe.

Schubert, S. J., Lee, C. W., de Araujo, G., Butler, S. R., & Taylor, G. (2016). The effectiveness of eye movement desensitization and reprocessing therapy to treat symptoms following trauma in Timor Leste. *Journal of Traumatic Stress, 29*, 141–148.

Schweitzer, R., Greenslade, J., & Kagee, A. (2007). Coping and resilience in refugees from the Sudan: A narrative account. *Australian & New Zealand Journal of Psychiatry, 41*, 282–288.

Schweitzer, R., Melville, F., Steel, Z., & Lacherez, P. (2006). Trauma, post-migration living difficulties, and social support as predictors of psychological adjustment in resettled Sudanese refugees. *Australian and New Zealand Journal of Psychiatry, 40*, 179–187.

Snodgrass, J. G., Most, D. E., & Upadhyay, C. (2017). Religious ritual is good medicine for indigenous Indian conservation refugees. *Current Anthropology, 58*(2), 257–274.

Steel, Z., Chey, T., Silove, D., Marnane, C., Bryant, R. A., & Van Ommeren, M. (2009). Association of torture and other potentially traumatic events with mental health outcomes among populations exposed to mass conflict and displacement. *Journal of the American Medical Association, 302*, 537–549.

Stepakoff, S., Hubbard, J., Katoh, M., Falk, E., Mikulu, J. B., Nkhoma, P., & Omagwa, Y. (2006). Trauma healing in refugee camps in Guinea: a psychosocial program for Liberian and Sierra Leonean survivors of torture and war. *American Psychologist, 61*, 921–932.

Thompson, C. T., Vidgen, A., & Roberts, N. P. (2018). Psychological interventions for post-traumatic stress disorder in refugees and asylum seekers: A systematic review and meta-analysis. *Clinical Psychology Review, 63*, 66–79.

UNHCR. (2001). *The 1951 Convention relating to the status of refugees and its 1967 protocol.* Geneva, Switzerland: UNHCR.

UNHCR. (2016). Information on UNHCR Resettlement. Retrieved from http://www.unhcr.org/en-us/information-on-unhcr-resettlement.html

UNHCR. (2018, October 21). *Figure at a glance: Statistical yearbooks.* Retrieved from http://www.unhcr.org/en-us/figures-at-a-glance.html

UNHCR. (2018). *The Refugee Convention (1951).* Retrieved from https://www.unhcr.org/4ca34be29.pdf

U.S. Department of State (2018, October 22). The reception and placement program. Retrieved from https://www.state.gov/j/prm/ra/receptionplacement/index.htm

Vang, C. Y., & Trieu, M. M. (2014). *Invisible newcomers: Refugees from Burma/Myanmar and Bhutan in the United States.* Washington, DC: Asian & Pacific Islander American Scholarship Fund & Association for Asian American Studies.

Vrana, S. R., Campbell, T. A., & Clay, R. (2013). Survey of national consortium of torture treatment program therapies about the assessment, diagnosis, and treatment of the psychological sequelae of torture. *Traumatology, 19*, 144–153.

Warr, S. (2010). Counselling refugee young people: An exploration of therapeutic approaches. *Pastoral Care in Education, 28*, 269–282.

Zayfert, C. (2008). Culturally competent treatment of posttraumatic stress disorder in clinical practice: An ideographic, transcultural approach. *Clinical Psychology: Science and Practice, 15*, 68–73.

9

Bringing Psychotherapy to Immigrants

Hamid Mirsalimi

Immigration has been a life-defining experience in the lives of millions of individuals, couples, and families. This chapter focuses primarily on challenges and strategies in bringing psychotherapy to immigrant populations in the United States, although many of the problems and barriers are likely to be experienced by immigrants to other countries as well. Information presented here is informed by both the cited literature and my experience of providing psychotherapy to hundreds of immigrant individuals, couples, and families; examples of such experiences are presented in this chapter and have been modified and individuals de-identified to maintain confidentiality. This chapter does not focus on refugee issues since that topic is the focus of Chapter 8.

It is important to note at the outset that there is tremendous diversity among immigrants, and one cannot refer to "immigrants" as if they are a singular group. Not only do immigrants have various countries of origin, but there is a great deal of within-group variability even among immigrants with the same national origin. Diversity in levels of education, socioeconomic status, acculturation, and enculturation (Jackson, 2003), as well as social and political points of view, are some of the variables that contribute to within-group variability in immigrant communities.

The Scope and Description of the Problem

According to the 2010 U.S. Census, there are about 39.9 million foreign-born individuals in the United States (U.S. Census Bureau, 2011); the great majority of that population is estimated to be immigrants (American Psychological Association [APA], 2012). Not only do immigrants face the tremendous stress of immigration and adjustment challenges to the new country, but "across the nation, immigrants have become the subject of negative media coverage (Massey & Sánchez, 2010; Suárez-Orozco, Louie, & Suro, 2011), hate crimes (Leadership Conference on Civil Rights Education Fund, 2009), and exclusionary political legislation (Carter, Lawrence, & Morse, 2011)" (APA, 2012, p. 3). Given the above, it is clear that immigrants are likely to have unique mental health challenges and treatment needs. At times the challenges are profound and many treatment needs are not sufficiently addressed, making the community of immigrants an underserved community as a whole.

To guide our discussion of unmet mental health treatment needs of immigrant communities, it is useful to consider Bronfenbrenner's ecological systems theory (Bronfenbrenner, 1986). Bronfenbrenner argued that to understand the individual, one needs to understand the ecological system within which the individual operates. Bronfenbrenner proposed five interrelated systems that impact the individual: (a) microsystem, which includes the individual, family, school, peers, and work; (b) mesosystem, which is the connecting, interfacing system between various microsystems (i.e., interacting influences of the individual, family, school, and work; e.g., what happens at home can influence school performance of a child and vice versa); (c) exosystem, which includes the extended family, religious community, social and mental health agencies or practitioners, legal services, government agencies, community health and welfare services, friends of family, and neighbors; (d) macrosystem, which includes cultural attitudes and ideologies, gender, race, ethnicity, region, and class; and (e) chronosystem, which involves sociohistorical circumstances and patterns of environmental events over the life course. Mental health professionals would do well to consider all of the above interrelated systems in order to adequately understand and address mental health needs of immigrants.

A number of issues create barriers to the needs of immigrant communities in receiving adequate psychotherapeutic services. Some of these challenges include language limitations, financial challenges, intimate partner violence (IPV), trust issues, cultural variables regarding disclosure and other issues impacted by acculturation, lack of knowledge about what psychotherapy is and how it can be beneficial, stigma regarding seeking psychotherapy, systemic issues including insurance limitations, fear of involvement with immigration authorities, lack of knowledge about which provider to contact for what purpose, differences in symptom expression, lack of cultural sensitivity or knowledge on the part of providers, lack of adequate literature and research regarding therapeutic needs of various immigrant communities, and limitations posed by state licensure agencies. These issues will be discussed in more detail next.

Barriers to Service Delivery

Language Barriers

A major barrier in providing psychotherapy to immigrants is language limitations (Kim et al., 2011). Psychotherapy, a discipline that relies heavily on communication, is tremendously impacted by communication difficulties. These difficulties may be subtle or profound. Subtle language difficulties may present themselves when a word with two meanings is used in communication. While immigrant patients may be aware of the first meaning, they may not be aware of the second meaning, which can cause miscommunication.

Some immigrants have a limited vocabulary that allows them to appear as if they are speaking somewhat fluently using the limited set of words. The listener, for example the psychotherapist, may assume that because individuals speak English fairly well, their command of vocabulary is much better than is actually the case. The psychotherapist may therefore use more sophisticated language, which may be misunderstood by the immigrant patient.

Many newly arrived adult immigrants rely on their children to communicate with authority figures. Having children translate during a psychotherapy session poses confidentiality and power differential issues that often make it impossible for the adult to benefit from therapeutic services. In addition, issues addressed and information discussed are often inappropriate for the child. The use of a translator also poses confidentiality concerns, particularly since the translator is likely to be a member of the small community of immigrants who speak that language.

Financial Barriers

Psychotherapy tends to be experienced as an expensive therapeutic modality, particularly when individuals do not understand how it can be of use to them. In a study by Kaltman et al. (Kaltman, Hurtado de Mendoza, Gonzales, & Serrano, 2014), cost emerged as the most salient factor, ahead of a preference for a bilingual provider, in trauma-related mental health services among Latina immigrants. Many individuals who immigrate to the United States with limited financial resources tend to live frugally and only spend money on necessities. Psychotherapy is viewed by many immigrants as a luxury they cannot afford. The high cost of psychotherapy becomes even more surprising to newly arrived immigrants who tend to use the exchange rate to understand the true cost of goods and services.

Due to such financial limitations, it is often the case that when immigrants seek psychotherapy for themselves, the issues tend to have lasted longer and the symptoms have become more entrenched. This is often the case both in terms of individual concerns (e.g., depression and anxiety) and marital and family issues. Immigrants are more likely to seek psychotherapy and be open to pay for such services when either there are concerns about their children or there are major marital conflicts.

Insurance Barriers

Given limited financial resources, many immigrants either do not have medical insurance or do not have adequate insurance (Hearst, Ramirez, & Gany, 2010). If immigrants buy insurance, they often buy the least expensive insurance plans, which are essentially only good for catastrophic coverage. Those plans often do not include general psychotherapy benefits, or if they do they provide very limited coverage. Given that many such policies are health maintenance organization (HMO) plans, individuals tend to have a very limited choice of providers. While this is a problem for many sectors of the society, the problem is particularly consequential for immigrants, who may need a provider who understands their background and speaks their language. If such a psychotherapist exists in their community but is not participating in their HMO, they face the choice of either paying privately or not receiving psychotherapy. From time to time an individual whose English is very limited and is persistent may persuade the insurance company to make a single case agreement with a psychotherapist who speaks the language; however, insurance companies tend to be very resistant to allowing such single case agreements. In those rare cases that they do, the payment rate, number of sessions allowed, and required paperwork are often prohibitive variables that may discourage the psychotherapist from making the single case agreement. In addition, many immigrants are not aware that such a possibility with their insurance provider may even exist.

IPV Issues

IPV is another barrier to receiving psychotherapeutic services for some immigrants (Reina & Lohman, 2015). Many IPV perpetrators often reject or threaten their spouse if the spouse is interested in receiving psychotherapy for fear of loss of control over the victim. This is likely to be more pronounced in immigrants from male-dominated societies in which women's rights are very limited. While IPV is certainly not limited to immigrant families, its consequences tend to be more harmful due to the limited support available to many immigrants, who may not have any family in the United States. This issue often involves financial difficulties as well since the offending partner often exerts economic control, limiting the ability of the spouse to seek any outside help, including psychotherapy. Depending on their immigration status, IPV victims may be afraid of deportation and hence may be exploited for this very reason. The fact that immigration applications are very typically filed for the entire family, or both spouses, means that if one person is deemed ineligible, the application may be rejected for all family members. In such cases, IPV victims may hesitate to contact the police for fear that if their spouse is arrested, the entire family's chance of receiving permanent resident status and later citizenship may be in jeopardy. Mental health professionals should be aware that documented immigrants who are IPV victims are allowed to self-petition for permanent resident status under the provision of the Violence Against Women Act (VAWA); this will allow them to petition for permanent residency independent of their spouse's application ("Information on the Legal Rights," 2018). Undocumented immigrants who are IPV victims can petition for nonimmigrant status visa through the U.S. Citizenship and Immigration Status Department (USCIS) ("Victims of Criminal Activity," 2018). Immigrant victims of IPV, similar to other victims, should be informed about women's domestic abuse shelters, as well as information about how they can learn about their legal rights. A list of pro bono legal service providers can be found through the U.S. Department of Justice website ("List of Pro Bono Legal Service Providers," 2018).

Cultural Variables Regarding Disclosure Issues

The cultural attitude of many immigrants that what happens in the family stays in the family poses another barrier to immigrants receiving psychotherapy. The idea that an individual, couple, or family would seek the help of a complete stranger, and then disclose the most intimate aspects of their lives, is a notion that is foreign to many immigrants (Chen, Lai, & Yang, 2013; Nguyen & Anderson, 2005). The problem is often exacerbated by the fact that many immigrants who are not aware of our ethical and legal obligations toward confidentiality have a difficult time trusting that their information will be kept confidential.

For many immigrants this is a double-edged sword, since they may not seek psychotherapy from a psychotherapist who does not speak their language (believing that they cannot truly communicate with the psychotherapist) and is not familiar with their cultural background (for the fear that the psychotherapist would not understand cultural issues), but they may also feel resistant to seeing a psychotherapist from their own immigrant community for the fear that the psychotherapist may not maintain confidentiality.

Fear of Involvement with Immigration Authorities

Undocumented immigrants may be harmed by a variety of issues, including sexual and physical violence, labor abuses, and limited employment opportunities (Ramirez & Monk, 2017). A barrier to providing mental health services to undocumented immigrants is the fear that their undocumented status may somehow be disclosed to the authorities; that fear is at times extended to psychotherapists. While mental health professionals may think that such a fear represents a paranoid cognition, it is important to place this issue in the context of what Bronfenbrenner refers to as an exosystemic issue: the legal system within which individuals find themselves. Of course, to a large extent this fear stems from a lack of knowledge about psychotherapy; however, it is not inconceivable that when seeking professional help, immigration status can surface either through electronic medical records, insurance filings, consultation, or other means. Regardless, mental health professionals need to be aware of such fears when working with undocumented immigrants, who may not differentiate them from the rest of a society in which they have experienced prejudice, discrimination, and marginalization. Mental health providers who are not culturally competent should consider that they may be unwittingly engaging in discrimination and marginalization themselves.

Trust Issues Regarding Political Matters

Trust issues can pose a barrier in the providing psychotherapy to immigrant communities (Sandhu et al., 2013). Many immigrants come from backgrounds of political oppression and persecution within a dictatorial political system. Growing up in such an environment, individuals learn to self-censor, abstaining from disclosing their true thoughts and feelings. Psychotherapy requires engagement in the opposite behavior since we expect our patients to talk about their struggles. Mental health professionals need to be aware that whether immigrant patients are consciously aware of this tendency toward not trusting and not disclosing, or if they are holding such attitudes unconsciously, creating an effective therapeutic alliance will require more effort and patience.

Lack of Knowledge About Psychotherapy

One of the major barriers to providing psychotherapy to immigrant populations is their lack of knowledge about psychotherapy, how it works, and how it can be beneficial. Such attitudes are impacted by the level of acculturation and acculturative stress (Rogers-Sirin, 2013). Many immigrants come from collectivistic backgrounds in which seeking support from family and community elders is the norm. As previously mentioned, individual psychotherapy, which involves seeking support and guidance from a stranger, is often counter to cultural norms. In addition, the notion that through psychotherapy people can learn about their options, explore unconscious motives, and arrive at personally derived decisions is often strange to many individuals who have not been exposed to psychotherapy. Many immigrants expect that if they have sought the help of a doctor, they will be told what to do within one or two visits; hence, the idea that psychotherapy is a longer-term process is often viewed as unusual and ineffective. These issues have been exacerbated by radio and television shows in which a mental health professional provides a quick recommendation to resolve the caller's problems. Such shows have made it seem as if psychotherapy involves a very quick diagnosis of the problem and a few suggestions to resolve it.

Stigma About Psychotherapy

Unfortunately, stigma related to receiving psychotherapy continues to exist and presents another barrier for immigrants receiving psychotherapeutic services (Kung, 2016). Many immigrants, particularly those who grew up in developing countries, believe that only patients with severe and persistent mental illness need mental health (including psychotherapeutic) services. Hence, they are concerned that if they seek psychotherapy, they will be labeled as mentally ill. Fear of losing the family's honor presents another barrier. For example, some Arab women worry that if the community finds out they are receiving mental health services, it may damage their marital prospects, increase the likelihood of divorce, or be used as leverage for their husbands to obtain a second wife (Al-Krenawi & Graham, 2000). Hence, stigma about psychotherapy is one of the reasons why, by the time some immigrants seek psychotherapy, their problems are more severe and entrenched.

Lack of Knowledge About Provider Types

People often take their knowledge of when to contact what type of provider for granted, but such knowledge is not always common among many immigrants who are unfamiliar with the host country's health care system. As is the case for much of the population, the provider most immigrants seek for mental health treatment is the primary care physician. It is often concerning to find out that a primary care physician has prescribed medication for the mental health concerns of an immigrant whose suffering is due to immigration and other contextual issues in need of psychotherapy. A newly arrived European immigrant woman with limited English contacted me recently stating that school officials had complained about the acting-out behavior of her nine-year-old son. She reported that the boy, whose English is also very limited, had not displayed behavior problems up to that point. The school officials suggested that he might have attention-deficit disorder/hyperactivity (ADHD). Unclear about what to do next, and assuming that ADHD is a neurological problem, she had contacted a neurologist, who had prescribed a stimulant medication. This individual was dismayed at the very brief assessment, which essentially involved answering a few questions about her child's behavior. Concerned about putting her nine-year-old son on medication, she had refused to give him the medication without further assessment. She was very happy to learn that there are psychologists who do ADHD assessments. She took her son for testing; the results confirmed that the issues were language and contextually based and had a lot to do with the stress of immigration. It is very important for mental health professionals to be aware of this lack of knowledge on the part of many immigrants about when to seek what provider type and what their options are. Educating the immigrant about the options is a very important step.

Differences in Symptom Expressions Across Cultures

Some mental health problems manifest in different symptoms across cultures (Helman, 2007). For example, in many Asian and Middle Eastern cultures depression is initially expressed in terms of physical aches and pains. Some immigrants who feel shame about having mental health problems downplay their symptoms and have found other explanations for them that are not mental health related (e.g., "I am not depressed, I just need to work less and sleep more; but I have to work long hours to provide for my family"). Psychotherapists would do well not to accept these initial explanations and should explore symptoms in more detail and depth.

Lack of Cultural Sensitivity on the Part of the Psychotherapist

Given all the aforementioned barriers, it is a big step when an immigrant seeks out and enters psychotherapy; hence, one of the most unfortunate situations is when, due to lack of cultural sensitivity of the psychotherapist (Hook, Davis, Owen, Worthington, & Utsey, 2013), the immigrant is alienated by psychotherapy itself. This is often the case when well-meaning providers make suggestions and recommendations that are contrary to the patient's cultural norms. For example, a number of female Middle Eastern immigrants have shared with me that a previous psychotherapist repeatedly urged them to divorce their husbands. Given that divorce has very negative cultural, economic, and social consequences in Middle Eastern societies, and divorcing is seriously frowned upon, it is often not seen as a viable option except in the most extreme of circumstances. Hence, a psychotherapist who insists that divorce is the only way to proceed, and may be critical of the patient for not choosing that option, not only is taking choice away from the patient but also is missing a critical cultural understanding. Under such circumstances patients often terminate treatment prematurely, missing out on badly needed mental health services.

Another example of a barrier to starting or continuing psychotherapy caused by a lack of cultural sensitivity is failing to recognize within-group diversity in immigrant populations. Some immigrants are savvy consumers of psychotherapy while others are not; some are quite affluent while others are not; some are quite educated while others are not; and some are quite liberal while others are not. Many immigrants have experienced prejudice and have been stereotyped. The fear that a provider may be stereotyping them or may be prejudiced against them is a tremendous barrier to seeking treatment. For example, a number of Middle Eastern immigrant men have expressed sadness and disbelief to me that simply by virtue of the fact that they are Middle Eastern men, a mental health provider assumed they were controlling husbands. Consciously or unconsciously holding such stereotypes is a sure way of damaging the therapeutic alliance with immigrant patients.

Lack of Adequate Literature and Research

Another barrier in providing psychotherapy to immigrants is the lack of adequate literature and research regarding the needs of various immigrant populations. Accurate literature and research are necessary to facilitate knowledge and cultural sensitivity. While there is an increasing availability of multicultural guidelines for mental health professionals (APA, 2017), empirically supported research leading to treatment recommendations is sparse.

Limitations Posed by State Licensure Boards

Another barrier for immigrants to receive psychotherapy is created by state licensing boards. Currently in the United States mental health professionals are only allowed to practice within the state in which they are licensed. As long as there are a sufficient number of mental health professionals in every state, this may not be an issue; however, at times there are few or no mental health professionals who are from a particular cultural and language background in a particular state. While patients may have access to a psychotherapist with a similar language and cultural background in another state, they cannot utilize the services of that professional due to licensing restrictions that prevent psychotherapists from providing tele-mental health services across state lines. The Association of State and Provincial Psychology Boards is making efforts toward interjurisdictional practice of psychology, but until their efforts come to fruition, this barrier continues to prevent many immigrants from receiving needed help.

Creating Cultural Competency

Suggestions regarding creating cultural competency in working with immigrant populations are often based on models developed for ethnic minorities. Hence, further literature and research into specific cultural competencies in working with immigrants is needed. Several pieces of literature are helpful as a starting point in that effort. *Crossroads: The Psychology of Immigration in the New Century* (APA, 2012), Pamela Hays's ADDRESSING model (Hays, 2016), and *Multicultural Guidelines: An Ecological Approach to Context, Identity, and Intersectionality* (APA, 2017) are three useful documents to consider. *Crossroads* (APA, 2012) will be referenced in the following pages. Hays's ADDRESSING model highlights the importance of considering age and generational influences, developmental disabilities, disability acquired later in life, religion and spiritual orientation, ethnicity/race identity, socioeconomic status, sexual orientation, indigenous heritage, national origin, and gender when working with individuals from diverse backgrounds. *Multicultural Guidelines* (APA, 2017) will be discussed in some detail next.

Multicultural Guidelines (APA, 2017), which incorporate Bronfenbrenner's ecological systems model (1986), were developed to provide a framework for the provision of multiculturally competent services, including practice, research, consultation, and education. The multicultural guidelines discuss a five-layered ecological model as well as 10 specific guidelines. The five layers of the model are:

Level 1: Bidirectional model of self-definition and relationships
Level 2: Community, school, and family context
Level 3: Institutional impact on engagement
Level 4: Domestic and international climate
Level 5: Outcomes.

The 10 guidelines, and their specific relevance to immigrants, will be discussed next. While they specifically reference psychologists, they could easily apply to all mental health professionals.

Guideline 1

> Psychologists seek to recognize and understand that identity and self-definition are fluid and complex and that the interaction between the two is dynamic. To this end, psychologists appreciate that intersectionality is shaped by the multiplicity of the individual's social context. (APA, 2017, p. 16)

The fluidity of identity and self-definition is particularly relevant to immigrants since acculturation, which influences identity and self-definition, is a continuous, evolving, and dynamic process. While challenges to identity and self-definition are much more intense for newly arrived immigrants, they continue to impact future generations of immigrants since they are multigenerational processes. For example, while recently arrived Hispanic immigrants are likely to experience many identity and self-definition challenges, their children and grandchildren still need to come to terms with their minority status, being the subject of stereotypes and prejudices that go along with belonging to a minority group, and family cultures that are different from that of the majority. Even grandchildren are likely to be impacted. Hispanic immigrants are at times frustrated because many people automatically assume that they, or their parents or grandparents, must have been undocumented immigrants and, therefore, are viewed by some as less of an American. Similarly, in the current political climate, even native-born children of Iraqi, Syrian, Afghani, and Iranian parents have to come to terms with their identity as the children of immigrants against whom there is a tremendous degree of prejudice (Khanlou, Koh, & Mill, 2008).

The theoretical framework on trauma proposed by Janoff-Bulman (1992) is a useful tool in understanding the experience of many immigrants. It is important to preface this by saying that many immigrants show a great deal of resilience and are not traumatized by the immigration process; regardless, the experience of immigrating is quite stressful, albeit not always traumatic. Janoff-Bulman defines trauma as an experience that involves the shattering of previously held assumptions. She focuses on three assumptions in particular: The world is benevolent, the world is meaningful, and the self is worthwhile. All three of these assumptions can be challenged through the process of immigration. For example, many immigrants face prejudice and discrimination for the first time in their lives after arriving to the host country. Hence, an experience that was previously unknown to them becomes a challenge with which they have to contend. Experiences of discrimination and prejudice often undermine an individual's self-definition and self-esteem. These experiences are particularly impactful when they are not overt; that is, in the absence of knowing that someone is prejudiced against them, immigrants are often impacted by an unconscious experience of somehow being flawed and less than others. Because ethnic minority families are likely to be aware of such prejudices, they may prepare their children for such experiences. That is not the case for newly arrived immigrants, who do not expect to be stereotyped and prejudiced. Such experiences challenge not only the sense of self-worth but also the other assumptions of benevolence and meaningfulness of the world.

Guideline 2

> Psychologists aspire to recognize and understand that as cultural beings, they hold attitudes and beliefs that can influence their perceptions of and interactions with others as well as their clinical and empirical conceptualizations. As such, psychologists strive to move beyond conceptualizations rooted in categorical assumptions, biases, and/or formulations based on limited knowledge about individuals and communities. (APA, 2017, p. 26)

We all hold beliefs about people from various backgrounds. Developing cultural competency involves the recognition of and attention to this fact as opposed to the belief that we are somehow immune to such cultural influences. Soon after agreeing to provide psychotherapy to an immigrant, it is important to sit back and reflect on what might be our preconceived notions about an individual from that background. Further reflecting on where our prejudicial and stereotyping beliefs may be coming from, and keeping in mind that there is tremendous within-group diversity among any category of people, are important steps toward guarding against harmful stereotyping. In addition, psychotherapists need to recognize that such efforts toward self-awareness need to be ongoing while we provide treatment to the immigrant client.

Guideline 3

> Psychologists strive to recognize and understand the role of language and communication through engagement that is sensitive to the lived experience of the individual, couple, family, group, community, and/or organizations with whom they interact. Psychologists also seek to understand how they bring their own language and communication to these interactions. (APA, 2017, p. 34)

An example that illustrates this point is the type of communication needed in working with some immigrant families. As members of the more egalitarian culture of the United States, mental health professionals tend to value direct and honest communication, and are likely to promote such a communication approach in their psychotherapy practices. However, many people from different cultural backgrounds, particularly those from collectivistic societies, do not share the value of direct communication. A degree of deference toward elders and authority figures is expected in many such societies. Psychotherapists may conceptualize that the inability of family members to express their thoughts and feelings directly to each other is at the heart of the presenting problem; hence, they may decide to teach family members to talk more directly to one another. While the intention of such an intervention is good, it may alienate elders, who will take offense if they are spoken to and confronted very honestly and directly by family members. Hence, the effort to teach more direct and honest communication needs to be balanced by an effort not to lose therapeutic alliance with elders and other authority figures in the family. That is not to say that direct communication should never be promoted; rather, such an effort should be slowly and respectfully made. Also, directly disagreeing or confronting parents in front of their children may be viewed as disrespectful and undermining their authority; such disagreements and confrontations may need to be made in individual sessions instead.

In addition to the above, psychotherapists should be aware that they may lose rapport if they, themselves, engage in direct communication with the immigrant. To guard against losing rapport, particular attention needs to be paid to issues of respect, allowing the client to "save face," and providing alternatives rather than being too critical of how an immigrant believes, feels, or behaves. There are of course times (e.g., child or spousal abuse) that a very direct confrontation is necessary. In deciding when to be confrontational and when to temper the approach, it is important to keep in mind that the loss of therapeutic alliance is likely to result in premature termination, which can be very harmful to the individual immigrant, the couple, or the bigger system.

Guideline 4

> Psychologists endeavor to be aware of the role of the social and physical environment in the lives of clients, students, research participants, and/or consultees. (APA, 2017, p. 40)

The resources available in the environment provide tools that individuals use to build their lives. In communities where financial, educational, and environmental resources are scarce, coping and building lives become more challenging than in communities that enjoy better resources (APA, 2017). Many immigrants live in communities in which resources are more limited. Psychotherapists should familiarize themselves with such lack of resources and factor such issues into their formulation and treatment planning. An example of such an issue is the struggle of an immigrant woman who does not have any help with childcare or may not have the bus fare to attend psychotherapy sessions and may be too embarrassed to disclose such information. Lack of knowledge about why the patient has missed sessions may lead to formulating such a patient's behavior as resistance to therapy, which is clearly a mistake. Hence, psychotherapists should familiarize themselves with social, economic, and other contextual/environmental challenges in the lives of their immigrant patients in order to provide more effective therapy.

Guideline 5

> Psychologists aspire to recognize and understand historical and contemporary experiences with power, privilege, and oppression. As such, they seek to address institutional barriers and related inequities, disproportionalities, and disparities of law enforcement, administration of criminal justice, educational, mental health, and other systems as they seek to promote justice, human rights, and access to quality and equitable mental and behavioral health services. (APA, 2017, p. 45)

The issue of human rights, particularly as it pertains to Latin American undocumented immigrants, has received a great deal of attention in recent years. Efforts by the current administration to separate children from their parents at the U.S. southern border and potentially deporting DACA (Deferred Action for Childhood Arrivals) recipients, and speaking negatively about immigrants as if the majority of them are criminals, have had a chilling effect in the lives of many immigrants. The impact of those policies and the rhetoric of administration officials have not been limited to South American immigrants, as all immigrant populations have been affected; many immigrants feel they are looked down upon and marginalized. Hence, those measures are likely to have a direct effect on the mental health of immigrant populations. For example, consider potential mental health challenges that U.S.-born school-aged children whose parents are undocumented face every time they go to school: the anxiety that their parents may be arrested and deported by the time they return home can lead to a state of constant distress (Blitzer, 2017). Also, imagine the level of distress that undocumented children have to endure every time they go to school and worry that they themselves may be arrested and deported by Immigration and Customs Enforcement (ICE) officers who may arrest them at school (Green,

2018). Psychotherapists can engage in political advocacy efforts in order to influence policies that undermine the mental health of immigrant populations. Mental health professionals can also encourage and provide consultation to schools to engage in a set of welcoming, anxiety-reducing efforts for their immigrant students (Center for Applied Linguistics, 2018); they can also provide pro bono services for immigrant families, or engage in outreach activities in immigrant communities. Inside the therapy office, psychotherapists can provide immigrant patients with information about legal services (including free legal aid), work with debilitating anxiety that patients may be experiencing, promote better coping strategies, and provide understanding and caring about feelings of worry, helplessness, and hopelessness by being a witness to their suffering.

Guideline 6

> Psychologists seek to promote culturally adaptive interventions and advocacy within and across systems, including prevention, early intervention, and recovery. (APA, 2017, p. 60)

The effectiveness of psychotherapeutic interventions is profoundly impacted by considering what approach works for whom (Roth & Fonagy, 2005). That is also true in providing psychotherapy to immigrant populations. Many immigrants prefer a more directive therapeutic approach than an indirect approach. In addition, many immigrants who are unfamiliar with psychotherapy can benefit from outreach and psychoeducation.

Guideline 7

> Psychologists endeavor to examine the profession's assumptions and practices within an international context, whether domestically or internationally based, and consider how this globalization has an impact on the psychologist's self-definition, purpose, role, and function. (APA, 2017, p. 65)

As the report suggests:

> [W]ith regard to understanding psychological processes and behaviors, it is important for psychologists to seek to understand that individualism, self-reliance, self-efficacy, self-actualization, and self-care do not connote the only model in which human development and positive functioning can occur. In

> many cultures, self-psychology and group and interpersonal processes are interpreted differently (Roland, 2006). (APA, 2017, p. 71)

Consider the theory of codependence (Weinhold & Weinhold, 2008). While codependence in its extreme form is problematic regardless of the cultural background, in its less extreme forms it is far more normative in collectivistic societies than in individualistic ones (Inclan & Hernandez, 1992). For example, in collectivistic societies a lot more emphasis is placed on the needs of the group than those of the individual, as opposed to more individualistic societies in which the rights of the individual are considered more important than the needs of the group. Hence, what is considered codependent in individualistic societies is often viewed as normative interdependence in collectivistic cultures (Kwon, 2001). Awareness of our biases and roots of our assumptions about what tendencies are pathological, and what psychotherapeutic approaches are helpful, is an important step toward developing cultural competency.

Guideline 8

> Psychologists seek awareness and understanding of how developmental stages and life transitions intersect with the larger biosociocultural context, how identity evolves as a function of such intersections, and how these different socialization and maturation experiences influence worldview and identity. (APA, 2017, p. 76)

Our understanding of developmental stages and life cycle transitions is a product of our cultural contexts. For example, while it is normative for the majority of American teens to leave home around the age of 18 (particularly as they go away to college), such a practice is not typical for recent Muslim immigrant teens, in whose cultures it is normative to stay in the parental home until marriage. In fact, it has been argued that the whole concept of "teen" is culturally constructed (Lesko, 2012). The intersection of immigrant parents' cultural beliefs and typical life cycle transitions in the United States around the age of 18 may cause a great deal of family turmoil due to differential rates of acculturation between parents and their children. Another example of a multigenerational conflict within a family due to differential rates of acculturation is co-sleeping habits of children with their parents. Owens (2004) discussed cross-cultural differences in sleep behaviors in children. She reported that while the prevalence of regular bed sharing of parents and their children in urban mainland China was as high as 55.8%, that rate among Americans is only 15%. Consider a Chinese family who immigrates to the United States. Parents and their children may not experience much family conflict until their children have children of their own. Differences of opinion between parents and their adult children regarding co-sleeping practices may emerge; such conflicts point to differential rates of acculturation that only manifest during life cycle transitions. Mental health professionals need to recognize such cross-cultural differences and guard against formulating differences as pathologies. Only by understanding multiple cultural frameworks can therapists help families navigate these multicultural and cross-generational differences.

Guideline 9

> Psychologists strive to conduct culturally appropriate and informed research, teaching, supervision, consultation, assessment, interpretation, diagnosis, dissemination, and evaluation of efficacy as they address the first four levels of the *Layered Ecological Model of the Multicultural Guidelines.* (APA, 2017, p. 83)

Although a course in diversity is a part of the curriculum of many psychology graduate programs, it is rare to see a course offering in the psychology of immigrants and immigration. Such a course, or at least inclusion of psychology of immigrants and immigration in general diversity courses, would be very beneficial in the training of future psychotherapists and psychotherapy supervisors. Such a course could cover the need for multiple frameworks in our understanding of reality, postmodern philosophy and its application to psychology, as well as cultural influences of what is considered healthy versus pathological.

Likewise, psychotherapy outcome research that is designed, conducted, analyzed, interpreted, and reported with cultural sensitivity toward specific immigrant populations is needed to shed light on how immigrant patients can best be understood and helped. Such research can be fascinating and complicated by multigenerational differences within immigrant families and communities. The development of culturally sensitive questionnaires and other assessment tools would help in accurate diagnosis and treatment planning for immigrant patients.

Guideline 10

> Psychologists actively strive to take a strength-based approach when working with individuals, families, groups, communities,

> and organizations that seek to build resilience and decrease trauma within the sociocultural context. (APA, 2017, p. 88)

Why do different cultures have differing belief systems and practices? Among a variety of answers that need to be considered, one is that the belief system and practice have been adaptive for that society. That is an important realization because it helps us to guard against pathologizing belief systems of immigrants that are different from ours. When faced with such differences, psychotherapists would benefit from considering what may be adaptive in the differing cultural perspective, and how, within the context of the immigrant's background, such beliefs may help with resiliency. Of course, immigrants still have to adapt to the cultures and practices of their host countries, but psychotherapists can help their patients recognize that the issue at hand is often not what is correct and what is incorrect when it comes to cultural differences, but what is adaptive and what is not adaptive given the new environment.

Effective Strategies and Empirically-Supported Treatments

There is unfortunately a dearth of information regarding empirically supported treatments in working with immigrant populations. What is available is often an application of previously established empirically supported treatment research with suggestions for their adaptation in the treatment of various immigrant groups, or extending what is empirically known about ethnic minorities to immigrant populations. For example, Domenech Rodríguez, Baumann, and Schwartz (2011) have proposed a cultural adaption of Parent Management Training—Oregon Model (Forgatch & Patterson, 2010) for Spanish-speaking Latino parents. Similarly, Hurwich-Reiss et al. (Hurwich-Reiss, Rindlaub, Wadsworth, and Markman, 2014) have proposed a cultural adaptation of a family-strengthening intervention for low-income Spanish-speaking families. And Pearl (2008) has described the application of the Parent–Child Interaction Therapy (Herschell, Calzada, Eyberg, & McNeil, 2002) to the treatment of a single Arab-American family exposed to domestic violence. Each of these represent suggestions for the application of previously established empirically supported treatments to new groups, as opposed to empirically supported interventions that are specifically developed with the culture of the particular group in mind. Since such adaptations represent the state of the majority of our cross-cultural interventions at this time, it is important to at least make the adaptations in the most accurate and culturally sensitive way possible.

A promising model of culturally adapting evidence-based practices to immigrant families and ethnic minorities has been proposed by Hwang (2016).

The model, which was initially proposed for working with Asian Americans (Hwang, 2006) and then expanded to other immigrant and ethnic minority groups, has two components. Hwang describes the first component, psychotherapy adaptation and modification framework (PAMF; Hwang, 2006), as a top-down and theory-driven psychotherapy adaptation of already established theories and evidence-based, empirically supported treatment approaches. The second component of Hwang's model, formative method for adapting psychotherapy (FMAP; Hwang, 2009) is described as a bottom-up community-based adaptation.

PAMF consists of six domains to which psychotherapists should pay attention (Hwang, 2006):

1. Dynamic issues and cultural complexities (e.g., address clients' multiple identities)
2. Orientation (e.g., orient client to therapy)
3. Cultural beliefs (e.g., integrate cultural strengths and healing practices into treatment)
4. Client–therapist relationship (e.g., join the client by inquiring into family background and migration history)
5. Cultural differences in expressing and communication (e.g., understand ethnic differences in expression of distress)
6. Cultural issues of salience (e.g., be aware of shame and stigma).

FMAP (Hwang, 2009) consists of five phases:

1. Generating knowledge and collaborating with stakeholders (e.g., attending to when to individualize, when to generalize, and when to consider culture)
2. Integrating generated information with theory and empirical and clinical knowledge (e.g., ensuring that cultural adaptations are grounded in cultural belief systems)
3. Reviewing culturally adapted clinical interventions by stakeholders and future revisions (e.g., conduct focus groups to assess the impression of community-based immigrants regarding the interventions)
4. Testing the culturally adapted intervention
5. Synthesizing stakeholder feedback and finalizing the culturally adapted intervention.

As previously stated, although the focus of Hwang's research has been on cultural adaptations of theory, research, and practice for Asian Americans, the approach and recommendations are general enough to apply to a variety of immigrant and ethnic minority populations. The tables provided in Hwang's 2006 and 2009 articles provide very useful summaries of the models.

Future Steps

Given the tremendous variety of immigrants' backgrounds, and the dearth of literature and research, there is much work to be done. As previously mentioned, the great majority of empirically supported treatment models for immigrants are adaptations of already established empirically supported treatments that are based on research on the non-immigrant population. While that approach is a good first step, it is not sufficient. Hwang (2016) has argued that the field needs to make a shift from what Resnicow, Baranowski, Ahluwalia, and Braithwaite (1999) referred to as surface structure adaptions to deep structure adaptions. Examples of surface-level adaptions are providing ethnically matched psychotherapies, conducting psychotherapy in the client's language, and locating clinics in areas accessible to immigrant groups. Examples of deep structure adaptions include incorporating beliefs and values of the culture into psychotherapy; understanding how immigrants perceive the cause, course, and treatment of mental illnesses; and incorporating the influence of religious beliefs and traditional family structures and dynamics into psychotherapy. More specifically, deep structure adaptations include developing psychotherapeutic approaches that attend to issues of communalism, respect for elders, beliefs about connections to ancestors and history, and a focus on intuition and experience as opposed to empiricism (Resnicow et al., 1999). Hwang asserts that "deep structure adaptations are much more difficult to understand, conceptualize, and implement" (Hwang, 2016, p. 290). In fact, these deep structure adaptations are what need to be considered, conceptualized, explored, researched, taught, and implemented in our future work with immigrant populations.

Beyond adaptation, psychotherapy research needs to focus on models that are developed for specific immigrant populations. For example, it is one approach to use prolonged exposure to treat post-traumatic stress disorder in immigrants from war-ravaged countries, and an entirely different approach to research and create a therapeutic model that is based on existential struggles related to war trauma (see Chapter 8) for that particular group of immigrants.

Finally, it is important to consider Maslow's hierarchy of needs as it pertains to the mental health needs of immigrants. When basic physiological needs (for food, water, warmth, and rest) and safety needs (for safety, security, and shelter) are not met, it is not likely (except in severe cases) that the immigrant would seek psychotherapy. The current zeitgeist of negative attitudes toward immigrants, and the political uncertainty faced by many of them, has created an atmosphere in which one of the most effective interventions by psychotherapists to help immigrant mental health is to engage in political advocacy on their behalf. Such efforts help immigrant populations to experience a sense of hope, safety, and security, which in turn can pave the way for implementation of effective psychotherapeutic interventions. Actively and visibly engaging with immigrant communities through political advocacy efforts would help immigrants perceive psychotherapists as supporters, advocates, and resources in their lives. In addition, a systems approach with a team of psychologists, psychiatrists, primary care physicians, social workers, volunteers, charities, businesses, teachers, and schools, working together to facilitate the transition of immigrants, is needed in order to address their multitudes of needs and promote better mental health in immigrant communities.

References

Al-Krenawi A., & Graham, J. R. (2000). Culturally sensitive social work practice with Arab clients in mental health settings. *Health & Social Work, 25*(1), 9–22.

American Psychological Association. (2012). *Crossroads: The psychology of immigration in the new century*. Report of the APA Presidential Task Force on Immigration. Retrieved from http://www.apa.org/topics/immigration/immigration-report.pdf

American Psychological Association. (2017). *Multicultural guidelines: An ecological approach to context, identity, and intersectionality*. Retrieved from http://www.apa.org/about/policy/multicultural-guidelines.pdf

Blitzer, J. (2017, March 23). After an immigration raid, a city's students vanish. *New Yorker*. Retrieved from https://www.newyorker.com/news/news-desk/after-an-immigration-raid-a-citys-students-vanish

Bronfenbrenner, U. (1986). Ecology of the family as a context for human development. *American Psychologist, 32*, 513–531.

Carter, A., Lawrence, M., & Morse, A. (2011). 2011 Immigration related laws, bills, and resolutions in the states: Jan. 1–March 31, 2011. Washington, DC: National Conference of State Legislatures. Retrieved from http://www.ncsl.org/research/immigration/immigration-laws-and-bills-spring-2011.aspx

Center for Applied Linguistics. (2018, October 17). Promoting a culture of welcome for refugees in schools: Approaches and opportunities. Retrieved from http://www.welcomingrefugees.org/sites/default/files/documents/resources/Welcoming%20Schools%20PPT.pdf

Chen, F., Lai, G. Y., & Yang, L. (2013). Mental illness disclosure in Chinese immigrant communities. *Journal of Counseling Psychology, 60*(3), 379–391.

Domenech Rodríguez, M. M., Baumann, A. A., & Schwartz, A. L. (2011). Cultural adaptation of an evidence based intervention: From theory to practice in a Latino/a community context. *American Journal of Community Psychology, 47*(1/2), 170–186.

Forgatch, M. S., & Patterson, G. R. (2010). The Oregon model of parent management training (PMTO): An intervention for antisocial behavior in children and adolescents. In J. Weisz & A. Kazdin (Eds.), *Evidence-based psychotherapies for children and adolescents* (2nd ed., pp. 85–102). New York, NY: Guildford Press.

Green, E. L. (2018, May 30). For immigrant students, a new worry: A call to ICE. *New York Times*. Retrieved from https://www.nytimes.com/2018/05/30/us/politics/immigrant-students-deportation.html

Hays, P. A. (2016). *Addressing cultural complexities in practice: Assessment, diagnosis, and therapy*. Washington, DC: American Psychological Association.

Hearst, A., Ramirez, J., & Gany, F. (2010). Barriers and facilitators to public health insurance enrollment in newly arrived immigrant adolescents and young adults in New York State. *Journal of Immigrant & Minority Health, 12*(4), 580–585.

Helman, C. G. (2007). *Culture, health, and illness*. Oxford, UK: Oxford University Press Inc.

Herschell, A., Calzada, E., Eyberg, S. M., & McNeil, C. B. (2002). Parent–child interaction therapy: New directions in research. *Cognitive and Behavioral Practice, 9*, 9–16.

Hook, J. N., Davis, D. E., Owen, J., Worthington, E. J., & Utsey, S. O. (2013). Cultural humility: Measuring openness to culturally diverse clients. *Journal of Counseling Psychology, 60*(3), 353–366.

Hurwich-Reiss, E., Rindlaub, L. A., Wadsworth, M. E., & Markman, H. J. (2014). Cultural adaptation of a family strengthening intervention for low-income Spanish-speaking families. *Journal of Latina/o Psychology, 2*(1), 21–36.

Hwang, W. (2006). The psychotherapy adaptation and modification framework: Application to Asian Americans. *American Psychologist, 61*(7), 702–715.

Hwang, W. (2009). The formative method for adapting psychotherapy (FMAP): A community-based developmental approach to culturally adapting therapy. *Professional Psychology: Research and Practice, 40*(4), 369–377.

Hwang, W. (2016). Culturally adapting evidence-based practices for ethnic minority and immigrant families. In N. Zane, G. Bernal, & F. L. Leong (Eds.), *Evidence-based psychological practice with ethnic minorities: Culturally informed research and clinical strategies* (pp. 289–308). Washington, DC: American Psychological Association.

Inclan, J., & Hernandez, M. (1992). Cross-cultural perspectives and codependence: The case of poor Hispanics. *American Journal of Orthopsychiatry, 62*(2), 245–255.

Information on the legal rights available to immigrant victims of domestic violence in the United States and facts about immigrating on a marriage-based visa fact sheet. (2018, October 12). Retrieved from https://www.uscis.gov/news/fact-sheets/information-legal-rights-available-immigrant-victims-domestic-violence-united-states-and-facts-about-immigrating-marriage-based-visa-fact-sheet

Jackson, Y. (2003). Research in ethnic minority communities: Cultural diversity issues in clinical psychology. In M. C. Roberts & S. S. Ilardi (Eds.), *Handbook of research methods in clinical psychology* (pp. 376–395). Malden, MA: Blackwell Publishing.

Janoff-Bulman, R. (1992). *Shattered assumptions: Towards a new psychology of trauma*. New York, NY: Free Press.

Kaltman, S., Hurtado de Mendoza, A., Gonzales, F. A., & Serrano, A. (2014). Preferences for trauma-related mental health services among Latina immigrants from Central America, South America, and Mexico. *Psychological Trauma: Theory, Research, Practice, and Policy, 6*(1), 83–91.

Khanlou, N., Koh, J. G., & Mill, C. (2008). Cultural identity and experiences of prejudice and discrimination of Afghan and Iranian immigrant youth. *International Journal of Mental Health & Addiction, 6*(4), 494–513.

Kim, G., Loi, C. X., Chiriboga, D. A., Jang, Y., Parmelee, P., & Allen, R. S. (2011). Limited English proficiency as a barrier to mental health service use: A study of Latino and

Asian immigrants with psychiatric disorders. *Journal of Psychiatric Research*, *45*, 104–110. doi:10.1016/j.jpsychires.2010.04.031

Kung, W. W. (2016). Culture- and immigration-related stress faced by Chinese American families with a patient having schizophrenia. *Journal of Marital & Family Therapy*, *42*(3), 409–422.

Kwon, S. (2001). Codependence and interdependence: Cross-cultural reappraisal of boundaries and relationality. *Pastoral Psychology*, *50*(1), 39–52.

Leadership Conference on Civil Rights Education Fund. (2009). Confronting the new faces of hate: Hate crimes in America: 2009. Retrieved from http://www.civilrights.org/publications/ hatecrimes/lccref_hate_crimes_report.pdf

Lesko, N. (2012). *Act your age! A cultural construction of adolescence*. New York, NY: Routledge.

List of pro bono legal service providers. (2018). Retrieved from https://www.justice.gov/eoir/list-pro-bono-legal-service-providers

Massey, D. S., & Sánchez, R. M. (2010). *Brokered boundaries: Creating immigrant identity in anti-immigrant times*. New York, NY: Russell Sage Foundation.

Nguyen, Q. C. X., & Anderson, L. P. (2005). Vietnamese Americans' attitudes toward seeking mental health services: Relation to cultural variables. *Journal of Community Psychology*, *33*, 213–231.

Owens, J. A. (2004). Sleep in children: Cross-cultural perspectives. *Sleep and Biological Rhythms*, *2*, 165–173.

Pearl, E. S. (2008). Parent–child interaction therapy with an immigrant family exposed to domestic violence. *Clinical Case Studies*, *7*(1), 25–41.

Ramirez, N., & Monk, G. (2017). Crossing borders: Narrative therapy with undocumented Mexican women on a journey beyond abuse and violence. *Journal of Systemic Therapies*, *36*(2), 27–38.

Reina, A., & Lohman, B. (2015). Barriers preventing Latina immigrants from seeking advocacy services for domestic violence victims: A qualitative analysis. *Journal of Family Violence*, *30*(4), 479–488.

Resnicow, K., Baranowski, T., Ahluwalia, J. S., & Braithwaite, R. L. (1999). Cultural sensitivity in public health: Defined and demystified. *Ethnicity & Disease*, *9*, 10–21.

Rogers-Sirin, L. (2013). Segmented assimilation and attitudes toward psychotherapy: A moderated mediation analysis. *Journal of Counseling Psychology*, *60*(3), 329–339.

Roland, A. (2006). Across civilizations: Psychoanalytic therapy with Asians and Asian Americans. *Psychotherapy: Theory, Research, Practice, Training*, *43*(4), 454–463.

Roth, A., & Fonagy, P. (2005). *What works for whom: A critical review of psychotherapy research*. New York, NY: Guilford Press.Sandhu, S., Bjerre, N., Dauvrin, M., Dias, S., Gaddini, A., Greacen, T., . . . Priebe, S. (2013). Experiences with treating immigrants: A qualitative study in mental health services across 16 European countries. *Social Psychiatry & Psychiatric Epidemiology*, *48*(1), 105–116.

Suárez-Orozco, M., Louie, V., & Suro, R. (Eds.). (2011). *Writing immigration: Scholars and journalists in dialogue*. Berkeley, CA: University of California Press.

U.S. Census Bureau. (2011). Selected social characteristics in the United States: Foreign-born. 2011 American Community Survey 1-year estimates. Retrieved from https://factfinder.census.gov/faces/tableservices/jsf/pages/productview.xhtml?pid=ACS_10_1YR_S0501&prodType=table

Victims of criminal activity: U nonimmigrant status. (2018, October 12). Retrieved from https://www.uscis.gov/humanitarian/victims-human-trafficking-other-crimes/victims-criminal-activity-u-nonimmigrant-status/victims-criminal-activity-u-nonimmigrant-status

Weinhold, B., & Weinhold, J. (2008). *Breaking free of the codependence trap*. Novato, CA: New World Library.

10

Providing Psychotherapy in Rural Areas

*Tracy J. Cohn and Pei-Chun Tsai**

"Why does rural mental health matter?" This is a question many mental health clinicians may ask. Three important reasons why rural mental health matters are the following:

1. The provision of services to rural residents is an act of social justice, which can be defined as having "the goal to decrease human suffering and to promote human values of equality and justice" (Vasquez, 2012, p. 337).
2. Rural life is an aspect of multiculturalism.
3. Rural communities are composed of unique contextual stressors that impact rural clients differently than urban peers.

Rural mental health matters because of the differences between urban and rural populations in the quality of care received and the sequelae of mental health distress; thus, working in rural mental health is an act of social justice and advocacy, in serving a culture that is marginalized. Social justice and advocacy are key components of the professional identity of mental health professionals (Gelso, Nutt Williams, & Fretz, 2014). Rural life is also an aspect of our understanding of culture. Rural culture has distinct beliefs, values, and customs that are important contextual factors that impact the delivery of services, and ultimately impact the quality of care of those inhabitants in rural communities (Hastings & Cohn, 2013).

Operating from the framework that rural mental health care is a social justice issue and rural life represents a distinct culture, this chapter will first define "rural" and discuss the complexities of this definition, followed by findings regarding the structural, systemic, and cultural barriers to providing care in this context. This overview is followed by examining barriers to service delivery, ways to increase cultural competence in rural health care, effective strategies and empirically supported treatments, and finally suggestions for future steps.

* Both authors contributed equally to this chapter and authorship order reflects alphabetical listing.

The Scope and Description of the Problem

One of the struggles in discussing "rural" mental health is the absence of a consistent and clear definition of "rural" according to Smalley et al. (2010) and others (Hastings & Cohn, 2013). The U.S. Census Bureau and the Office of Management and Budget (OMB) offer two of the most commonly used definitions (Jameson & Blank, 2007). The U.S. Census Bureau defines rural as what remains after accounting for urban ("rural" implies sparse population, less dense, less built up, and at a distance) (Ratcliff, Burd, Holder, & Fields, 2016). In contrast to the U.S. Census Bureau definition, OMB considers counties with a population less than 50,000 as rural (Defining Rural Population, 2017). If using the OMB definition, about 15% of U.S. residents would be considered "rural," which is approximately 46.2 million people (Defining Rural Population, 2017) and represents 72% of the U.S. landmass (Kassel, 2018).

In general, the varying definitions of rural result in challenging conversations about rural health because "rural" can mean different things to different people. Moreover, the absence of a standard definition complicates the ability to advocate for rural communities, as will be highlighted throughout this chapter. Definitions of rural are exclusionary, generally failing to integrate frontier areas, which are thought to be the most remote of rural areas (six or fewer people per square mile; Health and Healthcare in Frontier Areas, 2018). For the purposes of this chapter, we will use the term "rural" in an inclusive sense (rural and frontier).

While it is challenging to define "rural," it is equally challenging to summarize the barriers and changes for mental health for 46.2 million people who live across the country. It is critical to acknowledge the diversity of those who live in rural areas. Casey Tieken, in an interview with Illing (2017), noted:

> There tend to be two overwhelming stereotypes that shape how people think about rural America. One of those is the Andy Griffith fantasy, in which rural America represents a simpler, better time, a very romanticized image of history. Then there's this other portrayal, which is kind of the *Deliverance*, backwoods redneck model. So two very opposite portrayals—one is romanticized, and the other is backward. (para. 8)

While one might be prone to think of stereotypes in discussing rural communities and rural residents, it is clear that there is great variation within rural communities. For instance, there is enormous variation between the lives and experiences of a resident in frontier Alaska and the rural southern United States, just as there is variation in the experience of a resident in rural Australia and the frontier lands of Wyoming. Mental health clinicians should be attentive to the idiographic experience of the individual and actively work against the stereotypes that so strongly permeate discourse on rural society. When one uses the word "rural" it means not only location and population density, but also a culture. Findings suggest that overall, rural residents experience the world differently than urban and suburban counterparts. For example, in a study of 1,700 participants (Hamel, Wu, & Brodie, 2017), the researchers concluded that the differences between rural and urban participants are defined by culture and not necessarily by financial differences. In that study, 68% of rural respondents reported that urban values were different from rural values, and yet only 20% of urban residents reported that rural values were different from urban. Rural residents are more likely than urban residents to report that they perceive immigrants as a burden to the country (42% and 16% respectively), that the federal government is more willing to help urban residents than rural residents (56%), and that Christian values are "under attack" (59%). Even individuals within rural areas have unique cultural experiences, however. While 78% of White respondents indicated that other rural residents shared their values, the number fell to 64% for rural Hispanic individuals and 55% for African Americans. Thus, while poverty is one aspect of rural life, it does not fully describe the experience of rural residents. Therefore, mental health practitioners should carefully consider how the culture of rural life can vary from state to state, community to community, and individual to individual.

Researchers have generally concluded that rural residents do not experience higher rates of mental health concerns than urban counterparts (Breslau, Marshall, Pincus, & Brown, 2014). Yet, rural residents are more likely to commit suicide than urban peers, a finding that is consistent for adolescents, veterans, and older adults (Fontanella et al., 2015; McCarthy et al., 2012). Rural residents are more likely to die prematurely, as defined as death before the age of 75, and have higher rates of morbidity and chronic health conditions (Eberhardt & Pamuk, 2004).

While rates of mental health concerns may be similar to urban residents, the experiences of residents in rural communities are profoundly different with regard to treatment and care around mental health (Mohatt, Adams, Bradley, & Morris, 2005). Findings indicate that rural residents are less likely to self-perceive a need for care (Rost, Fortney, Fischer, & Smith, 2002), and those who do perceive that they need care are subsequently less likely to access care (Wang et al., 2005) in comparison to urban peers. The quality of care that rural residents receive may be lower than those services provided in urban areas (Fortney, Rost, & Zhang, 1999; Kessler et al., 2004). Wang et al. (2005) argued that individuals in rural areas are more likely to receive poorer care than urban peers because of the lack of specialists in behavioral health.

While urban and rural residents have a similar incidence of mental health concerns, structural and systemic barriers exist in accessing care as well as the quality of care received. Bischoff et al. (2014) argued for examining access to mental health services by considering both the availability and acceptability of services. Acceptability of services, according to Mohatt, Adams, Bradley, and Morris (2005), reflects cultural beliefs around mental health and whether the care is an acceptable source of treatment, and these aspects will be addressed later in this chapter. Factors of availability are addressed next.

Barriers to Service Delivery

Availability of Services

Availability factors (Bischoff et al., 2014) associated with accessing mental health services in rural areas include (a) the role of poverty, (b) access to transportation, and (c) provider availability.

Individuals in rural communities tend to experience poverty at higher rates than urban peers (16.9% rural, 13.6% urban), with 23.5% of rural children living in poverty versus 20.5% of urban children (Farrigan, 2018). Rates of poverty are disproportionately higher for Blacks and African Americans (33.0%), American Indians and Alaska Natives (31.8%), and Latinx (25.9%) in comparison to rural White residents (14.6%). Rural residents are also less likely to have private or public insurance (Hoffman, Damico, & Garfield, 2011) in comparison to urban peers, and thus would be considered uninsured. Children in rural areas are 24 times more likely to have public-assisted insurance than children in urban areas (Pudelski, 2018), and 28.9% of rural adult residents have public insurance and 23.9% are uninsured (MacKinney et al., 2014).

Access to reliable transportation is a considerable challenge (Syed, Gerber, & Sharp, 2013), and when individuals do have access to transportation, they will often need to travel longer distances to access care than urban counterparts (Robinson et al., 2012), ultimately increasing the cost for care for residents and thus decreasing the chances they will access care. In addition, rural residents are more likely to be unemployed (Hertz, 2017), even when accounting for population density, in comparison to urban residents because of the limited opportunity for low-skilled jobs and the limited diversity of labor markets (Harrison & Bluestone, 1990), thus increasing financial barriers to care.

Even if a rural resident has the financial and physical means to access care, there may be few providers in the local area. Rural areas face a shortage of providers (Larson, Patterson, Garberson, & Andrilla, 2016). Sixty percent of health shortage areas, a designation by the U.S. federal government, are in rural communities (Shortage Areas, n.d.). The lack of providers in rural communities can be associated with overwhelmed providers with too many clients as well as with highly complex and challenging clients with limited resources and few referral options (Hastings & Cohn, 2013). Recruitment of providers to rural communities is particularly challenging, as freshly minted licensed mental health clinicians are frequently single, often carrying large student debt, and do not generally find the isolation and limited dating opportunities particularly appealing (Hastings & Cohn, 2013). Whereas individuals living in metropolitan areas may be able to make additional income through moonlighting at a hospital emergency room, adjunct teaching at a local community college, or building a small private practice, these opportunities may be more limited in rural settings given limited hospitals, distance to travel to community college or other educational institutions, and multiple relationships that may emerge in having a private practice while also working in a local agency.

Acceptability of Services

There has been a cognitive gap between how traditional psychotherapy may work from the lens of an urban training model and how it has been experienced by psychotherapists and clients in rural settings. The gap may reflect the omission of taking rural cultural reality and contextual factors into consideration. The interpersonal boundary in the rural community has a distinct feature compared to its urban counterpart. Several studies have indicated the rural communities tend to value close bonding to family and the local community, to regard religion/spirituality as their essential identity, and to adopt conservative gender role socialization (Aten, Mangis, & Campbell, 2010; Jayaram, Goud, & Srinivasan, 2011; Smalley et al., 2010). Considering the tight-knit character of rural communities, individuals may describe themselves as "living in a fishbowl," reflecting the high visibility and lack of anonymity in the community (Hastings & Cohn, 2013; Smalley et al., 2010). Moreover, rural residents are inclined to value independence and self-sufficiency, in part due to adaptation to their living and working environment (Dyck & Hardy, 2013; Stewart, Jameson, & Curtin, 2015). Based on the rural cultural reality and its intersection with contextual stressors (e.g., limitation of available and acceptable resources), the following section depicts three different dimensions of the barriers to service delivery in the rural community: (a) clients' help-seeking attitudes and behaviors, (b) psychotherapists in practice, and (c) training and supervision.

Barriers to Clients' Help-Seeking Attitudes and Behaviors

Public stigma (i.e., the negative attitude or belief held by the society toward individuals who were negatively affected by this) and self-stigma (i.e., the internalized negative messages from the public and the personal consequences of the negative messages) have been shown to have a detrimental association with individual help-seeking attitudes and behaviors (Corrigan, Morris, Michaels, Rafacz, & Rüsch, 2012; Vogel, Wade, & Haake, 2006). Empirical studies have shown that stigma has a negative impact on the treatment process and outcome, including working alliance (Owen, Thomas, & Rodolfa, 2013), missed appointments (Vega, Rodriguez, & Ang, 2010), symptom severity (Livingston & Boyd, 2010), and treatment adherence (Livingston & Boyd, 2010). The "fishbowl effect" may make it challenging to maintain privacy and confidentiality, which may amplify the negative impact of stigma on rural individuals. In particular, the fear of being judged by family members, neighbors, and friends, and a desire to avoid feelings of shame and embarrassment, may discourage rural residents from seeking psychotherapy (Bischoff et al., 2014; Larson & Corrigan, 2010; Robinson et al., 2012). Empirically, research has revealed that men and older adults in rural areas have a higher level of stigma in connection with help seeking compared to their counterparts in suburban or urban areas (Hammer, Vogel, & Heimerdinger-Edwards, 2013; Stewart et al., 2015). The influence of stigma may also extend to family members or caregivers of these clients. It is likely that strong family bonding may be the reason why rural residents experience the pressure of family stigma (i.e., prejudice or discrimination encountered by individuals because of their affiliation with a family member who has a mental illness) (Larson & Corrigan, 2008).

The acceptability of the treatment delivery method presents another challenge for help seeking in rural communities (U.S. Department of Health and Human Services, 2011). Psychotherapy in rural communities is usually perceived as a less preferable source of care in comparison to more informal support such as from one's family and local church (McBride Murry, Heflinger, Suiter, & Brody, 2011). Also, seeking a psychotherapist for help may be incongruent with a resident's value of being independent and self-sufficient. Moreover, the limited awareness and understanding of mental health and unfamiliarity about mental health resources may make rural residents feel uneasy with psychological services. Nover (2014) has revealed that rural clients may struggle with how to communicate their presenting issues to mental health professionals effectively and may be reluctant to disclose some of their unhealthy behaviors (e.g., smoking and drinking).

Barriers to Psychotherapists in Practice

Meta-analyses have confirmed that the quality of the therapeutic working alliance serves as a significant predictor of treatment outcomes (Del Re, Flückiger, Horvath, Symonds, & Wampold, 2012; Horvath, Del Re, Flückiger, & Symonds, 2011). However, in the clinical work, psychotherapists may encounter barriers that are associated with rural cultural reality and contextual factors. Individuals in a rural community may have distrust, resistance, and skepticism of psychotherapy, and they may initially view psychotherapists as "outsiders" (Bradley, Werth, Hastings, & Pierce, 2012; Hastings & Cohn, 2013). To build the working alliance with clients, psychotherapists may need to consider making themselves knowledgeable about and visible in the community (Bischoff et al., 2014), even though navigating the fine line between professional relationship and personal privacy can be an emotion-laden experience for some psychotherapists (Hastings & Cohn, 2013).

For psychotherapists, contextual factors (e.g., close interpersonal boundaries and the fishbowl effect) may present an inevitable dilemma in the areas of ethics and reconciliation of values conflicts. Regarding ethical dilemmas, the challenges of dual or multiple relationships and competence are cited as two of the most common ones by many rural psychotherapists (Bradley et al., 2012; Hastings & Cohn, 2013). Compared to psychotherapy practice in urban or suburban settings, dual or multiple relationships are inevitable for many clinicians who practice in rural communities considering the availability (e.g., limited clinicians in the rural area) and accessibility (e.g., long traveling distance and time cost) of the resources (Hastings & Cohn, 2013). In addition, clinicians who reside in rural settings often need to balance their professional role (i.e., a clinician) and their social role (i.e., an engaged community member) (Barnett, 2017). Moreover, competence presents a doubled-edged ethical dilemma for many psychotherapists (Bradley, Werth, & Hastings, 2011). On the one hand, the limited available psychotherapists and referral resources along with the broad and complex scope of clients' presenting concerns may require psychotherapists to serve as generalists. On the other hand, therapists have limited time and energy to expand and deepen their scope of competence. Psychotherapists are likely to run the risk of practicing beyond their competence level or of feeling overwhelmed by the need to develop many other areas of expertise.

Also, the dilemma of values conflicts has trapped many psychotherapists in clinical work. Research has shown that psychotherapists' personal values/worldviews concerning social, environmental, or political topics (e.g., gun rights, environmental impact of mining, legislation permitting gay marriage) often run counter to rural cultural values/reality (e.g., hunting and mining as a family career for multiple generations, conservative religious beliefs) (Bradley et al., 2012; Hastings & Cohn, 2013). Providers might choose to suppress their authentic voice/freedom of speech to avoid therapeutic relationship ruptures and a negative reputation in the community (Bradley et al., 2012). But doing so may complicate the therapeutic relationship, given that providers may have to channel some mental energy to manage their inner reactions to values conflicts in sessions, and this may undermine their capacity to be fully present with the clients in the moment. Also, the trust may be broken if clients become aware later in treatment that the provider has omitted (or perhaps faked) his or her values and beliefs.

Barriers in Training and Supervision

Unconscious adoption of an urban training model may lead to a gap between the traditional theoretical framework and clinical practice. In rural practice, it is unrealistic to assume that referral resources will be readily available and one will be able to consistently maintain clear boundaries (Fifield & Oliver, 2016; McNichols, Witt, & Gatewood, 2016). Because of the limited available and accessible mental health treatment resources in rural communities, coupled with the complexity and broad scope of presenting issues, trainees may practice beyond their competence and developmental training levels, which could be a concern for clients' treatment, trainees' self-efficacy, and supervisors' professional liability. In addition, due to the limited availability of supervisors and practicum sites, trainees may not always receive adequate supervision and training. For example, some practicum sites may not always have licensed mental health professionals available to serve as doctoral-level trainees' clinical supervisors. Also, professional and personal boundaries may not be clearly distinguishable given the features of high visibility, close interpersonal boundaries, and relatively limited community resource options (e.g., shops, restaurants, daycare centers, recreational places) in rural areas. Navigating dual or multiple relationships can be challenging for trainees, considering they may live, study, and work in the same community, campus, or school as do their clients (e.g., a client may take a course taught by the trainee or live in the same off-campus apartment complex as the trainee). In addition, dual or multiple relationships in training and supervision (e.g., the same clinical supervisor also serves as practicum instructor and academic advisor for a trainee) may exacerbate the power differential and place trainees in a vulnerable position.

Creating Cultural Competency

While rurality has not been viewed as a critical cultural component in the discussion of multiculturally informed care and social justice, even for clients not physically living in rural areas, rural heritage may continue playing an essential role in their presenting issues, such as family dynamics, religion/spirituality, gender role conflict, identity development, coping, and interpersonal relationships. If psychotherapy only sees the trees (i.e., the surface level of presenting concerns) but dismisses the forest (i.e., the root or rural cultural/contextual factors), this is likely to result in missing the whole picture (i.e., biased understanding in case conceptualization). In this case, psychotherapists might have "rural-blindness," similar to the ideology of "color-blindness," implying a lack of the cultural awareness and tendency to blame clients for their adversity because of contextual stressors.

This section will illustrate how to create cultural competence through the levels of knowledge, awareness, and skill, respectively, which may apply not only to psychotherapists in rural settings but also to non-rural psychotherapists who may work with clients who are influenced by rural cultural values. Also, the implications for psychotherapists and training programs will be discussed. We hope that the increase of cultural competency will enhance the therapeutic working alliance, help-seeking attitudes, mental health literacy in rural communities, and ultimately the effectiveness and quality of the treatment and treatment delivery (e.g., acceptability of the services).

Knowledge

On the knowledge level, many studies have suggested that psychotherapists acquire background knowledge about rural daily life and the impact of religion/spirituality, family dynamics, and environmental conditions on clients' presenting concerns (McNichols et al., 2016). In particular, Bischoff et al. (2014) suggested that learning about the function and composition of the community (e.g., shops, recreation places, community events, social resources, and communication patterns) would enable psychotherapists to be perceived as members of the local community. By doing so, prospective clients are likely to feel more comfortable with psychotherapists, which in turn may increase the likelihood of seeking out services from them. Also, it is noteworthy that religion/spirituality is rooted in many rural clients' cultural identity, not only guiding their daily life but also affecting their help-seeking attitudes and behaviors. For example, Aten et al. (2010) found that rural fundamentalists might hold strict gender roles related to their literal interpretation of scripture and may believe their depressive symptoms are a result of unresolved sin.

Instead of attributing the presenting concerns to cultural deficits or barriers in rural settings, psychotherapists may need to consider whether they also are linked to the contextual factors. For example, psychotherapists are advised to learn that contextual factors (e.g., poverty, limited resources and job opportunities) may contribute to some clients' presenting concerns (e.g., unemployment). As another example, Correll, Cantrell, and Dalton (2011) found that the challenge in changing rural clients' unhealthy behaviors (e.g., smoking) might be related to their family's vocational identity (i.e., generations have worked in the tobacco field).

Finally, clinicians may need to be mindful of the heterogeneity of rural settings. While viewing rurality as a cultural factor, it is also vital for psychotherapists to explore the potential impact of intersectionality between rurality and other cultural factors (e.g., rural ethnic minority or rural sexual minority individuals). The Housing Assistance Council's nationwide survey (2012) on communities from 2006 to 2010 suggested that rural ethnic minorities consistently report higher poverty rates than the overall national minority population. In addition, empirical studies revealed that racial minorities and LGBT clients in rural settings often experience greater disadvantages and discrimination than their urban counterparts (Taylor & Ruiz, 2017; Willging, Salvador, & Kano, 2006).

Awareness

On the awareness level, psychotherapists are encouraged to continually reflect upon and confront their cultural values, assumptions, biases, stereotypes, and privileges (Owens, Watabe, & Michael, 2013). Psychotherapists usually possess greater privileges in education and socioeconomic status compared to their rural clients. Therapists must be mindful of their unconscious assumptions (e.g., assuming rural individuals have lower socioeconomic status or conservative religious beliefs). They should keep an open mind and take an emic perspective to view issues from the client's perspective.

Regarding training and supervision, instructors and supervisors can facilitate students' rural culture awareness in several ways. For example, faculty may consider infusing rurality in the multicultural dialogue among different courses (e.g., ethics, practicum, and assessment). As another example, adding cultural immersion experiential activities (e.g., attending social events) can expand trainees' cultural awareness. Clinicians in practice should be conscious about the ways they present themselves in front of the clients (e.g., how they dress and whether they use the title of Dr. or first name).

Skill

On the skill level, incorporating the roles of community member, collaborator, and mental health advocate in one's personal and professional identity may help psychotherapists transform contextual stressors into potential opportunities while working with clients in rural settings. In particular, the identity as a community member reflects a sense of belongingness and commitment to the local rural setting that can help build feelings of comfort, trust, and the working alliance with clients. Research has suggested that small talk about local events and appropriate self-disclosure in sessions may enhance trust in these relationships (Bischoff et al., 2014; Slama, 2004). Research has shown that maintaining therapeutic neutrality or vagueness in self-disclosure might be perceived as a sign of devaluing one's belief or a message of distrust to rural clients (Aten et al., 2010; Willging et al., 2006).

As a mental health advocate, one may adopt the mentality of "if clients don't come to us, we can reach out to them." In other words, psychotherapists may provide outreach and psychoeducation in local communities to promote mental health awareness and knowledge, which in turn may help reduce the stigma of help seeking, increase mental health literacy, and maximize the use and effectiveness of psychotherapy.

Effective Strategies and Empirically-Supported Treatments

Rural communities are ripe for innovative interventions that can address the systemic, structural, and cultural obstacles of rural mental health delivery. Innovative techniques can focus on training and education as well as on integrating empirically supported interventions into treatment.

Training and Education

Training and educational opportunities abound in rural clinical practice. The federal government has been an active agent in addressing rural health disparities. First, the Health Resources and Services Administration (HRSA) has designated funding for training graduate psychology students, known as Graduate Psychology Education (GPE) programs. The GPE grants allow doctoral-level trainees to focus on developing skills in integrated behavioral health care that focus on underserved populations, including rural residents (Behavioral Health, 2018).

HRSA also provides student loan repayment up to $50,000 under the National Health Service Corps (NHSC). A two-year commitment is required, with the opportunity to extend the commitment time in order to receive additional student loan repayment monies. The NHSC targets licensed providers in several disciplines of behavioral health (i.e., social workers, marriage and family therapists, counselors) to provide services in underserved communities at NHSC-approved service sites, including but not limited to rural areas (Apply for Loan Repayment, n.d.).

University training programs in psychology have also worked toward training practitioners to have a focus on advocacy and social justice (Mallinckrodt, Miles, & Levy, 2014), including the University of Tennessee, Knoxville. Building off the ideas of Fassinger and O'Brien (2000), the training model moves away from a deficit-based conceptualization of pathology and focuses instead on contextualizing client distress and developing practitioner advocacy (Ph.D. Program—Counseling Psychology, n.d.). Other university training programs offer specialized training in rural mental health, including Radford University in rural southwest Virginia. As one of four foci, the program offers specialized training in assessment and treatment of addictive disorders in rural settings, rural program evaluation, and rural health psychology (Counseling Psychology Radford University, n.d.).

Interventions

Developing empirically supported treatments (ESTs) and testing them for rural residents pose considerable challenges (Rural Behavioral Health, 2011). First, ESTs are often developed and tested on urban residents; thus, the intervention may not translate to a rural setting, where resources are scarce, transportation is limited, and limited finances may impede interventions that require frequent sessions, frequent assessments, or post-intervention follow-ups. Even though difficult, ESTs must be tested to ensure that they are translatable to rural practice.

The Rural Health Information Hub (n.d.a) offers ESTs that can be filtered by level of evidence, state, and topic, allowing providers to determine which interventions are culturally appropriate to their setting. Several identified interventions seem particularly salient to rural residents.

Veterans

A sizeable portion of rural residents have served in the military. Estimates suggest that 35% of current and former veterans reside in rural areas (Fortney et al., 2015), so interventions targeted for veterans also respond to the need for services in these underserved communities. Egede et al. (2015), in a randomized controlled study of the efficacy of telemedicine, concluded that behavioral health delivered via an electronic medium (live and internet-based) was as effective as in-person treatment for a sample of 241 veterans with depression. This finding is highly relevant, given that access to care for rural residents poses a significant obstacle. Fortney et al. (2015) postulated that tele-psychiatry and tele-counseling can solve both the "equity problem" in unequal access to care for rural residents in comparison to urban residents as well as the "capacity problem" in that more providers, specifically those living in urban areas, would be accessible to rural residents.

While not specific solely to the veteran population, researchers have suggested that tele-mental health may help resolve aspects of access to care (Nelson & Bui, 2010), with appropriately trained providers in urban and metropolitan areas providing services in rural and remote communities. In addition to access to care, as tele-mental health becomes more mainstream and clients are able to connect to mental health clinicians from their homes, the stigma and acceptability associated with being "seen" at the doctor's office may dissipate. Finally, the ability to receive supervision and consult with expert clinicians may further increase clients' access to cutting-edge treatments that otherwise may take a longer time to trickle down to rural communities (Wood, Miller, & Hargrove, 2005). Perhaps the newest area of emerging technology is the role of mobile tele-mental health, where cellphones can be used to access providers instantaneously, and cellphone apps can be used to gather feedback on the client's level of functioning (Chan, Torous, Hinton, & Yellowless, 2014).

Individuals with Chronic Disease

The Chronic Disease Self-Management Program (CDSMP), an intervention developed at Stanford University, is a 6-week workshop designed for individuals with chronic conditions such as HIV, diabetes, and depression. Research has been conducted for over 20 years on the intervention, and recent findings by Smith et al. (2017) suggest that although better technology is needed for adequate service delivery, that the CDSMP model is adaptable to rural communities.

African American Families with Children

Kogan et al. (2016) found in a sample of 465 African American youth living in rural areas that the Strong African American Families program (SAAF), which focused on increasing self-regulation and decreasing problematic behaviors, showed a statistically significant effect. SAAF was developed to "address the lack of ecologically appropriate preventive interventions for rural African American Youth" (Kogan et al., p. 249).

Affordability of Nutritious Food

One tool that has been effective, at least anecdotally, for both students and practitioners is a cookbook for individuals using Supplemental Nutrition Assistance Program (SNAP). SNAP, also called food stamps, provides 46.2 million individuals in the United States with approximately $126 each month for food. The free pdf, called "Good and Cheap," offers recipes and tips for managing eating on four dollars a day (Brown, 2014).

Models of Care

While particular interventions have been identified as efficacious, models of care have also been identified as efficacious, especially as these models may address barriers to care in rural areas. Integrated care shows particular promise. Schmit, Watson, and Fernandez (2018) found a statistically significant difference for the effectiveness of integrated behavioral and primary care among a sample of 196 individuals. Fortney at al. (2015) noted that there is "rigorous scientific evidence from 80 randomized controlled trials that have demonstrated that practice-based collaborative care improves depression/anxiety outcomes in facilities that have on-site mental health specialists" (p. 529). Moreover, the researchers noted that practice-based collaborative care is not as effective in rural communities if there is not an onsite mental health staff (Fortney et al., 2013).

The federal government has taken steps to increase access to cost-effective care. One in six residents in rural communities receive health care services through an HRSA-funded health care center (United States, Health Resources and Services Administration, 2018). These HRSA-supported health care centers have been found to reduce health care costs (United States, Health Resources and Services Administration, 2018) and reduce inpatient admissions using an integrated model of care of dental, behavioral health, and primary care. HRSA-supported health care centers offer a rich resource for rural residents who may struggle to access care due to limited financial resources, lack of insurance, or the absence of providers. Existing community agencies can apply to become federally qualified health centers.

Mobile health clinics show promise in addressing long travel times to access care. Converted vans and trucks can help address the long travel typically associated with accessing care in rural communities. The mobile unit model is a model of service delivery offered by the Rural Health Information Hub (Rural Health Information Unit, n.d.b) that helps address access to care, including transportation and funding. Findings by Yu, Hill, Ricks, Bennet, and Oriol (2017) indicate that mobile health clinics may offer cost savings and cost-effective care by keeping individuals out of the emergency room and addressing issues before they become chronic.

Future Steps

Although this chapter illustrates the backdrop of delivering psychological service in rural settings, more effort is still needed in research, clinical work, training, and systems/policy to help increase the visibility and attention of this topic. Though the existing research has discussed the barriers and advantages for psychotherapists to work in rural settings (Bradley et al., 2012; Fifield & Oliver, 2016; Hastings & Cohn, 2013), future researchers may want to take a further step to conduct comprehensive needs assessments from the perspectives of the clients, caregivers, and training programs. Also, while it is critical to better understand barriers in the service delivery, future researchers are encouraged to explore rural cultural strengths (e.g., support and emotional connection with family, religion/spirituality, and community, resiliency in coping) and their impact on psychological service delivery. Also, more research is needed to investigate the clinical implications of the interplay between rurality and other cultural dimensions. Specifically, it is worth exploring the unique adversity (e.g., discrimination) that may be encountered by these individuals as well as culturally adaptive coping strategies and interventions. Furthermore, the development of a comprehensive conceptual theory framework of rural cultural psychotherapy will add value to guide clinical practice moving forward.

Regarding clinical work, psychotherapists must continue advancing their rural cultural awareness, knowledge, and skills. In the face of contextual barriers in rural practice, psychotherapists are encouraged to expand their personal and professional identity (e.g., roles of community member, collaborator, and mental health advocator) and acknowledge their value as mental health providers in rural areas.

With regard to training for rural practice, one common challenge faced by rural mental health care providers and related graduate programs is the recruitment and retention of faculty members and students. Potential solutions may include marketing the strengths and unique values of rural practice, offering financial support, and providing career development opportunities such as clinical experience in integrated care settings, multidisciplinary collaboration, specialty training in treating individuals with trauma and substance abuse, crisis management, and training in outreach to the community. In addition, departmental training clinics may consider becoming hubs of support and professional development for rural community-based clinicians, such as offering continuing education workshops and providing collaboration to include peer supervision and consultation.

This topic should receive greater recognition at the systemic level. Some professional associations (e.g., National Association for Rural Mental Health, http://www.apa.org/practice/programs/rural/resources.aspx; National Rural Health Association, https://www.ruralhealthweb.org/; National Advisory Committee on Rural Health & Human Services, https://www.hrsa.gov/advisory-committees/rural-health/index.html) at the national level have been working on the consolidation of rural resources (e.g., research/publication, telehealth, and health associations and federal agencies). However, there still a need for more information on the development of culturally responsive interventions as well as practical support for personal and professional development (e.g., continuing education focused on rural practice, supervision, and integrated care).

In addition, state and local policymakers may actively advocate for and allocate more administrative and financial resources to aid psychotherapy delivery in rural settings. In particular, adding administrative staff and case manager positions in rural mental health clinics could be a great support for psychotherapists. The rationale is that psychotherapists in rural settings usually spend a considerable amount of their work hours managing administrative paperwork or connecting clients to local resources, which may compromise the time and depth of actual intervention that rural clients so clearly need (Bradley et al., 2011; Hastings & Cohn, 2013).

Rural communities represent more than physical locations; they represent cultures that have distinct challenges and opportunities related to the delivery of psychological services. This chapter highlighted challenges of accessibility and acceptability for rural health care. It focused on innovative techniques and interventions that have been developed to overcome common obstacles to care. Ideally, with additional resources to help address both systemic and structural barriers to care, rural residents will be able to have greater accessibility to and quality of care.

References

Apply for Loan Repayment. (n.d.). Retrieved from https://nhsc.hrsa.gov/loan-repayment/apply-loan-repayment/index.html

Aten, J. D., Mangis, M. W., & Campbell, C. (2010). Psychotherapy with rural religious fundamentalist clients. *Journal of Clinical Psychology*, *66*(5), 513–523.

Barnett, J. E. (2017). Unavoidable incidental contacts and multiple relationships in rural practice. In O. Zur (Ed.), *Multiple relationships in psychotherapy and counseling: Unavoidable, common and mandatory dual relations in therapy* (pp. 97–107). New York, NY: Routledge.

Behavioral Health. (2018, May 1). Retrieved from https://bhw.hrsa.gov/grants/mentalbehavioralhealth

Bischoff, R. J., Reisbig, A. M. J., Springer, P. R., Schultz, S., Robinson, W. D., & Olson, M. (2014). Succeeding in rural mental health practice: Being sensitive to culture by fitting in and collaborating. *Contemporary Family Therapy, 36*(1), 1–16.

Bradley, J. M., Werth, J. L., & Hastings, S. L. (2011). Social justice advocacy in rural communities: Practical issues and implications. *The Counseling Psychologist, 40*(3), 363–384.

Bradley, J. M., Werth Jr., J. L., Hastings, S. L., & Pierce, T. W. (2012). A qualitative study of rural mental health practitioners regarding the potential professional consequences of social justice advocacy. *Professional Psychology: Research and Practice, 43*(4), 356–363.

Breslau, J., Marshall, G. N., Pincus, H. A., & Brown, R. A. (2014). Are mental disorders more common in urban than rural areas of the United States? *Journal of Psychiatric Research, 56*, 50–55.

Brown, L. (2014). *Eat well on $4/day good and cheap*. Retrieved from https://books.leannebrown.com/good-and-cheap.pdf

Chan, S. R., Torous, J., Hinton, L., & Yellowlees, P. (2014). Mobile tele-mental health: Increasing applications and a move to hybrid models of care. *Healthcare, 2*(2), 220–233.

Correll, J. A., Cantrell, P., & Dalton, W. T. (2011). Integration of behavioral health services in a primary care clinic serving rural Appalachia: Reflections on a clinical experience. *Families, Systems, & Health, 29*(4), 291–302.

Corrigan, P. W., Morris, S. B., Michaels, P. J., Rafacz, J. D., & Rüsch, N. (2012). Challenging the public stigma of mental illness: A meta-analysis of outcome studies. *Psychiatric Services, 63*(10), 963–973.

Counseling Psychology Radford University. (n.d.). Retrieved from https://www.radford.edu/content/chbs/home/psychology/programs/counseling/Curriculum.htmlDefining Rural Population. (2017, January). Retrieved from https://www.hrsa.gov/rural-health/about-us/definition/index.html

Del Re, A. C., Flückiger, C., Horvath, A. O., Symonds, D., & Wampold, B. E. (2012). Therapist effects in the therapeutic alliance–outcome relationship: A restricted-maximum likelihood meta-analysis. *Clinical Psychology Review, 32*(7), 642–649.

Dyck, K. G., & Hardy, C. (2013). Enhancing access to psychologically informed mental health services in rural and northern communities. *Canadian Psychology/Psychologie Canadienne, 54*(1), 30–37.

Eberhardt, M., & Pamuk, E. (2004). The importance of place of residence: Examining health in rural and nonrural areas. *American Journal of Public Health, 94*(10), 1682–1686.

Egede, L. E., Acierno, R., Knapp, R. G., Lejuez, C., Hernandez-Tejada, M., Payne, E. H., & Frueh, B. C. (2015). Psychotherapy for depression in older veterans via telemedicine: A randomised, open-label, non-inferiority trial. *Lancet Psychiatry, 2*(8), 693–701.

Farrigan, T. (2018, April 18). Rural poverty & well-being. Retrieved from https://www.ers.usda.gov/topics/rural-economy-population/rural-poverty-well-being/

Fassinger, R. E., & O'Brien, K. M. (2000). Career counseling with college women: A scientist-practitioner-advocate model of intervention. In D. Luzzo (Ed.), *Career counseling of college students: An empirical guide to strategies that work* (pp. 253–266). Washington, DC: American Psychological Association.

Fifield, A. O., & Oliver, K. J. (2016). Enhancing the perceived competence and training of rural mental health practitioners. *Journal of Rural Mental Health, 40*(1), 77–83.

Fontanella, C. A., Hiance-Steelesmith, D. L., Phillips, G. S., Bridge, J. A., Lester, N., Sweeney, H. A., & Campo, J. V. (2015). Widening rural-urban disparities in youth suicides, United States, 1996–2010. *JAMA Pediatrics, 169*(5), 466–473.

Fortney, J. C., Pyne, J. M., Mouden, S. B., Mittal, D., Hudson, T. J., Schroeder, G. W., . . . Rost, K. M. (2013). Practice-based versus telemedicine-based collaborative care for depression in rural federally qualified health centers: A pragmatic randomized comparative effectiveness trial. *American Journal of Psychiatry, 170*(4), 414–425.

Fortney, J. C., Pyne, J. M., Turner, E. E., Farris, K. M., Normoyle, T. M., Avery, M. D., . . . Unützer, J. (2015). Telepsychiatry integration of mental health services into rural primary care settings. *International Review of Psychiatry, 27*(6), 525–539.

Fortney, J., Rost, K., & Zhang, M. (1999). The impact of geographic accessibility on the intensity and quality of depression treatment. *Medical Care, 37*, 884–893.

Gelso, C. J., Nutt Williams, E., & Fretz, B. R. (2014). An introduction to counseling psychology. In C. J. Gelso, E. Nutt Williams, & B. R. Fretz, *Counseling psychology* (3rd ed., pp. 3–23). Washington, DC: American Psychological Association.

Hamel, L., Wu, B., & Brodie, M. (2017). *The health care views and experiences of rural Americans: Findings from the Kaiser Family Foundation/Washington Post Survey of Rural America*. Retrieved from http://files.kff.org/attachment/Report-The-Health-Care-Views-and-Experiences-of-Rural-Americans

Hammer, J. H., Vogel, D. L., & Heimerdinger-Edwards, S. (2013). Men's help seeking: Examination of differences across community size, education, and income. *Psychology of Men & Masculinity, 14*(1), 65–75.

Harrison, B., & Bluestone, B. (1990). *The great U-turn: Corporate restructuring and the polarizing of America*. New York, NY: Basic Books.

Hastings, S. L., & Cohn, T. J. (2013). Challenges and opportunities associated with rural mental health practice. *Journal of Rural Mental Health, 37*(1), 37–49.

Health and Healthcare in Frontier Areas Introduction—Rural Health Information Hub. (2018, June 7). Retrieved from https://www.ruralhealthinfo.org/topics/frontier#definition

Hertz, T. (2017, July 6). Rural employment and unemployment. Retrieved from https://www.ers.usda.gov/topics/rural-economy-population/employment-education/rural-employment-and-unemployment/

Hoffman, C., Damico, A., & Garfield, R. (2011). *Research brief: Insurance coverage and access to care in primary care shortage areas*. Washington, DC: Henry J. Kaiser Family Foundation.

Horvath, A. O., Del Re, A. C., Flückiger, C., & Symonds, D. (2011). Alliance in individual psychotherapy. *Psychotherapy, 48*(1), 9–16.

Housing Assistance Council. (2012). *Poverty in rural America*. Retrieved from http://www.ruralhome.org/manager/uploads/Povertyruralamerica.pdf

Illing, S. (2017, April 24). "Rural America" doesn't mean "white America"—here's why that matters. Retrieved from https://www.vox.com/platform/amp/conversations/2017/4/24/15286624/race-rural-america-trump-politics-media

Jameson, J. P., & Blank, M. B. (2007). The role of clinical psychology in rural mental health services: Defining problems and developing solutions. *Clinical Psychology: Science and Practice, 14*, 283–298.

Jayaram, G., Goud, R., & Srinivasan, K. (2011). Overcoming cultural barriers to deliver comprehensive rural community mental health care in southern India. *Asian Journal of Psychiatry, 4*(4), 261–265.

Kassel, K. (2018, April 26). Rural economy. Retrieved from https://www.ers.usda.gov/data-products/ag-and-food-statistics-charting-the-essentials/rural-economy

Kessler, R. C., Berglund, P. A., Glantz, M. D., Koretz, D. S., Merikangas, K. R., Walters, E. E., & Zaslavsky, A. M. (2004). Estimating the prevalence and correlates of serious mental illness in community epidemiological surveys. In R. W. Manderscheid & M. J. Henderson (Eds.), *Mental health, United States, 2002* (pp. 155–164). Rockville, MD: Center for Mental Health Services, Substance Abuse and Mental Health Services Administration. DHHS Pub. No. (SMA) 3938.

Kogan, S. M., Lei, M.-K., Brody, G. H., Futris, T. G., Sperr, M., & Anderson, T. (2016). Implementing family-centered prevention in rural African American communities: A randomized effectiveness trial of the Strong African American Families program. *Prevention Science, 17*(2), 248–258.

Larson, E. H., Patterson, D. G., Garberson, L. A., & Andrilla, C. A. (2016). Data brief: Supply and distribution of the behavioral health workforce in rural America. Rural Health Research Center. Retrieved from http://depts.washington.edu/fammed/rhrc/wp-content/uploads/sites/4/2016/09/RHRC_DB160_Larson.pdf

Larson, J. E., & Corrigan, P. (2008). The stigma of families with mental illness. *Academic Psychiatry, 32*(2), 87–91.

Larson, J. E., & Corrigan, P. W. (2010). Psychotherapy for self-stigma among rural clients. *Journal of Clinical Psychology, 66*(5), 524–536.

Livingston, J. D., & Boyd, J. E. (2010). Correlates and consequences of internalized stigma for people living with mental illness: A systematic review and meta-analysis. *Social Science & Medicine, 71*(12), 2150–2161.

MacKinney, A. C., Coburn, A. F., Lundblad, J. P., McBride, T. D., Mueller, K. J., & Watson, S. D. (2014). Access to rural health care—A literature review and new synthesis. Retrieved from http://www.rupri.org/wp-content/uploads/Access-to-Rural-Health-Care-A-Literature-Review-and-New-Synthesis.-RUPRI-Health-Panel.-August-2014-1.pdf

Mallinckrodt, B., Miles, J. R., & Levy, J. J. (2014). The scientist-practitioner-advocate model: Addressing contemporary training needs for social justice advocacy. *Training and Education in Professional Psychology, 8*(4), 303–311.

McBride Murry, V., Heflinger, C. A., Suiter, S. V., & Brody, G. H. (2011). Examining perceptions about mental health care and help-seeking among rural African American families of adolescents. *Journal of Youth and Adolescence, 40*(9), 1118–1131.

McCarthy, J. F., Blow, F. C., Ignacio, R. V., Ilgen, M. A., Austin, K. L., & Valenstein, M. (2012). Suicide among patients in the Veterans Affairs Health System: Rural–urban differences in rates, risks, and methods. *American Journal of Public Health, 102*(S1), S111–S117.

McNichols, C., Witt, K. J., & Gatewood, D. C. (2016). The successes of experienced rural counselor supervisors and their recommendations for rural mental health. *Journal of Rural Mental Health, 40*(3–4), 139–153.

Mohatt, D. F., Adams, S. J., Bradley, M. M., & Morris, C. D. (2005). *Mental health and rural America: 1994–2005, an overview and annotated bibliography*. Rockville, MD: U. S. Department of Health and Human Services, Health Resources and Services Administration, Office of Rural Health Policy.

Nelson, E. L., & Bui, T. (2010). Rural telepsychology services for children and adolescents. *Journal of Clinical Psychology, 66*(5), 490–501.

Nover, C. H. (2014). Implementing a mental health and primary care partnership program in Placer County, California. *Social Work in Health Care, 53*(2), 156–182.

Owen, J., Thomas, L., & Rodolfa, E. (2013). Stigma for seeking therapy: Self-stigma, social stigma, and therapeutic processes. *The Counseling Psychologist, 41*(6), 857–880.

Owens, J. S., Watabe, Y., & Michael, K. D. (2013). Culturally responsive school mental health in rural communities. In C. S. Clauss-Ehlers, Z. N. Serpell, & M. D. Weist (Eds.), *Handbook of culturally responsive school mental health: Advancing research, training, practice, and policy* (pp. 31–42). New York, NY: Springer Science + Business Media.

Ph.D. Program—Counseling Psychology. (n.d.). Retrieved from https://psychology.utk.edu/grad/spa_model.php

Pudelski, S. (2018, January 17). Report: Children in rural communities more likely to rely on CHIP and Medicaid. Retrieved from https://ccf.georgetown.edu/2017/11/16/report-children-in-rural-communities-more-likely-to-rely-on-chip-and-medicaid/

Ratcliff, M., Burd, C., Holder, K., & Fields, A. (2016). Defining rural at the U.S. Census Bureau. *American Community Survey and Geography Brief.* Retrieved from https://www2.census.gov/geo/pdfs/reference/ua/Defining_Rural.pdf

Robinson, W. D., Springer, P. R., Bischoff, R., Geske, J., Backer, E., Olson, M., . . . Swinton, J. (2012). Rural experiences with mental illness: Through the eyes of patients and their families. *Families, Systems, & Health, 30*(4), 308–321.

Rost, K., Fortney, J., Fischer, E., & Smith, J. (2002). Use, quality, and outcomes of care for mental health: The rural perspective. *Medical Care Research and Review, 59*(3), 231–265.

Rural Behavioral Health Programs and Promising Practices. (2011). Department of Health and Human Resources, Health Resources and Services Administration. Retrieved from https://www.hrsa.gov/sites/default/files/ruralhealth/pdf/ruralbehavioralmanual05312011.pdf

Rural Health Information Hub. (n.d.a). Retrieved from http://www.ruralhealthinfo.org/

Rural Health Information Unit. (n.d.b). Mobile unit model—Rural services integration toolkit. Retrieved from https://www.ruralhealthinfo.org/toolkits/services-integration/2/care-coordination/mobile-unit

Schmit, M. K., Watson, J. C., & Fernandez, M. A. (2018). Examining the effectiveness of integrated behavioral and primary health care treatment. *Journal of Counseling & Development, 96*(1), 3–14.

Shortage Areas. (n.d.). Retrieved from https://datawarehouse.hrsa.gov/topics/shortageAreas.aspx

Slama, K. M. (2004). Toward rural cultural competence. *Minnesota Psychologist, 53*(2), 6–13.

Smalley, K. B., Yancey, C. T., Warren, J. C., Naufel, K., Ryan, R., & Pugh, J. L. (2010). Rural mental health and psychological treatment: A review for practitioners. *Journal of Clinical Psychology, 66*(5), 479–489.

Smith, M. L., Towne, S. D., Herrera-Venson, A., Cameron, K., Kulinski, K. P., Lorig, K., . . . Ory, M. G. (2017). Dissemination of chronic disease self-management education (CDSME) programs in the United States: Intervention delivery by rurality. *International Journal of Environmental Research and Public Health, 14*(6), 638–652.

Stewart, H., Jameson, J. P., & Curtin, L. (2015). The relationship between stigma and self-reported willingness to use mental health services among rural and urban older adults. *Psychological Services, 12*(2), 141–148.

Syed, S. T., Gerber, B. S., & Sharp, L. K. (2013). Traveling towards disease: Transportation barriers to health care access. *Journal of Community Health, 38*(5), 976–993.

Taylor, Z. E., & Ruiz, Y. (2017). Contextual stressors and the mental health outcomes of Latino children in rural migrant-farmworker families in the midwest. *Journal of Rural Mental Health, 41*(4), 284–298.

United States, Health Resources and Services Administration. (2018, August). *HRSA health center program.* Retrieved from https://bphc.hrsa.gov/about/healthcenterfactsheet.pdf

U.S. Department of Health and Human Services. (2011). Rural behavioral health programs and promising practices. Retrieved from https://www.hrsa.gov/sites/default/files/ruralhealth/pdf/ruralbehavioralmanual05312011.pdf

Vasquez, M. J. T. (2012). Psychology and social justice: Why we do what we do. *American Psychologist, 67*(5), 337–346.

Vega, W. A., Rodriguez, M. A., & Ang, A. (2010). Addressing stigma of depression in Latino primary care patients. *General Hospital Psychiatry, 32*(2), 182–191.

Vogel, D. L., Wade, N. G., & Haake, S. (2006). Measuring the self-stigma associated with seeking psychological help. *Journal of Counseling Psychology, 53*(3), 325.

Wang, P. S., Lane M., Olfson M., Pincus, H. A., Wells, K. B., & Kessler, R. C. (2005). Twelve-month use of mental health services in the United States: Results from the National Comorbidity Study Replication. *Archives of General Psychiatry, 62*, 629–640.

Willging, C. E., Salvador, M., & Kano, M. (2006). Brief reports: Unequal treatment: Mental health care for sexual and gender minority groups in a rural state. *Psychiatric Services, 57*(6), 867–870.

Wood, J. A. V., Miller, T. W., & Hargrove, D. S. (2005). Clinical supervision in rural settings: A telehealth model. *Professional Psychology: Research and Practice, 36*(2), 173–179.

Yu, S. Y., Hill, C., Ricks, M. L., Bennet, J., & Oriol, N. E. (2017). The scope and impact of mobile health clinics in the United States: A literature review. *International Journal for Equity in Health, 16*, 1–12.

11

Responding to the Mental Health Needs of Underserved Latin Americans

Héctor Fernández-Álvarez, Maria del Pilar Grazioso, Diana Kirszman, Meri Lubina, and Rodney Goodyear

Latin America extends from Tierra del Fuego in Argentina in the south to the U.S.–Mexican border in the north and includes several Caribbean islands. Access to mental health services in this vast region ranges from exceptionally good, at least for the middle class (e.g., Buenos Aires has the highest concentration of psychotherapists in the world; Alonso & Klinar, 2014), to very poor, which is the circumstance for much of the population. Yet the need for those services is strong given the effects that endemic poverty and the histories of colonization and racism (Wade, 2010) as well as war, violence, and even genocide (Oettler, 2006) have had on Latin Americans' mental health. The World Bank (2015) identified regional, poor mental health as an obstacle to Latin American economic development.

This chapter begins with a brief overview of mental health care needs in the region and the barriers to addressing those needs. It discusses the importance of cultural competence and evidence-based practices and the attention placed on them. It then presents the work that is carried out by one nongovernmental organization, Fundación Aiglé (in English, "Aiglé Foundation"), to address some of these issues and concludes with suggestions that further address the needs of underserved Latin Americans.

The Scope and Description of the Problem

By focusing on a region as large as Latin America, our perspective is necessarily more molar than that of the authors of the other chapters in this volume. They focus, for example, on specific underserved subpopulations, including racial and ethnic minorities, war civilians and refugees, immigrants, and rural populations. But all of these subpopulations, and more, are encompassed within Latin

America. Therefore, it makes sense to focus in this section on several of the more pervasive factors affecting the mental health of Latin Americans.

Affluence level is one of those. The average annual income for the countries in this region is below the world average (Central Intelligence Agency, 2018), and poverty is significantly associated with common mental disorders (Lund et al., 2010). In fact, this association between poverty and mental health has been confirmed in studies conducted in Latin America, including those in Chile (Araya, Rojas, Fritsch, Acuna, & Lewis, 2001) and in Colombia (Harpham, Snoxell, Grant, & Rodriguez, 2005).

Violence also has been a pervading factor, although the type of violence and the extent to which people have been traumatized by it varies by country or subregion. Some violence has occurred through systematic political repression or civil war, as was the case, for example, in Argentina's "dirty war" (Suarez-Orozco, 1991; 30,000 killed); in the decades-long, genocidal persecution of indigenous people in Guatemala (Oettler, 2006; 200,000 killed); and in the El Salvadoran civil war (75,000 killed). Other violence has been the result of lawlessness: With 8% of the world's population, Latin America accounts for about a third of its murders (Luhnow, 2018).

Finally, Latin America is a region that continues to address the consequences of its history of conquests of indigenous peoples and slavery of people of African descent. Wade (2010) observed that "Indigenous people and Africans . . . had different locations in the colonial order, both socially and conceptually. Indigenous people were, officially, to be protected as well as exploited; Africans were slaves" (p. 26). But the oppression that both groups experienced has left a legacy of what Brave Heart, Chase, Elkins, and Altschul (2011) have termed "historical trauma," with its associated sequelae.

Barriers to Service Delivery

Affluence levels affect not only the prevalence of common mental disorders but also treatment availability, through both the ability of individuals to pay for services and the adequacy of their countries' treatment infrastructures. Saxena, Thornicroft, Knapp, and Whiteford (2007) observe, for example, that comprehensive mental health systems with balanced community-based and hospital resources tend to be present in higher-income countries where financial resources have been matched as well by political will. But few Latin American countries have achieved this. Most, in fact, devote more than 50% of their generally small mental health budgets to psychiatric hospitals (Pan American Health Association [PAHA], 2013).

Some progress has been made in response to the 1990 Caracas Declaration that delegates of 11 Latin American nations adopted (Levav, Restrepo, & de Macedo, 1994). It called for reducing reliance on psychiatric hospitals as the primary means of psychiatric treatment and instead developing a more comprehensive network of providers focusing to a greater extent on prevention. Caldas de Almeida and Horvitz-Lennon (2010) report that by 2005, and largely in response to that Declaration, three fourths of the countries reporting in the region had a national mental health plan and had enacted mental health legislation. But despite this progress, they also report that in Latin America "59% of people with depression, 64% of people with bipolar disorder, 63% of people with anxiety disorders, and 37% of people with nonaffective psychoses do not have access to any kind of mental health treatment, either in primary or specialty care settings" (p. 220).

One contributor to this treatment gap is the limited availability of mental health service providers. PAHA (2013) reported, for example, that there were only 1.2 psychiatrists per 100,000 people in Central America, Mexico, and the Latin Caribbean and 2.9 per 100,000 in South America. This contrasts with the United States or the United Kingdom, where the ratios are 12.4/100,000 and 14.6/100,000 respectively (World Health Organization, 2014).

In response, some universities have developed multipronged initiatives to increase the availability of service providers. For example, the Universidad del Valle de Guatemala (with which two of this chapter's authors are affiliated) has developed undergraduate programs in psychology and graduate training programs in counseling and counseling psychology. Those programs prepare practitioners to deliver culturally responsive treatment services. Graduates are prepared as well to work with local and indigenous communities to develop prevention programs. Moreover, and consistent with the university's community empowerment perspective, faculty have developed a train-the-trainers program that enables those communities to increase treatment capacity by preparing and overseeing the work of paraprofessionals. Multipronged, university-based initiatives such as these can be an important means for increasing treatment access in the region.

Finally, poverty and the relatively lower education levels across the region (see Cruces, Domenech, & Gasparini, 2014) affect attitudes about mental illness and the extent to which people attach stigma to receiving treatment. These attitudes reduce help-seeking behavior (Saxena et al., 2007). Andrade et al. (2014), for example, concluded from their study of people in 24 countries that the two biggest barriers to treatment seeking are low perceived need and attitudinal barriers. They suggested population-level initiatives to increase mental health literacy.

Creating Cultural Competency

Multicultural competence (Fouad et al., 2009) is essential to all psychotherapy, but it is especially so in Latin America, with its very large range of racial, ethnic, and cultural groups (Arredondo et al., 2014). That importance is underscored by the strong empirical link between multicultural competence and both treatment effectiveness and strength of the working alliance (Tao, Owen, Pace, & Imel, 2015).

Yet the dominant psychotherapy models have been largely imported from other countries or regions. For example, Argentinian psychotherapists have relied primarily on European models, particularly psychoanalysis, whereas psychotherapists in other regions of Latin America, particularly Central America, have been much more influenced by North American models (Fernández Álvarez, Grazioso, & Kirszman, 2018). Bernal and Sáez-Santiago (2006) make the important argument, though, for ensuring that treatments for Latina/o populations are culturally centered. Their own culturally centered model attends to such dimensions as language, concepts, metaphors and idioms, and the client's social and cultural contexts. Both liberation psychology and the model development efforts of Fundación Aiglé address dimensions in this model.

Liberation Psychology

Liberation psychology is focused on Bernal and Sáez-Santiago's dimension of social and cultural contexts. It was developed, in fact, as a response to the effects that various forms of oppression had on Latin Americans' mental health, effects to which available models of psychotherapy were giving too little attention.

Ignacio Martín-Baró is credited as liberation psychology's originator (Marín, 1991). The lesson he took from his experiences in the community as a Jesuit priest and from his exposure to the Latin American Catholic Church's liberation theology movement was that mental illness often is a result of a group's history of oppression (Tate, Rivera, Brown, & Skaistis, 2014). Although he was trained as a social psychologist, he concluded that Western psychology was limited in what it could offer poor, oppressed people.

Martín-Baró and his contemporaries developed a new epistemology (Martín-Baró, 1994) that assumed an equivalence between power and knowledge, with knowledge enabling people to gain control of their own existence and capabilities. Clients learn "not only what reality is, but what it is not, and within it, work towards what it should be" (Martín-Baro, 2006, p. 12). People achieve this new perspective on reality by deconstructing the messages that the dominant social structures (churches, schools, the media, and so on) deliver about the nature of their world. Liberation psychologists assert that helping oppressed people requires an explicitly political stance. This might mean, for example, that a psychotherapist would discuss with clients the political contexts in which they live, the effects of those contexts on them and others, and kinds of advocacy and social action that might be both possible and appropriate.

A Salvadoran counter-insurgency unit assassinated Martín-Baró and seven others in 1989. Yet his ideas have continued to affect practice, especially by community psychologists (e.g., Kagan, Burton, Duckett, Lawthom, & Siddiquee, 2011). Liberation psychology can offer valuable insights for psychotherapists anywhere, particularly for those working with oppressed populations. Its perspective requires sensitivity to the effects that power and politics have on clients and a commitment to making societies more just. Comas-Díaz, Lykes, and Alarcón (1998) also would admonish psychotherapists to engage in self-reflection and to learn to "think culturally about their own social situatedness as professionals, contributing to the recognition of their own limitations due to training and their own positions as powerful others" (p. 785). This means identifying their blind spots related to values, politics, and oppression; gaining new understandings of the impact of economic and ecological injustice; and making a commitment to revisiting dominant discourse (Burton, 2015).

Fundación Aiglé's Focus on Cultural Competence

Fundación Aiglé's founders were and remain heavily influenced by principles of liberation psychology, which are embedded in the organizational model and which inform many of its goals and initiatives. When Aiglé's members enter the Clinical Assistential Network, they commit both to devoting some portion of their time to providing services to people with limited social and financial resources and to developing and maintaining multicultural competence.

Aiglé's premise is that the most effective psychotherapists in Latin America will work from a model that is both culturally responsive to clients and sufficiently flexible to adapt to their needs, values, and expectations. Aiglé's signature treatment model, the integrative model of psychotherapy (MIP for its initials in Spanish; Fernández-Álvarez, 2008), responds to those criteria. The model was developed with international visits and input from, among others, John Norcross, Michael Lambert, and Larry Beutler. That input always has been tempered by an awareness of the unique characteristics and needs of our Latin American clientele.

The MIP continually evolves, informed by experience with clients and by emerging research. Aiglé supports that research by its participation in the practice-oriented research global movement (see Youn, Xiao, & Castonguay,

2016). Aiglé's journal and recent publications attest to our participation in these research initiatives.

It is important to note that research-based treatment innovations from other countries do not always apply in Latin America. For example, U.S.- and European-derived empirically supported treatments are not always compatible with the beliefs and worldviews of the primarily rural and ethnically diverse populations we serve. They also do not address the social justice and advocacy stances that are essential to adequately address the needs of the underserved in the region. These points provide a useful segue, then, to the next section, which addresses the meaning and importance of empirically supported treatments in the Latin American context.

Effective Strategies and Empirically-Supported Treatments

Models of treatment do not appreciably differ from one another in effectiveness (Benish, Imel, & Wampold, 2008; Wampold & Imel, 2015), but psychotherapists themselves do. Some consistently outperform their counterparts—and, more worrisome, some have a higher-than-average number of their clients deteriorate during treatment with them (see, e.g., Goldberg et al., 2016; Okiishi, Lambert, Nielsen, & Ogles, 2003). One of the more important predictors of psychotherapists' effectiveness is their ability to establish strong alliances with their clients. In fact, the best psychotherapists establish strong alliances across a broader range of clients than other psychotherapists (Baldwin, Wampold, & Imel, 2007).

A number of factors contribute to quality of the therapeutic alliance. One that we noted earlier was client-perceived multicultural competence (Tao et al., 2015). Another is the ability to provide clients with a rationale for treatment that is congruent with their values and beliefs, and then to use rituals or techniques consistent with that treatment rationale (see Wampold & Imel, 2015). Comas-Diaz (2006) was implicitly speaking to this point when she argued for adapting our dominant models of psychotherapy so that they are consistent with Latino clients' expectations and values. The MIP is one such adaptation.

Psychotherapists who use the MIP employ a constructivist epistemology to understand client problems and then design tailored treatment plans (Fernández-Álvarez, Consoli, & Gómez, 2016). The model's primary emphasis is cognitive behavioral, though it also integrates psychodynamic, humanistic-existential, and systemic elements and stresses cultural competence. The interventions focus on developing coping strategies, contingency management, skills training, and other resources that allow clients to readily transfer changes into daily decision making. These strategies are designed to take into consideration the client's resources and expectations.

Psychotherapists in Aiglé's treatment network employ the MIP, which also is taught in the training programs that Aiglé offers and through consultation and supervision. In the next section, we describe Aiglé, its mission, and the use of the MIP in one program that was explicitly designed to address the treatment needs of underserved populations.

Supervision is a key mechanism in Aiglé's workforce development efforts (Fernández-Alvarez et al., 2019) and therefore the dissemination of the MIP. Aiglé-trained psychologists supervise graduate students in the postgraduate training program that the Universidad Nacional de Mar del Plata runs in collaboration with Aiglé. That program has cohorts of up to 35 students, graduates about 250 students per year, and now has approximately 2,000 alumni. Faculty in that program are psychologists who have been trained with the MIP. All psychotherapists who have participated in Aiglé training and who belong to the Fundación Aiglé Assistance Network are encouraged to join a supervision group network in which they receive MIP-focused supervision in groups of three to six practitioners via videoconferencing for a predetermined time (e.g., one or two years).

Aiglé's Therapeutic Assistance Program for People with Limited Resources

We have been discussing Fundación Aiglé but have not yet described it in detail. Aiglé is a nongovernmental organization that now is in its 42nd year of providing direct service, training mental health professionals (see, e.g., Fernández Álvarez et al., 2018), and facilitating clinical research. *Aiglé* is "a classical Greek word that means 'shining,' 'radiant,' or even 'illumination' " (Gómez & Esnal, 2015, p. 9) and is the name for the torch that Olympic athletes carry. It is sketched as an image, the torch of life, providing clients with a sign that despite their problems, they eventually can reach a place of peace. To kindle this light, relational connections are required as well as encouraging spirituality in oneself and others.

Based in Buenos Aires, Fundación Aiglé has developed an increasingly wider reach by way of networks and affiliates across Latin America and in Spain. The Aiglé Guatemala Project (Proyecto Aiglé Guatemala in Spanish) in Guatemala City is an affiliated organization that provides treatment and outreach services and maintains an ongoing commitment to training and research. Aiglé also partners with several universities, including the Universidad del Valle de Guatemala, offering graduate training at the master's and doctoral level, and the Universidad

Nacional de Mar del Plata, with which it has maintained a training program that is now offered both online across Latin America and in 10 cities in Argentina.

During the past 20 years, Aiglé has capitalized on its training and service networks to provide mental health services to vulnerable populations in communities with limited resources and restricted services through PATER. PATER is a program named for the Spanish-language acronym for Therapeutic Assistance Program for People with Limited Resources. It was born of Aiglé professionals' shared commitment to addressing the needs of these vulnerable populations. Although PATER clients are expected to pay a minimal fee, no one is turned away because of inability to pay.

The public mental health services networks in Argentina and in the region have limited resources and so attend primarily to emergencies and acute situations related to severe psychopathology. PATER works in concert with and as a complement to that public system by (a) providing services to low-income people who would profit from psychotherapy and (b) referring clients who present with severe and acute problems. Client referrals come primarily through collaborative agreements with nongovernmental groups, including community help organizations that offer services to orphans, victims of maltreatment and abuse, hospices, and churches.

Aiglé staff constantly market PATER and other of its programs through presentations in the community and via social media. This includes visits to institutions with residential populations (e.g., hospices, residences for minors and youth who have suffered abuse or maltreatment) as well as agencies that serve underprivileged persons who need ambulatory psychological help. Aiglé also distributes two online publications without cost, both as a public service and as a marketing strategy: One is a magazine that targets the social service community with mental health–focused articles (www.revistaandaresaigle.org); the other is a professional journal that targets psychologists (*Revista Argentina de Clínica Psicológica*; http://www.clinicapsicologica.org.ar/index.php).

Students in the Aiglé /Universidad Nacional de Mar del Plata graduate program treat approximately 60% of the PATER clients during their practic. Other psychotherapists in the Aiglé network, most of whom have been trained in Aiglé programs, treat the remaining 40%. Because supervision is a foundational component of PATER, all psychotherapists are supervised, whether they are students or practicing clinicians. Depending on their level of training and whether they are trained on site or online, trainees participate in supervision through group, live, distance (with the use of technology), and peer supervision. They participate much less frequently in one-on-one supervision, usually in response to critical or urgent situations. Furthermore, supervision of supervisors' sessions is included in the program. Psychotherapists report that their participation in PATER enriches their clinical experiences by putting them in contact with people whose social circumstances and cultural backgrounds often differ from those of the clients with whom they otherwise work.

Client Assessment

Demand for PATER services often exceeds capacity, so decisions are made to balance the needs of those seeking help against available treatment resources. This demands effective screening processes, beginning with an assessment of clients' subjective distress and problem severity to determine the program can address their needs. That admissions assessment relies both on clinical observation and the use of standardized instruments, focused initially on determining whether clients meet our criterion of demonstrating moderate to severe levels of dysfunction. Fundación Aiglé encourages those who exhibit only minor dysfunction to seek help in a different type of agency. It also initiates measures to offer security for those who are at high risk, typically connecting them directly with appropriate public psychiatric services. When a client seems suited for psychotherapeutic intervention, additional assessment is conducted that includes a more extensive psychological evaluation, complementary medical assessments, and a social assessment by an Aiglé social worker.

Most tests and inventories in our psychological batteries have strong psychometric properties; however, few have been standardized in Latin America, which forces us to work cautiously. We have made it a priority to culturally adapt those measures for use in our countries, re-standardizing them when possible. This has been the case of the SCL-90, the Beck Depression Inventory II, and others. Furthermore, we have developed our own adaptations with the Inventory of Interpersonal Problems (Horowitz, Rosenberg, Baer, Ureño, & Villaseñor, 1988) and the Dimensional Approach to Personality Pathology (Livesly, 2006). We have also developed some measures, such as an instrument to assess hypochondria.

Treatment

PATER's goals are to improve clients' functioning and increase their competencies in personal, social, and work interactions. We initially contract to work with clients for up to 15 sessions, conducted in intervals determined by each client's needs. Clients may leave treatment sooner if they reach their goals in fewer sessions but are informed that they have the option of returning later to complete their allotted number of sessions if that should be necessary. Treatment can be extended for an additional 15 sessions if the client has been progressing but has not yet achieved the treatment goals after the initial 15 sessions. Thirty sessions is the expected maximum for any client. Should more extended treatment be needed, there is a case review and the client may be referred to another Aiglé program or to another agency. We do our best to screen at the outset but sometimes miss client problems that would dictate longer treatment. Also, clients sometimes encounter unanticipated life circumstances that prolong the need for treatment.

We monitor all client treatment using the OQ-45.2 (Lambert, 2015). We have conducted research to adapt this instrument to our context, and so we have a measure with solid psychometric properties. If the client's initial score is greater than the cut score (50), the OQ is administered every three sessions. If the score is less than 50, it is administered every five sessions. Therapists use the OQ data to monitor therapeutic process, supported by their supervisors, who routinely use those data in supervision. We also conduct an assessment at the end of treatment and at a later follow-up.

Psychotherapists use the MIP as their treatment approach. They supplement their treatment with a psychoeducation program that is tailored to the client's needs and requires the client to complete assignments between sessions. Our treatment approach has evolved over the two decades we have offered this program. For example, PATER therapists initially used a manualized approach, but it was later modified to allow them to tailor their work to a particular client's needs and to draw from a broader range of techniques than the manualized treatment had allowed. We also have capitalized on technological advances as they have occurred, incorporating into our treatment, for example, the use of texting, videoconferencing, and apps such as WhatsApp (see Fernández-Álvarez et al., 2019). We anticipate that these technologies will enable us to continue to expand PATER to reach more clients.

Unique Features of Working with PATER Clients

PATER clients experience barriers to participating in treatment that our more typical, privileged clients usually do not. For example, transportation problems and difficulties obtaining the necessary time off from work or from other responsibilities can affect their attendance. Their often-turbulent life circumstances can also redirect their attention from the work of psychotherapy. We have found as a result that psychotherapists must be prepared to work with and around these barriers and to invest additional effort to sustain clients' adherence to treatment. Dealing with these and other issues that PATER clients present can also elicit countertransference (e.g., becoming impatient or perhaps overprotective) that the required supervision can help therapists to manage.

We have found, too, that PATER clients can confuse the processes and goals of our services with those of agencies that provide humanitarian aid or social assistance. That can affect both their participation and their levels of satisfaction. It has become important, then, for us to explicitly educate them about what to expect in their psychotherapy.

Program Impacts

We treat approximately 300 clients per year through PATER. Although this is miniscule compared to those who need treatment, it still represents 300 people (and, over a 20-year period, many more) who otherwise would not have been served. But we believe that the value of the program extends beyond what its clients receive. In particular, PATER provides a model that other nongovernmental agencies in Latin America can adapt to their own circumstances. It is also having demonstrable effects on how psychotherapy is practiced: The MIP has become broadly adopted across Latin America, and the cultural responsiveness that is at its core has been informed, and is continually refined, by our experiences with PATER.

Variations of PATER have had important local impacts and the potential as well to be models for other programs. For example, in 2013 Fundacion Aiglé conducted a needs assessment among the population served by Fundacion Pobre de Asis (a community agency) that led us in 2014 to develop and implement a social skills training program. This program targets unemployed adults older than 40 years who are under significant economic and social constraints so they can rejoin the workforce. It focuses on enhancing clients' interpersonal and communication competencies and helping them to become more effective at resolving conflicts, particularly those related to power and hierarchical relationships. The program helps clients to differentiate among passive, aggressive, and assertive behaviors and teaches social skills in public situations and relational skills (Michelson, 1987).

PATER clients often have been marginalized, are vulnerable, lack resources, and are from cultures different from our own. For example, more PATER clients are from immigrant backgrounds than is true of those who receive Aiglé's other services. An advantage of requiring supervision for all therapists is the opportunities it has afforded Fundación Aiglé's leadership to be reflective about how these factors of marginalization, resource deficits, and diverse cultures affect treatment and to develop deeper understandings of how we can be more responsive to them. We also have recognized how important a stance of cultural humility is to the quality of the therapist–client relationships (Hook, Davis, Owen, Worthington, & Utsey, 2013). We are committed to ensuring that we transmit these evolving understandings of cultural competence to students in the Aiglé-affiliated graduate programs and to all PATER therapists through the supervision we require.

Training and supervision follows Comas-Díaz, Lykes, and Alarcón's (1998) advice and helps supervisees develop greater self-awareness about their motivations for working with underserved populations, as well as their values and attitudes. This requires that they be open to leaving their comfort zones and to revising their personal and professional identities.

Future Steps

Psychotherapy continues to have promise for underserved populations in Latin America. But for that promise to be realized, clients must have access to treatment and mechanisms must be in place to support the therapists who provide those services. Many psychotherapists are required to travel, sometimes considerable distances, to work with these vulnerable populations, and the compensation is typically low. Although younger professionals might be drawn to this work as a social commitment, their motivation or ability to continue doing so tends to diminish over time.

These and other barriers to access to quality mental health services in Latin America ultimately must be addressed at national policy levels, taking into consideration the wide diversity that vulnerable populations entail. This would include, for example, developing adequate and relevant, cultural, treatment infrastructures as well as national and regional workforce development programs that select and train therapists who value and pursue cultural competence as well as cultural humility. But until those policies and stances begin to have an appreciable impact, the most significant initiatives are likely to come from nongovernmental organizations or training programs that are committed to addressing underserved populations following social justice and transformative paradigms.

Most of us on this writing team are affiliated with Aiglé (and two were founders), which was established during a period of turmoil and political repression in Argentina. In the decades since, we have been witness to the struggles of many Latin Americans, including those related to humanitarian crises, poverty, and the demoralizing weight of prejudice and injustice. It is our hope, then, that what we have learned in offering PATER will be useful as a model that other nongovernmental organizations, professionals, and training programs can adapt to their own circumstances.

We also hope that the workforce development we provide through our publications, graduate training programs, and supervision networks will provide useful models as well. And finally, we hope that our MIP (Fernández-Alvarez,

2008) will not only be useful in its own right, but also stimulate the development of other treatment models that are responsive to Latin American clients' needs.

References

Alonso, M. M., & Klinar, D. (2014). *Los psicólogos en argentina. Relevamiento cuantitativo 2013* [Psychologists in Argentina. Quantitative Survey 2013]. VI Congreso Internacional de Investigación y Práctica Profesional en Psicología XXI Jornadas de Investigación Décimo Encuentro de Investigadores en Psicología del MERCOSUR. Facultad de Psicología—Universidad de Buenos Aires.

Andrade, L. H., Alonso, J., Mneimneh, Z., Wells, J. E., Al-Hamzawi, A., Borges, G., . . . Florescu, S. (2014). Barriers to mental health treatment: Results from the WHO world mental health surveys. *Psychological Medicine, 44*(6), 1303–1317.

Araya, R., Rojas, G., Fritsch, R., Acuña, J., & Lewis, G. (2001). Common mental disorders in Santiago, Chile: Prevalence and socio-demographic correlates. *British Journal of Psychiatry, 178*(3), 228–233.

Arredondo, P., Gallardo-Cooper, M., Delgado-Romero, E. A., & Zapata, A. L. (2014). *Culturally responsive counseling with Latinas/os*. Alexandria, VA: American Counseling Association.

Baldwin, S. A., Wampold, B. E., & Imel, Z. E. (2007). Untangling the alliance–outcome correlation: Exploring the relative importance of therapist and patient variability in the alliance. *Journal of Consulting and Clinical Psychology, 75*, 842–852.

Benish, S. G., Imel, Z. E., & Wampold, B. E. (2008). The relative efficacy of bona fide psychotherapies for treating post-traumatic stress disorder: A meta-analysis of direct comparisons. *Clinical Psychology Review, 28*(5), 746–758.

Bernal, G., & Sáez-Santiago, E. (2006). Culturally centered psychosocial interventions. *Journal of Community Psychology, 34*(2), 121–132.

Brave Heart, M. Y. H., Chase, J., Elkins, J., & Altschul, D. B. (2011). Historical trauma among indigenous peoples of the Americas: Concepts, research, and clinical considerations. *Journal of Psychoactive Drugs, 43*(4), 282–290.

Burton, M. (2015). Economy and planet: A blind spot for community psychology? *Universitas Psychologica, 14*(4), 1339–1345.

Caldas de Almeida, J. M., & Horvitz-Lennon, M. (2010). Mental health care reforms in Latin America: An overview of mental health care reforms in Latin America and the Caribbean. *Psychiatric Services, 61*(3), 218–221.

Central Intelligence Agency. (2018). *World fact book*. Retrieved from https://www.cia.gov/library/publications/the-world-factbook/rankorder/2004rank.html

Comas-Diaz, L. (2006). Latino healing: The integration of ethnic psychology into psychotherapy. *Psychotherapy: Theory, Research, Practice, Training, 43*(4), 436–453.

Comas-Díaz, L., Lykes, M. B., & Alarcón, R. D. (1998). Ethnic conflict and the psychology of liberation in Guatemala, Peru, and Puerto Rico. *American Psychologist, 53*(7), 778–792.

Cruces, G., Domenech, C. G., & Gasparini, L. (2014). *Inequality in education: Evidence for Latin America*. Documento de Trabajo, No. 135, Universidad Nacional de La Plata, Centro de Estudios Distributivos, Laborales y Sociales (CEDLAS), La Plata. Retrieved from https://www.econstor.eu/bitstream/10419/127654/1/cedlas-wp-135.pdf

Fernández-Álvarez, H. (2008). Integration in psychotherapy: An approach from Argentina. *Journal of Psychotherapy Integration*, *18*(1), 79–86.

Fernández-Álvarez, H., Consoli, A. J., & Gómez, B. (2016). Integration in psychotherapy: Reasons and challenges. *American Psychologist*, *71*(8), 820–830.

Fernández Álvarez, H., Grazioso, M., & Kirszman, D. (2018). Distance supervision in the Aiglé Foundation's Latin American psychotherapy training program. *Journal of Clinical Psychology/In Session*, *75*(2), 282–291.

Goldberg, S. B., Rousmaniere, T., Miller, S. D., Whipple, J., Nielson, S. L., Hoyt, W. T., & Wampold, B. E. (2016). Do psychotherapists improve with time and experience? A longitudinal analysis of outcomes in a clinical setting. *Journal of Counseling Psychology*, *63*, 1–11.

Gómez, B., & Esnal, J. (2015). Sculpting psychotherapy integration in Argentina: The Aiglé Project 1977–2016. *Psychotherapy Bulletin*, *50*(4), 9–13.

Harpham, T., Snoxell, S., Grant, E., & Rodriguez, C. (2005). Common mental disorders in a young urban population in Colombia. *British Journal of Psychiatry*, *187*(2), 161–167.

Hook, J. N., Davis, D. E., Owen, J., Worthington Jr, E. L., & Utsey, S. O. (2013). Cultural humility: Measuring openness to culturally diverse clients. *Journal of Counseling Psychology*, *60*(3), 353–366.

Horowitz, L. M., Rosenberg, S. E., Baer, B. A., Ureño, G., & Villaseñor, V. S. (1988). Inventory of Interpersonal Problems: Psychometric properties and clinical applications. *Journal of Consulting and Clinical Psychology*, *56*(6), 885–892.

Kagan, C., Burton, M., Duckett, P., Lawthom, R., & Siddiquee, A. (2011). *Critical community psychology*. Chichester, West Sussex, UK: Wiley.

Lambert, M. J. (2015). Progress feedback and the OQ-system: The past and the future. *Psychotherapy*, *52*(4), 381–390.

Levav, I., Restrepo, H., & de Macedo, C. G. (1994). The restructuring of psychiatric care in Latin America: A new policy for mental health services. *Journal of Public Health Policy*, *15*(1), 71–85.

Livesley, W. J. (2006). The Dimensional Assessment of Personality Pathology (DAPP) approach to personality disorder. In S. Strack (Ed.), *Differentiating normal and abnormal personality* (2nd ed., pp. 401–425). New York, NY: Springer.

Luhnow, D. (2018, Sept. 20). Latin America is the murder capital of the world. *Wall Street Journal*. Retrieved from https://www.wsj.com/articles/400-murders-a-day-the-crisis-of-latin-america-1537455390

Lund, C., Breen, A., Flisher, A. J., Kakuma, R., Corrigall, J., Joska, J. A., . . . Patel, V. (2010). Poverty and common mental disorders in low- and middle-income countries: A systematic review. *Social Science & Medicine*, *71*(3), 517–528.

Marín, G. (1991). Ignacio Martín-Baró, S. J. (1942–1989): Obituary. *American Psychologist*, *46*(5), 532.

Martín-Baró, I. (1994). *Writings for a liberation psychology*. Cambridge, MA: Harvard University Press.

Martín-Baró, I. (2006). Hacia una psicología de la liberación. *Psicología Sin Fronteras: Revista Electrónica de Intervención Psicosocial y Psicología Comunitaria*, *1*(2), 7–14.

Michelson, L. (1987). *Las habilidades sociales en la infancia [Social habilities in childhood]*. Madrid, Spain: Martinez Roca.

Oettler, A. (2006). *Guatemala in the 1980s: A genocide turned into ethnocide?* German Institute of Global and Area Studies Working Paper 19. Retrieved from https://www.econstor.eu/bitstream/10419/47795/1/605209480.pdf

Okiishi, J., Lambert, M. J., Nielsen, S. L., & Ogles, B. M. (2003). Waiting for supershrink: An empirical analysis of therapist effects. *Clinical Psychology & Psychotherapy, 10*(6), 361–373.

Pan American Health Organization. (2013). *WHO-AIMS: Report on mental health systems in Latin America and the Caribbean*. Washington, DC: World Health Organization. Retrieved from https://www.paho.org/hq/dmdocuments/2013/ENG-WHOAIMSREG-(For-Web-Apr-2013).pdf

Saxena, S., Thornicroft, G., Knapp, M., & Whiteford, H. (2007). Resources for mental health: Scarcity, inequity, and inefficiency. *Lancet, 370*(9590), 878–889.

Suarez-Orozco, M. M. (1991). The heritage of enduring a" dirty war:" Psychosocial aspects of terror in Argentina, 1976–1988. *Journal of Psychohistory, 18*(4), 469–505.

Tao, K. W., Owen, J., Pace, B. T., & Imel, Z. E. (2015). A meta-analysis of multicultural competencies and psychotherapy process and outcome. *Journal of Counseling Psychology, 62*(3), 337–350.

Tate, K. A., Rivera, E. T., Brown, E. M., & Skaistis, L. (2014). Foundations for liberation: Social justice, liberation psychology, and counseling. *Revista Interamericana de Psicologia/Interamerican Journal of Psychology, 47*(3), 373–382.

Wade, P. (2010). *Race and ethnicity in Latin America*. New York, NY: Pluto Press.

Wampold, B. E., & Imel, Z. E. (2015). *The great psychotherapy debate: The evidence for what makes psychotherapy work*. New York, NY: Routledge.

World Bank. (2015). *Poor mental health, an obstacle to development in Latin America* Retrieved from http://www.worldbank.org/en/news/feature/2015/07/13/bad-mental-health-obstacle-development-latin-america

World Health Organization. (2014). *Global Health Observatory data repository*. Retrieved from http://apps.who.int/gho/data/node.main.MHHR?lang=en

Youn, S. J., Xiao, H., & Castonguay, L. G. (2016). Practice oriented research: Clinical implications and benefits. *Psychotherapy Bulletin, 51*(1), 24–26.

SECTION 4

OVERLOOKED OR “INVISIBLE” PEOPLES

12
Delivering Mental Health Services to Children and Adolescents

Ric G. Steele

The Scope and Description of the Problem

Recent survey and epidemiological data indicate that as many as 20% of children and adolescents in the United States have a mental, behavioral, or developmental disorder that causes significant impairment (Angold et al., 2002; Bitsko et al., 2016; Merikangas et al., 2010). These figures are generally consistent with worldwide estimates of child and adolescent mental health problems (Costello, Egger, & Angold, 2005; Polanczyk, Salum, Sugaya, Caye, & Rohde, 2015). Further, approximately half of the lifetime cases of mental health disorders in the United States originate before the age of 14, and three quarters originate before the age of 24 (Kessler et al., 2005). Mental health concerns that develop during childhood or adolescence are among the costliest in the World Health Organization's estimates of the global burden of disease (see Costello et al., 2005). Thus, the accurate identification and treatment of mental health disorders in children and adolescents is critical.

Despite the relatively high proportion of children and adolescents with significant mental health needs, the number of youths receiving psychological or mental health services remains low (Gudiño, Lau, Yeh, McCabe, & Hough, 2009). For example, in a large sample of rural adolescents, Angold et al. (2002) reported that about 36% of those with mental health diagnoses had received mental health care within the past three months. Similarly, Merikangas et al. (2010, 2011) reported that between one half and one third of children and adolescents with identified diagnosed mental disorders had accessed mental health services in the past year. Children and adolescents with externalizing problems (e.g., attention-deficit/hyperactivity disorder [ADHD], behavioral problems) were more likely to receive services than adolescents with other disorders (e.g., anxiety, eating disorders, substance use disorders).

Barriers to Service Delivery

The literature identifies a number of structural, perceptual, and contextual barriers to mental health care for youths (Reardon et al., 2017). Unlike adults, who may seek mental health services when they deem them necessary, children and adolescents are usually dependent on adult caregivers (e.g., parents, teachers, other caregivers) to facilitate those services for them. Thus, the agent responsible for the care of the person in need (and not necessarily the person in need of care) is tasked with determining whether and how to access services. The addition of this "gatekeeper" (see Stiffman, Pescosolido, & Cabassa, 2004) represents a key difference in how children or adolescents access mental health services and compounds many of the barriers that other underserved groups face.

As described by Owens et al. (2002) and Reardon et al. (2017), *structural barriers* to service utilization for children include lack of insurance coverage, transportation problems, insufficient mental health services in the community, and lack of knowledge of appropriate referral sources. Owens et al. found that about 20% of parents reported at least one structural barrier to mental health services, including expense, distance to services, wait time, or transportation. Other structural barriers include opportunity costs (e.g., missing work to attend child's treatment session), instrumental barriers (e.g., insufficient childcare), and interference with other beneficial activities (e.g., participation on sports teams). As discussed later in this chapter (and at greater length in Chapter 5), such structural barriers may differentially affect children and adolescents from families with lower incomes.

Perceptual barriers include beliefs about the nature and severity of the problem, the acceptability of mental health services (i.e., stigma), and beliefs about the role of psychological services in addressing the identified problem (Owens at al., 2002; Reardon et al., 2017). Because children and youth typically access mental health services through an adult gatekeeper, perceptual barriers may play a particularly significant role in the delivery of psychological services. Owens et al. reported that about one quarter of parents endorsed perceptual barriers related to the problem itself (e.g., "problems were not serious"), and one third reported at least one barrier related to the role of mental health services (e.g., "treatment would not help," "worried about what family/friends would say").

Structural and perceptual barriers may be particularly salient among children and adolescents from ethnic minority communities and among lower-income children and adolescents. For example, Angold et al. (2002) reported that African American adolescents in their sample were roughly half as likely as Caucasian youth to receive specialty mental health services for depressive symptoms. However, they reported that African American youth were just as likely as Caucasian youth to receive mental health care in the school system.

Whether this pattern is due to structural barriers (e.g., economic constraints, access to community-based services) or perceptual barriers (e.g., stigma concerning mental health treatment in the community) cannot be known from the data presented. However, consistent evidence suggests that African American parents hold less positive views about mental health services and report more stigma associated with mental health services than European American parents (e.g., Turner, Jensen-Doss, & Heffer, 2015).

Creating Cultural Competency

Children and adolescents inhabit complex ecological systems in which multiple adults can serve as gatekeepers to various services, including mental health care. Uri Bronfenbrenner is well known for his conceptualization of the ecological systems that can impact youth development as well as health and mental health service delivery (see Steele & Alyward, 2009). Understanding these ecological systems and having the skills necessary to provide services within these contexts represent indispensable cultural competencies for working with children and adolescents. Indeed, these complex and sometimes interacting ecological systems can facilitate or impede effective mental health service delivery, depending on the quality of the communication or coordination of services among different providers/gatekeepers.

Consistent with a cultural competence framework, training guidelines for child and adolescent psychotherapists address the importance of understanding developmental differences that exist within and across individuals in this population, and across developmental domains (social, emotional, cognitive) within individuals (see, e.g., Palermo et al., 2014; Roberts et al., 1998). Although uneven development across domains of functioning can exist among adults, it is more normative to encounter such discrepancies in children and youth. Simeonsson and Rosenthal (2001) noted that "age usually is not a central issue in the provision of psychological services to adults. However, every facet of clinical work with children is influenced by developmental factors" (p. 20). To deliver effective intervention for youths, the clinician must appreciate the specific developmental levels of the client, and how the various systems noted above support or inhibit therapeutic change in the context of developmental level.

Beyond employing a developmental perspective, mental health professionals must also ensure that the interventions they select for clients are effective for the intended population. An ongoing debate is the degree to which cultural adaptations enhance treatment outcomes in clients from ethnic minority groups (see Bernal, Jiménez-Chafey, & Domenech Rodríguez, 2009). Adaptations may include treatment content, structure, and/or delivery (Chu, Leino, Pflum, & Sue,

2016), and there is some evidence that culturally adapted treatments for children are superior to those that are not culturally adapted (e.g., Hall, Ibaraki, Huang, Marti, & Stice, 2016). However, other literature points to equivalent effect sizes between adapted and non-adapted interventions among minority youths (Huey & Polo, 2017).

In light of these equivocal results, psychotherapists must be careful in their approach to selecting culturally sensitive interventions for children and adolescents. In the best case, a psychotherapist will identify a culturally adapted intervention with a strong evidence base that is appropriate for the client's presenting problem(s) (see Huey & Polo, 2017, for examples). However, in the absence of a culturally adapted intervention with a strong evidence base, the use of non-adapted evidence-based interventions is recommended (Huey & Polo, 2008, 2017; Kotchick & Grover, 2008). In such cases, Kotchick and Grover (2008) and Chu et al. (2016) note the importance of taking a flexible approach to treatment delivery, structure, and content while adhering to the active ingredients of the intervention. The psychotherapist should also directly address culture as a context for the client's experience of psychotherapy.

Effective Strategies and Empirically-Supported Treatments

Recent meta-analyses (e.g., Weisz et al., 2017) provide ample evidence of the general efficacy of psychological interventions delivered to children and adolescents, with aggregated effect sizes in the "medium" range, which is generally consistent with effect sizes obtained for pharmacological interventions for youths (Locher et al., 2017). More important than the overall effect size, however, is the degree to which specific treatments "work" for specific presenting problems in children and youths. For example, Weisz et al. (2017) noted significant differences in observed effect sizes across problem type (e.g., ADHD, anxiety, conduct problems, depression) and informant (i.e., child, parent, teacher report). This is not terribly surprising, given that "success" from a child or adolescent's perspective might be quite different from a parent's or teacher's view of "success." Thus, a nuanced look at empirically supported and practice-based programs is necessary to identify the most promising approaches for youth.

Early Childhood (0 to 5)

Most frequently, preschool-aged children are referred to clinic for treatment of disruptive behavior problems, including subclinical behavioral noncompliance, oppositional defiant disorder, disruptive or self-injurious behaviors due to autism spectrum disorder and/or intellectual disabilities, and/or disruptive behavior in school or daycare settings (e.g., biting, hitting). Internalizing problems—though perhaps less common at this age—are also possible and frequently manifest with elements of noncompliance or aggression. Both because of the child's relatively limited metacognitive abilities and because of the specific roles of parents/caregivers in the child's life, behavioral interventions are often selected for this age group.

Generally, behavioral interventions for young children manipulate the environment to change the contingencies surrounding both desired and undesired behaviors. Modeling and direct instruction are often included to help the youngster develop skills necessary to meet developmental milestones or behavioral expectations. Specific behavioral parent management interventions include Helping the Noncompliant Child (McMahon & Forehand, 2003), Parent-Child Interaction Therapy (PCIT; Hembree-Kigin & McNeil, 1995), Defiant Children (Barkley, 1997), and others. Common themes across these approaches include the use of clear directives, positive reinforcement to encourage desired behaviors, and withdrawal of reinforcement (e.g., "time out") to remove or limit the possibility of environmental reinforcement of undesired behaviors. The use of positive reinforcement can also increase child self-esteem and improve parent–child relationships, making these approaches appropriate for disruptive behavior in the context of internalizing problems (i.e., depression, anxiety).

Although perhaps less well documented than behavioral interventions, child-centered play therapy (CCPT) also has support for efficacy among young children (Bratton, Ray, Rhine, & Jones, 2005). Based in Rogerian (client-centered) psychotherapy, CCPT posits that therapeutic change in children is a result of a nonjudgmental relationship (i.e., with the psychotherapist) that will facilitate the child's growth and maturity, enhance the child's mental health and coping skills, and foster the child's self-direction toward fulfilling her or his needs. Bratton et al. reported medium to large effect sizes for CCPT delivered by professionals and parents (i.e., filial therapy) for a range of presentations, including adjustment problems, adaptive behavior deficits, "personality" problems, internalizing symptoms, and some externalizing symptoms.

Middle Childhood (5 to 11)

Like their younger counterparts, youth in middle childhood continue to present with oppositional and disruptive behavior (including early onset conduct disorder) but also frequently present with symptoms of ADHD, anxiety, and depression. Along with the enhanced cognitive, affective, and social competencies and challenges that come with middle childhood, there is a broadening of the range of issues that may be the focus of therapeutic intervention. These new social and cognitive competencies also increase the range of therapeutic techniques that may be effective within this population. Psychotherapists who work with individuals in middle childhood must be prepared to work also with the expanding ecosystems that make up the lives of these youngsters.

Behavioral interventions continue to be appropriate for youths with disruptive behavior in this age group. However, given the expanded range of cognitive and behavioral abilities, as well as the range of environments that elementary school–aged children occupy, behavioral therapy must account for a wider range of possible reinforcers (and punishers) in environments that the psychotherapist and parents do not necessarily control. For example, the Coping Power program (Lochman & Wells, 2004) was originally developed as a school-based universal prevention program for aggressive school-aged children but has since been modified for individual (i.e., child + caregiver) delivery in a clinic setting. Coping Power employs behavioral (e.g., contingency management) and cognitive (e.g., problem solving) strategies to reduce children's propensity toward aggression and to increase pro-social skills. When employed in a group format, sessions afford the opportunity to practice skills with peers, enhancing the ecological validity of the intervention. Cognitive behavioral therapy (CBT) with parental involvement has also proven effective for ADHD symptoms in children (Daley et al., 2014), with better outcomes possible when CBT is accompanied by medical management from a qualified provider (MTA Cooperative Group, 2004). Materials are available to help integrate parents into the therapeutic process (e.g., Barkley, 2013).

Behavioral and cognitive behavioral interventions also can be appropriate for school-aged children presenting with internalizing symptoms (Ewing, Monsen, Thompson, Cartwright-Hatton, & Field, 2015). Treatment approaches such as those described by Kendall and Hedtke (2006), for example, employ cognitive strategies to decrease catastrophic or unrealistic thinking in children and behavioral strategies (e.g., graduated exposure) to address the physiological arousal that accompanies the feared stimulus. Both cognitive (e.g., coping statements) and behavioral (e.g., positive reinforcement) strategies can be valuable for reducing avoidance of the feared stimulus and encouraging adherence to the treatment plan. When using CBT to address anxiety, care must be taken to move at an appropriate therapeutic pace for the child's developmental level, and in designing exposures that generate sufficient (but not overwhelming) anxiety to effect the extinction of the fear response. As with CBT for externalizing problems, parent/caregiver involvement in treatment for anxiety disorders is usually necessary. The parent or caregiver must understand and agree to the treatment model and will assist with the child's exposure exercises during and between sessions.

Consistent with CBT for adults or adolescents with depressive symptoms, CBT for depressed children focuses on the thoughts and schemata that accompany or produce negative affect and restricted behavioral activation (Arnberg & Öst, 2014). One challenge in the implementation of CBT for school-aged children can be the child's metacognitive ability. Younger children and those with more limited abstract reasoning may find some cognitive tasks difficult. However, there is evidence that CBT can decrease negative thoughts and metacognitions in children (Normann, Lønfeldt, Reinholdt-Dunne, & Esbjørn, 2016). Various workbooks (e.g., Stallard, 2002) can provide structure to help youngsters to think about their thoughts and to appreciate the connections between thoughts, feelings, and behaviors. For children whose metacognitive skills may be insufficiently developed for cognitive therapy, Chu, Colognori, Weissman, and Bannon (2009) describe an adaptation of a behavioral activation intervention that may be effective for depressive symptoms.

School-aged children who have experienced abuse, neglect, or trauma may benefit specifically from trauma-focused CBT, which was developed to address the affective, cognitive, and behavioral sequelae of traumatic events (Cohen, Deblinger, Mannarino, & Steer, 2004). Trauma-focused CBT explicitly involves the family system in treatment, both as a means of assisting the child with the treatment components and as a means of contextualizing the traumatic event. Trauma-focused CBT provides opportunities to address specific symptoms of post-traumatic stress that sometimes result from trauma as well as more generalized symptoms of distress, including depressive symptoms. Morina, Koerssen, and Pollet (2016) reported medium to large effect sizes for trauma-focused CBT in comparison to alternative treatments and waitlist control conditions, respectively. Clinicians interested in using trauma-focused CBT can access online training materials through the Medical University of South Carolina (https://tfcbt2.musc.edu/).

Adolescence (12+)

Although G. Stanley Hall's (1904) characterization of adolescence as a season of "storm and stress" (p. 306) may no longer be accepted as universally true, is it recognized that adolescents must navigate a host of socioecological changes while also experiencing significant cognitive, physical, emotional, and social growth. Thus, it is not surprising that while still often presenting with the emotional and behavioral problems identified in childhood, adolescents are at increased risk for mood disorders, eating disorders, substance use disorders, suicidal ideation, and impulse-control disorders (Kessler et al., 2005).

The literature supports the continued use of behavioral and cognitive behavioral interventions for adolescents with a range of presenting problems, including suicidality and self-harm (e.g., Ewing et al., 2015; Morina et al., 2016; Ougrin, Tranah, Stahl, Moran, & Asarno, 2015; Weisz, McCarty, & Valeri, 2006). Although adolescent clients may take more of the responsibility for treatment than younger children, support from family/caregivers remains important in the implementation of behavioral and cognitive behavioral approaches generally, and is critical to the delivery of trauma-focused CBT for adolescents who have experienced trauma or abuse. As with younger children, an assessment of adolescents' metacognitive skills will help determine the degree to which cognitive interventions can be effective. Weisz et al. (2006) reported that non-CBT interventions for depression in adolescence (e.g., behavioral activation) can produce outcomes as robust as those that focus on changing cognitions.

Adolescents' socioecological contexts and their social development may suggest other psychotherapeutic approaches that can be beneficial for adolescents as well. For example, recent evidence suggests that interpersonal therapy (IPT) for adolescents can be effective (Cuijpers et al., 2011; Weisz et al., 2006). IPT is a brief, manualized intervention (Mufson, Moreau, Weissman, & Klerman, 1993) that addresses current stressors in adolescents' lives (e.g., grief, role disputes, transitions, and skills deficits) and provides adaptive strategies to address the identified problems. Given that IPT focuses on specific problems identified by the client, adolescents may view this form of psychotherapy as particularly salient. Shaffer and Pfeffer (2001) have noted that IPT is effective at decreasing adolescents' use of inappropriate means to communicate distress (e.g., their use of non-suicidal self-injury). However, a recent meta-analysis suggested that IPT had limited efficacy to address suicidality in this sample (Pu et al., 2017).

Given the likelihood of self-injury, suicidality, and substance use among adolescents, other psychotherapeutic approaches may be appropriate in this population. For example, Ougrin et al. (2015) noted that in addition to CBT, dialectical behavior therapy (DBT) is among the treatment approaches with the greatest demonstrated efficacy in their meta-analysis of interventions for suicidality and self-harm. Workbooks and skills manuals for DBT for adolescents are widely available (e.g., Miller, Rathus, & Linehan, 2006; Rathus & Miller, 2015). CBT and DBT share several common elements, including problem-solving, cognitive restructuring, and mood regulation skills that may reduce suicidal ideation and self-harm. Mindfulness-based techniques are also included in some variants of CBT (e.g., mindfulness-based cognitive therapy) and are routinely included in DBT. A recent meta-analysis found that mindfulness-based interventions (including Acceptance and Commitment Therapy [ACT]) can reduce adolescent stress, anxiety, and depressive symptoms either alone or in combination with other techniques (Kallapiran, Koo, Kirubakaran, & Hancock, 2015).

Finally, Lundahl and Burke (2009) found that motivational interviewing (MI) is an effective approach for reducing alcohol, marijuana, and other substance use and risky sexual behaviors and for engaging clients in treatment more generally. Though Lundahl and Burke did not examine the efficacy of MI specifically in adolescent samples, they found no age-related differences in effectiveness across developmental periods, including adolescence. Small to medium effect sizes for MI have been reported for adolescent substance use (Jensen et al., 2011) and health behaviors (Gayes & Steele, 2014). Given adolescents' increased risk for problematic substance use and health risk behaviors, as well as their potential ambivalence about these behaviors, MI can be an important tool in helping teens find motivation for behavior change.

General Implementation Issues

In addition to the implementation issues noted earlier with regard to specific therapeutic approaches, some general challenges associated with working with children and adolescents deserve note. For example, with school, extracurricular activities, parental and/or adolescent work schedules, and other activities, finding time when both child and caregiver can attend sessions can be challenging. This may be especially true in families in which the caregiver has hourly employment and may face negative economic consequences for repeated absences. Although it is appropriate to schedule sessions during school hours, many parents do not find repeated absences from school palatable. As a result, many child psychotherapists develop flexible office hours to accommodate evening or weekend appointment times, offer onsite childcare (for the child-client's siblings) so that parents can attend sessions, or offer services in more accessible settings (i.e., the child's school; see Chu et al., 2016).

Telehealth and teletherapy options have also been used to provide more flexibility for children and adolescents with good results (e.g., Bee et al., 2008; Cushing & Steele, 2010). Telehealth may have particular relevance for adolescents, who tend to be comfortable using digital technologies (e.g., Skype, FaceTime) as a primary means of communication (Boydell et al., 2014). Beyond telehealth and telepsychology, emerging evidence suggests that computer-based interventions for anxiety, depression, and chronic pain can be effective as adjunct or even first-line treatments (e.g., Ebert et al., 2015; Fisher, Law, Palermo, & Eccleston, 2015). The American Psychological Association (APA; 2013) has provided practice guidelines for the effective use of telehealth by mental health professionals. These guidelines address privacy/confidentiality, technical (e.g., internet speed), and jurisdictional issues and also encourage psychologists to obtain sufficient training to deliver treatment via remote technologies.

Because the delivery of psychological services for children and adolescents is most often facilitated by adult caregivers, youths' motivation to participate in the therapeutic process can be highly variable. This may be especially true for children with externalizing disorders, where the "problem" may be experienced more by the adult gatekeepers than by the child or adolescent in treatment. MI may be effective in helping adolescents find intrinsic motivation for psychotherapy or specific behavior change (e.g., substance use). However, for younger children, the service provider is tasked with enhancing motivation by other means (i.e., making therapy "fun"). One approach is to contextualize psychotherapy, therapeutic principles, or specific intervention components within child-friendly topic areas. For example, when delivering CBT for anger management, one might recast key therapeutic ingredients (e.g., cognitive restructuring, coping skills, relaxation training) as "Jedi skills" in order to engage a child who is an avid *Star Wars* fan. Many genres of literature or media of interest to children and teens can be used to illustrate psychological concepts (e.g., the Harry Potter series, *Hunger Games*) with great effect. It is incumbent on the psychotherapist to know the active ingredients of the intervention (and to be "current" on child/adolescent-friendly media) so as to ensure the flexible application of the approach with fidelity to the treatment model.

Future Steps

Although a robust literature exists to guide mental health clinicians in the delivery of effective interventions for children and youths, a number of issues limit the reach of our services. As noted earlier, structural and perceptual barriers remain in place for many children and adolescents in need of services. Internet-delivered interventions and telepsychology may alleviate some of these barriers for some potential clients, but the lack of access to a high-speed internet connection (i.e., to facilitate secure services that are compliant with the Health Insurance Portability and Accountability Act [HIPAA]) will remain a barrier for others. Co-location of psychological services in settings that are less foreign to children and families (e.g., schools, churches/mosques/synagogues, community centers, and primary care offices) may decrease barriers, particularly for individuals and families from traditionally underserved communities (Chu et al., 2016). Several models of such co-location have been described in the literature and serve as examples for professionals who work with children or adolescents (e.g., Tyler, Hulkower, & Kaminski, 2017).

Further, the lack of coordination of services and care across disciplines has been identified as a significant barrier to adequate mental health care. Brown, Green, Desai, Weitzman, and Rosenthal (2014) noted that as many as 40% of parents of children with mental health needs reported insufficient care coordination. Unmet coordination needs were especially high among children with anxiety disorders, conduct disorder, and autism spectrum disorder, and among those children and youth who were uninsured or insured by Medicaid only. Clinicians who work with children and families should consider ways to coordinate with other professionals from the youths' ecological systems (e.g., teachers, religious leaders, law enforcement officers, court officials, medical providers) to ensure optimal care.

A significant barrier to mental health services for children and adolescent is the lack of providers with specific competencies necessary for treatment of this vulnerable population, particularly in rural and low-income areas, and for individuals who are linguistically or ethnically isolated (Thomas, Ellis, Konrad, Holzer, & Morrissey, 2009). Moving forward, it will be important for training programs to consider how they can develop a workforce sufficient to meet these unmet needs. Various organizations have articulated specific functional and foundational competencies for working with children and youths. For example, both the Society of Pediatric Psychology (Palermo et al., 2014) and the Society of Clinical Child and Adolescent Psychology (Roberts et al., 1998) have developed specific training guidelines that are consistent with the functional competencies articulated by the Commission for the Recognition of Specialties and Proficiencies in Professional Psychology (CRSPPP; APA, n.d.). Further, the CRSPPP's Education and Training Guidelines (APA, 2012), provide a framework for initial development and continued professional development of competencies for psychologists intending to work with children and youths. As more training programs provide opportunities for trainees to develop these specialized competencies, and as more psychologists recognize the unmet need in this underserved population, perhaps the field can close this critical gap.

The field of mental health services for children and adolescents has grown tremendously over the past 20 years in terms of our understanding of what works (or what *can* work) and for whom. Yet the number of children with unmet mental health service needs remains substantial. Providers must continue to develop both their knowledge of "what works," as well as their competencies in delivering these effective treatments to ensure that those who do access treatment will benefit maximally. Further, clinicians must consider novel settings and delivery methods to reach youths with still unmet needs: Co-location of services, remote technologies, and partnerships with community agencies and other service providers may expand the reach of our services. Finally, improved bidirectional dialogue between researchers and providers will allow faster development of even more effective treatments for children and adolescents with a range of presenting problems. The field has grown, but it must continue to do so in order to meet the growing needs of children and adolescents now and in the future.

References

American Psychological Association. (n.d.). Recognized specialties and proficiencies in professional psychology. Retrieved from http://www.apa.org/ed/graduate/specialize/recognized.aspx

American Psychological Association. (2012). *Education and training guidelines: A taxonomy for education and training in professional psychology health service specialties*. Retrieved from http://www.apa.org/ed/graduate/specialize/taxonomy.pdf

American Psychological Association. (2013). Guidelines for the practice of telepsychology. *American Psychologist, 68*(9), 791–800.

Angold, A., Erkanli, A., Farmer, E. M., Fairbank, J. A., Burns, B. J., Keeler, G., & Costello, E. J. (2002). Psychiatric disorder, impairment, and service use in rural African American and white youth. *Archives of General Psychiatry, 59*(10), 893–901.

Arnberg, A., & Öst, L-G. (2014). CBT for children with depressive symptoms: A meta-analysis. *Cognitive Behaviour Therapy, 43*(4), 275–288.

Barkley, R. A. (1997). *Defiant children: A clinician's manual for assessment and parent training* (2nd ed.). New York, NY: Guilford Press.

Barkley, R. A. (2013). *Taking charge of ADHD: The complete, authoritative guide for parents* (3rd ed.). New York, NY: Guildford Press.

Bee, P. E., Bower, P., Lovell, K., Gilbody, S., Richards, D., Gask, L., & Roach, P. (2008). Psychotherapy mediated by remote communication technologies: A meta-analytic review. *BMC Psychiatry, 8*(1), 60.

Bernal, G., Jiménez-Chafey, M. I., & Domenech Rodríguez, M. M. (2009). Cultural adaptation of treatments: A resource for considering culture in evidence-based practice. *Professional Psychology: Research and Practice, 40*(4), 361–368.

Bitsko, R. H., Holbrook, J. R., Robinson, L. R., Kaminski, J. W., Ghandour, R., Smith, C., & Peacock, G. (2016). Health care, family, and community factors associated with mental, behavioral, and developmental disorders in early childhood—United States, 2011–2012. *Morbidity and Mortality Weekly Report, 65*, 221–226.

Boydell, K. M., Hodgins, M., Pignatiello, A., Teshima, J., Edwards, H., & Willis, D. (2014). Using technology to deliver mental health services to children and youth: A scoping review. *Journal of the Canadian Academy of Child and Adolescent Psychiatry, 23*(2), 87–99.

Bratton, S. C., Ray, D., Rhine, T., & Jones, L. (2005). The efficacy of play therapy with children: A meta-analytic review of treatment outcomes. *Professional Psychology: Research and Practice, 36*, 376–390.

Brown, N. M., Green, J. C., Desai, M. M., Weitzman, C. C., & Rosenthal, M. S. (2014). Need and unmet need for care coordination among children with mental health conditions. *Pediatrics, 133*, e530–e537.

Chu, B. C., Colognori, D., Weissman, A. S., & Bannon, K. (2009). An initial description and pilot of group behavioral activation therapy for anxious and depressed youth. *Cognitive and Behavioral Practice, 16*(4), 408–419.

Chu, J., Leino, A., Pflum, S., & Sue, S. (2016). A model for the theoretical basis of cultural competency to guide psychotherapy. *Professional Psychology: Research and Practice, 47*(1), 18–29.

Cohen, J. A., Deblinger, E., Mannarino, A. P., & Steer, R. A. (2004). A multisite, randomized controlled trial for children with sexual abuse-related PTSD symptoms. *Journal of the American Academy of Child & Adolescent Psychiatry, 43*(4), 393–402.

Costello, E. J., Egger, H., & Angold, A. (2005). 10-year research update review: The epidemiology of child and adolescent psychiatric disorders: I. Methods and public health burden. *Journal of the American Academy of Child & Adolescent Psychiatry, 44*(10), 972–986.

Cuijpers, P., Geraedts, A. S., van Oppen, P., Andersson, G., Markowitz, J. C., & van Straten, A. (2011). Interpersonal psychotherapy for depression: A meta-analysis. *American Journal of Psychiatry, 168*(6), 581–592.

Cushing, C. C., & Steele, R. G. (2010). A meta-analytic review of eHealth interventions for pediatric health promoting and maintaining behaviors. *Journal of Pediatric Psychology, 35*(9), 937–949.

Daley, D., Van der Oord, S., Ferrin, M., Danckaerts, M., Doepfner, M., Cortese, S., & Sonuga-Barke, E. J. S. (2014). Behavioral interventions for children and adolescents with attention deficit hyperactivity disorder: A meta-analysis of randomized controlled trials across multiple outcome domains. *Journal of the American Academy of Child & Adolescent Psychiatry, 53*(8), 835–847.

Ebert, D. D., Zarski, A. C., Christensen, H., Stikkelbroek, Y., Cuijpers, P., Berking, M., & Riper, H. (2015). Internet and computer-based cognitive behavioral therapy for anxiety and depression in youth: A meta-analysis of randomized controlled outcome trials. *PLoS One, 10*(3), e0119895.

Ewing, D. L., Monsen, J. J., Thompson, E. J., Cartwright-Hatton, S., & Field, A. (2015). A meta-analysis of transdiagnostic cognitive behavioural therapy in the treatment of child and young person anxiety disorders. *Behavioural and Cognitive Psychotherapy, 43*(5), 562–577.

Fisher, E., Law, E., Palermo, T. M., & Eccleston, C. (2015). Psychological therapies (remotely delivered) for the management of chronic and recurrent pain in children and adolescents. *Cochrane Database of Systematic Reviews, 3*, CD011118.

Gayes, L. A., & Steele, R. G. (2014). A meta-analysis of motivational interviewing interventions for pediatric health behavior change. *Journal of Consulting and Clinical Psychology, 82*(3), 521–535.

Gudiño, O. G., Lau, A. S., Yeh, M., McCabe, K. M., & Hough, R. L. (2009). Understanding racial/ethnic disparities in youth mental health services: Do disparities vary by problem type? *Journal of Emotional and Behavioral Disorders, 17*(1), 3–16.

Hall, G. C. N., Ibaraki, A. Y., Huang, E. R., Marti, C. N., & Stice, E. (2016). A meta-analysis of cultural adaptations of psychological interventions. *Behavior Therapy, 47*(6), 993–1014.

Hall, G. S. (1904). *Adolescence: Its psychology and its relation to physiology, anthropology, sociology, sex, crime, religion, and education* (Vols. I & II). Englewood Cliffs, NJ: Prentice-Hall.

Hembree-Kigin, T. L., & McNeil, C. B. (1995). *Parent-child interaction therapy.* New York, NY: Plenum Press.

Huey, S. J., & Polo, A. J. (2008). Evidence-based psychosocial treatments for ethnic minority youth. *Journal of Clinical Child and Adolescent Psychology, 37*, 262–301.

Huey, S. J., & Polo, A. J. (2017). Evidence-based psychotherapies with ethnic minority children and adolescents. In J. R. Weisz & A. E. Kazdin (Eds.), *Evidence-based psychotherapies for children and adolescents* (3rd ed., pp. 361–378). New York, NY: Guilford Press.

Jensen, C. D., Cushing, C. C., Aylward, B. A., Craig, J. T., Sorell, D. M., & Steele, R. G. (2011). Effectiveness of motivational interviewing interventions for adolescent substance use change: A meta-analytic review. *Journal of Consulting and Clinical Psychology, 79*, 433–440.

Kallapiran, K., Koo, S., Kirubakaran, R., & Hancock, K. (2015). Effectiveness of mindfulness in improving mental health symptoms of children and adolescents: A meta-analysis. *Child and Adolescent Mental Health, 20*(4), 182–194.

Kessler, R. C., Berglund, P., Demler, O., Jin, R., Merikangas, K. R., & Walters, E. E. (2005). Lifetime prevalence and age-of-onset distributions of DSM-IV disorders in the National Comorbidity Survey Replication. *Archives of General Psychiatry, 62*, 593–602.

Kendall, P. C., & Hedtke, K. A. (2006). *Cognitive-behavioral therapy for anxious children: Therapist manual*. Ardmore, PA: Workbook Publishing.

Kotchick, B. A., & Grover, R. L. (2008). Implementing evidence-based treatments with ethnically diverse clients. In R. G. Steele, T. D. Elkin, & M. C. Roberts (Eds.), *Handbook of evidence-based therapies for children and adolescents: Bridging science and practice* (pp. 487–504). New York, NY: Springer.

Locher, M. C., Koechlin, M. H., Zion, M. S. R., Werner, M. C., Pine, D. S., Kirsch, I., . . . Kossowsky, J. (2017). Efficacy and safety of SSRIs, SNRIs, and placebo in common psychiatric disorders: A comprehensive meta-analysis in children and adolescents. *JAMA Psychiatry, 74*(10), 1011–1020.

Lochman, J. E., & Wells, K. C. (2004). The Coping Power program for preadolescent aggressive boys and their parents: Outcome effects at the 1-year follow-up. *Journal of Consulting and Clinical Psychology, 72*(4), 571–578.

Lundahl, B., & Burke, B. L. (2009). The effectiveness and applicability of motivational interviewing: A practice-friendly review of four meta-analyses. *Journal of Clinical Psychology, 65*(11), 1232–1245.

McMahon, R. J., & Forehand, R. (2003). *Helping the noncompliant child: Family-based treatment for oppositional behavior* (2nd ed.). New York, NY: Guilford Press.

Merikangas, K. R., He, J-P., Brody, D., Fisher, P. W., Bourdon, K., & Koretz, D. S. (2010). Prevalence and treatment of mental disorders among US children in the 2001–2004 NHANES. *Pediatrics, 125*(1), 75–81.

Merikangas, K. R., He, J., Burstein, M., Swendsen, J., Avenevoli, S., Case, B., . . . Olfson, M. (2011). Service utilization for lifetime mental disorders in U.S. adolescents: Results of the National Comorbidity Survey-Adolescent Supplement (NCS-A). *Journal of the American Academy of Child & Adolescent Psychiatry, 50*(1), 32–45.

Miller, A. L., Rathus, J. H., & Linehan, M. M. (2006). *Dialectical behavior therapy with suicidal adolescents*. New York, NY: Guilford Press.

Morina, N., Koerssen, R., & Pollet, T. V. (2016). Interventions for children and adolescents with posttraumatic stress disorder: A meta-analysis of comparative outcome studies. *Clinical Psychology Review, 47*, 41–54.

MTA Cooperative Group. (2004). National Institute of Mental Health Multimodal Treatment Study of ADHD follow-up: 24-month outcomes of treatment strategies for attention-deficit/hyperactivity disorder. *Pediatrics, 113*(4), 754–761.

Mufson, L., Moreau, D., Weissman, M. M., & Klerman, G. L. (1993). *Interpersonal psychotherapy for depressed adolescents*. New York, NY: Guilford Publications.

Normann, N., Lønfeldt, N. N., Reinholdt-Dunne, M. L., & Esbjørn, B. H. (2016). Negative thoughts and metacognitions in anxious children following CBT. *Cognitive Therapy and Research, 40*(2), 188–197.

Ougrin, D., Tranah, T., Stahl, D., Moran, P., & Asarnow, J. R. (2015). Therapeutic interventions for suicide attempts and self-harm in adolescents: Systematic review and meta-analysis. *Journal of the American Academy of Child & Adolescent Psychiatry, 54*(2), 97–107.

Owens, P. L., Hoagwood, K., Horwitz, S. M., Leaf, P. J., Poduska, J. M., Kellam, S. G., & Ialongo, N. (2002). Barriers to children's mental health services. *Journal of the American Academy of Child & Adolescent Psychiatry, 41*(6), 731–738.

Palermo, T. M., Janicke, D. M., McQuaid, E. L., Mullins, L. L., Robins, P. M., & Wu, Y. P. (2014). Recommendations for training in pediatric psychology: Defining core competencies across training levels. *Journal of Pediatric Psychology, 39*(9), 965–984.

Polanczyk, G. V., Salum, G. A., Sugaya, L. S., Caye, A., & Rohde, L. A. (2015). Annual research review: A meta-analysis of the worldwide prevalence of mental disorders in children and adolescents. *Journal of Child Psychology and Psychiatry, 56*(3), 345–365.

Pu, J., Zhou, X., Liu, L., Zhang, Y., Yang, L., Yuan, S., . . . Xie, P. (2017). Efficacy and acceptability of interpersonal psychotherapy for depression in adolescents: A meta-analysis of randomized controlled trials. *Psychiatry Research, 253*, 226–232.

Rathus, J. H., & Miller, A. L. (2015). *DBT® skills manual for adolescents*. New York, NY: Guilford.

Reardon, T., Harvey, K., Baranowska, M. O'Brien, D., Smith, L., & Creswell, C. (2017). What do parents perceive are the barriers and facilitators to accessing psychological treatment for mental health problems in children and adolescents? A systematic review of qualitative and quantitative studies. *European Child & Adolescent Psychiatry, 26*(6), 623–647.

Roberts, M. C., Carlson, C. I., Erickson, M. T., Friedman, R. M., La Greca, A. M., Lemanek, K. L., . . . Wohlford, P. F. (1998). A model for training psychologists to provide services for children and adolescents. *Professional Psychology: Research and Practice, 29*(3), 293.

Shaffer, D., & Pfeffer, C. R. (2001). Practice parameter for the assessment and treatment of children and adolescents with suicidal behavior. *Journal of the American Academy of Child & Adolescent Psychiatry, 40*(7), 24S–51S.

Simeonsson, R. J., & Rosenthal, S. L. (2001). Developmental theories and clinical practice. In C. E. Walker & M. C. Roberts (Eds.), *Handbook of clinical child psychology* (3rd ed., pp. 20–33). New York, NY: Wiley.

Stallard, P. (2002). *Think good-feel good: A cognitive behavior therapy workbook for children and young people*. West Sussex, UK: John Wiley & Sons.

Steele, R. G., & Aylward, B. S. (2009). An overview of systems in pediatric psychology research and practice. In M. C. Roberts & R. G. Steele (Eds.), *Handbook of pediatric psychology* (4th ed., pp. 649–655). New York, NY: Guilford.

Stiffman, A. R., Pescosolido, B., & Cabassa, L. J. (2004). Building a model to understand youth service access: The gateway provider model. *Mental Health Services Research, 6*(4), 189–198.

Thomas, K. C., Ellis, A. R., Konrad, T. R., Holzer, C. E., & Morrissey, J. P. (2009). County-level estimates of mental health professional shortage in the United States. *Psychiatric Services, 60*(10), 1323–1328.

Turner, E. A., Jensen-Doss, A., & Heffer, R. W. (2015). Ethnicity as a moderator of how parents' attitudes and perceived stigma influence intentions to seek child mental health services. *Cultural Diversity and Ethnic Minority Psychology, 21*(4), 613–618.

Tyler, E. T., Hulkower, R. L., & Kaminski, J. W., (2017). *Behavioral health integration in pediatric primary care: Considerations and opportunities for policymakers, planners, and providers*. Retrieved from https://www.milbank.org/publications/

behavioral-health-integration-in-pediatric-primary-care-considerations-and-opportunities-for-policymakers-planners-and-providers/

Weisz, J. R., Kuppens, S., Ng, M. Y., Eckshtain, D., Ugueto, A. M., Vaughn-Coaxum, R., . . . Weersing, V. R. (2017). What five decades of research tells us about the effects of youth psychological therapy: A multilevel meta-analysis and implications for science and practice. *American Psychologist*, *72*(2), 79–117.

Weisz, J. R., McCarty, C. A., & Valeri, S. M. (2006). Effects of psychotherapy for depression in children and adolescents: A meta-analysis. *Psychological Bulletin*, *132*(1), 132–149.

13

Psychotherapy with the Underserved Older Adult Population

Susan Krauss Whitbourne and Bruna Martins

The Scope and Description of the Problem

The mental health needs of older adults present a significant set of challenges for the professionals who serve them, yet relatively few have expertise in geropsychology, the professional specialty that focuses on therapeutic approaches for use on aging individuals. Although a growing number of professional programs provide opportunities for training, these are still insufficient to meet the demand represented by the aging of the baby boom population (those born between 1945 and 1964).

Ageist views about the limited potential of older adults to benefit from psychotherapy lead many mental health training programs to focus their efforts on populations believed to be able to show improvement, even though in reality it is likely that graduates of these programs will find themselves treating adults who are in their 50s or beyond. Unfortunately, because of their lack of training in geropsychology, the treatments these professionals provide may fail to address a number of the concerns of their aging clients. According to the Institute of Medicine (2012), in the United States, instead of the 1,200 needed to meet the needs of older patients, only 75 medical professionals who specialize in aging trained in 2010. Fostering growth in interest among rising providers is crucial to closing this gap in future years.

Within the mental health field, the lack of providers is even more striking, as social workers make up only 9% of the geriatrics workforce, and merely 4% of aging specialists are health service psychologists. In fact, only 4% of psychologists nationwide specialize in geropsychology (Hoge, Karel, Zeiss, Alegria, & Moye, 2015). As a result, screening, diagnosis, and treatment of older adults often is managed by the patient's primary care provider (PCP), who may have limited training in appropriate mental health screening and/or lack of competency identifying and utilizing screening instruments appropriate for use with older adults. Among 10,000 aging patients in the United Kingdom, over 80% of those with depression never receive treatment, and 65% of people with dementia are not diagnosed (Royal College of Psychiatrists, 2009). Mental health care providers who see older adults may treat their patients based on the inaccurate assumptions that older adults suffer inevitable declines in mental health associated with aging and would benefit little from psychotherapy.

The purpose of this chapter is to provide an understanding of why these disparities in treatment provision exist and to give clinicians information about how they can prepare to address the concerns of older adult clients in their own practices. Prevalence and effective treatments for different mental health conditions in older adults are reviewed, and we provide suggestions for adapting therapeutic approaches for older adults via examples of modifications that are culturally competent. We then outline steps for how to bridge the geriatric mental health workforce gap.

Barriers to Service Delivery

A key factor that limits accessibility to mental health services for older adults is the relative lack of attention given to them by professionals, who may inaccurately believe that they can simply apply the therapeutic approach they use in their general practice. They may also regard their familiarity with aging individuals in their personal lives, or their own aging, as sufficient for understanding the needs of their older clients. The flaw in this logic should become evident if one considers psychological treatment with other specialized populations, such as individuals dealing with substance use disorders, eating disorders, or serious mental illness. It is doubtful that clinicians would embark on treatment with such patients without having received the training needed to provide appropriate care.

Ageism Among Mental Health Professionals

We maintain that lack of attention to older adults in the mental health professions can be attributed to "ageism," or the stereotyping and prejudice directed at individuals on the basis of their age (Butler, 1969). Unique to ageism, compared to other "isms," people can become a member of this group about whom they previously held negative views by doing nothing other than remaining alive. The predominant theory of ageism is, then, of the inevitability of death.

Unfounded assumptions about older adults further contribute to the problems of ageism among mental health professionals. The so-called social indicator model (Mroczek & Kolarz, 1998) assumes that older adults "should" be depressed due to the accumulation of physical infirmity, bereavement over the loss of significant others, and the need to live on a fixed income, which limits their access to housing, food, and travel. Mental health professionals who share this view believe, then, that aging must bring with it poor mental health. Such beliefs reinforce the idea that there is no need to treat depression in older adults because it is an inevitable byproduct of the normative aging process.

The implicit assumption that older adults are "too old to change," one component of ageism, further leads mental health professionals to place their emphasis on younger patients. Indeed, when licensed mental health clinicians were presented with a vignette describing a clinical case of a patient with the same symptoms who was either a younger or older adult, they reported the older patient as being less able to build a proper therapeutic relationship, having a poorer prognosis, and being less appropriate for psychotherapy (Helmes & Gee, 2003). Using the term "reluctant therapist" to describe this phenomenon, Robb, Chen, and Haley (2002) maintain that "acceptance of cultural stereotypes that portrayed joy evaporating with old age" (p. 2) is a potent factor affecting service delivery to older adults.

Despite reports by older adults of both physical and emotional benefits from sexual activity, there also seems to be an unwillingness for health care providers to address the sexual needs of older adults. Due to age-related stereotypes of older people being disinterested in sex, matters related to sexuality are seldom discussed in health care settings and sexual needs of older adults remain unmet. A review of attitudes toward sexual education of older adults found that most health care providers believe that assessment of sexuality and counseling in this population are beyond the scope of their field, and unfortunately this means that neither social workers, geriatricians, nurses, psychologists, nor health care trainees are asking these crucial questions of older adults (Haesler, Bauer, & Fetherstonhaugh, 2016).

Popular media outlets further contribute to the ageist attitudes that can translate into less-than-optimal treatment of older adults. Jokes about aging, news coverage that emphasizes accidents involving older drivers, and stereotypical media portrayals in film and television become part of a culture that makes older people appear incompetent, ridiculous, and out of touch. This illusory picture of older adults as "senile" propels negative stereotypes and stigma associated with their condition and age and normalizes pathological cognitive changes as an expectation rather than a sign of illness (Peel, 2014).

Worse still, the infantilizing of older adults in a patronizing and condescending manner by health care professionals further detracts from the regard others have of them as capable of managing their own affairs (Salari & Rich, 2001). In psychotherapy, such attitudes would lead to a self-fulfilling prophecy in which the autonomy and capabilities of older adult clients are downplayed, and mental health professionals do not offer the same options they offer to younger adults.

Internalization of Ageism by Older Adults

Negative portrayals of aging can also be internalized by the clients via "implicit ageism," a process by which ageist attitudes can adversely impact physical, cognitive, and emotional well-being and health behaviors (Levy, Slade, Kunkel, & Kasl, 2002). Indeed, reminding older adults of their age can result in greater stress responses (Levy, Hausdorff, Hencke, & Wei, 2000), slower walking speed in lab tasks (Hausdorff, Levy, & Wei, 1999), and memory impairments (Hess, Hinson, & Statham, 2004). The bias against older adults and their ability to use technology is another one that, unfortunately, aging individuals might apply to themselves and thus serve to reinforce the stereotype within themselves, leading to a self-fulfilling prophecy (Fowler, Gasiorek, & Giles, 2015).

The greatest reported barrier to engaging in psychotherapy is the belief held by older adults with anxiety and comorbid mood disorders that their symptoms were normal (Wuthrich & Frei, 2015). Older adults from cultures that stigmatize help seeking for psychological symptoms may be afraid to reveal their distress if they mistakenly assume that health care providers will regard them as having Alzheimer's disease or another neurocognitive disorder. Older adults may worry that if they confide to a medical professional that they are having psychological symptoms, they will be deprived of important freedoms such as being allowed to drive or live alone.

Creating Cultural Competency

Correcting misconceptions about the mental health needs of older adults grounded in available epidemiological data is the first step toward furthering cultural competency. Although adults are less likely than their younger counterparts to report experiencing serious mental distress (Substance Abuse and Mental Health Services Administration, 2017), there remain significant concerns in treating individuals in their later adult years (World Health Organization, 2017).

Epidemiology of Psychological Disorders in Older Adults

We review the prevalence and presentation of mental health disorders in older adults, and then discuss considerations in assessment and treatment of these disorders. Awareness of the links among normal aging changes, medical conditions, life experience, and expression of symptoms in older adults is required for mental health professionals to provide culturally competent treatment to patients in this age group.

Depression

Although the prevalence of a diagnosable mood disorder is lower in older than in younger adults, symptoms of depressive disorders remain of concern in the aging population. The rates of subclinical depression among older adults range from 20% of community-dwelling individuals to as high as 30% in medical settings (Whitbourne & Meeks, 2010). When screening for depression in older adults, mental health professionals should be aware that rather than acknowledging dysphoria, guilt, low self-esteem, and suicidal thoughts, older adults are more likely to seek treatment for physical symptoms, such as pain and abdominal disturbances (Amore, Tagariello, Laterza, & Savoia, 2007).

Even so, medical conditions and chronic disease can contribute to depressive symptoms in older adults, such as arthritis (Brooks et al., 2018), hip fracture (Lenze et al., 2007), diabetes (Campayo et al., 2010), metabolic syndrome (Almeida, Calver, Jamrozik, Hankey, & Flicker, 2009), stroke (Santos et al., 2009), and hypertension (Garcia-Fabela et al., 2009). Older adults may also experience depressive symptoms or disorder due to less obvious contributions such as tooth loss (Hugo, Hilgert, de Sousa Mda, & Cury, 2009), lack of sufficient vitamin D (Barnard & Colon-Emeric, 2010), and pain (Bierman & Lee, 2018). Fatigue and loneliness may play additional roles in increasing the risk of depression in older adults (Jaremka et al., 2010).

Bipolar Disorder

Rates of bipolar disorder are lower in older adults compared to the younger population (Depp & Jeste, 2004). A more passive coping style may contribute to the experience of depressive symptoms in older adults with bipolar disorder, suggesting that a potentially important route for treatment involves psychoeducation focusing on developing more adaptive coping strategies (Paans, Dols, Comijs, Stek, & Schouws, 2018).

Anxiety Disorders

Prevalence rates of anxiety disorders are lower in older than younger or middle-aged adults (15.3%) (Kessler et al., 2005). Gender differences in rates of anxiety disorders persist from younger adulthood, with older women being five times more likely than older men to be diagnosed with an anxiety disorder (Gum, King-Kallimanis, & Kohn, 2009). Prevalence rates for these disorders are highest for specific phobia (7.5%) and generalized anxiety disorder (3.6%). Older adults also have lower lifetime prevalence of agoraphobia and panic disorder (Kessler et al., 2005), although there are variations by racial and ethnic status (Jimenez, Alegria, Chen, Chan, & Laderman, 2010). The lower prevalence rates in older adults may reflect poorer training among clinicians in recognizing and diagnosing anxiety disorder symptoms in their older clients (Scogin, Floyd, & Forde,

2000), but, as is true for depressive disorders, anxiety disorder symptoms may present or coexist with medical conditions (Mehta et al., 2007), particularly in the case of panic attacks and agoraphobia (Sareen, Cox, Clara, & Asmundson, 2005). Unfortunately, there can be serious consequences of failure to recognize anxiety disorder symptoms, as older adults with anxiety symptoms have elevated mortality rates, with rates that are especially high in the Black older adult population (Brenes et al., 2007).

Stress and Trauma-Related Disorders

Post-traumatic stress disorder (PTSD) is another significant area of concern for mental health professionals working with older adults. Estimates are that at the age of 19, the prevalence of PTSD among Vietnam veterans was 15% (U.S. Department of Health and Human Services, 1999). With the aging of this cohort into their 60s, it is clear that PTSD rates remain high, particularly among those whose service took place in the theater of operations, with prevalence rates as high as 22% (Goldberg et al., 2016).

Among civilians exposed to the 9/11 terrorist attacks, older adults were more likely to experience PTSD than their younger counterparts (DiGrande et al., 2008). Natural disasters present another risk for PTSD among older adults, as was the case in a study of Hurricane Sandy (New Jersey) survivors, although high levels of social cohesion were found to buffer against the development of symptoms (Heid, Pruchno, Cartwright, & Wilson-Genderson, 2017).

Late-onset stress symptomatology (LOSS) is observed in aging veterans who were exposed to stressful combat situations in young adulthood. Symptoms of LOSS are similar to those of PTSD, but the progression is distinct in that LOSS develops late in life and is likely to involve symptoms related to depression, anxiety, sense of mastery, and life satisfaction (Potter et al., 2013). Symptoms related to the combat experiences (e.g., an increase in memories about the trauma) begin to emerge in later life, perhaps as a function of exposure to stresses associated with aging, such as retirement and health problems (Davison et al., 2006).

Substance Use Disorders

As of 2017, an estimated 15.4 million adults aged 65 and older (31.2%) had used an illicit drug at some point in their lives, with 2.8 million in the past year (5.7%) and 1.5 million in the past month (3.0%). Older adults are at significant risk for use and misuse of prescription psychotherapeutics as well as nonprescription pain relievers (Substance Abuse and Mental Health Services Administration, 2018). Alcohol use is virtually universal among older adults, with 82% of those 65 and older reporting lifetime use; over half (56.5%) have used alcohol in the past year, and a substantial portion within the past month (44.2%). The pattern of heavy (2.8%) and binge (11.5%) drinking within the past month in older adults remains surprisingly high given that these alcohol use patterns are associated with younger adults.

Symptoms of alcohol dependence account for an estimated 14% of older adults who receive medical attention in hospitals and emergency rooms. Alcohol use is also thought to be relatively prevalent in settings in which only older adults live, such as nursing homes and retirement communities. People with a history of problem drinking and those who retired involuntarily seem most likely to abuse alcohol after they retire (Kuerbis & Sacco, 2012).

Gaining Cultural Competency in Psychotherapy with Older Adults

This brief review of the cultural competence needed to understand specific disorders in older adults suggests that the first step needed for proper treatment is knowledge of the epidemiology of the major disorders seen in this age group. Additionally, culturally competent mental health professionals take a biopsychosocial approach to understanding the backdrop against which older adults present with these specific symptoms.

The normal aging process involves changes in physical health, cognition, relationships, and work role, any of which can interact with the individual's sense of identity (Whitbourne & Collins, 1998). Changes in response speed, memory, and communicative abilities further stimulate potential changes in identity. Social role changes of retirement, caregiving, and bereavement become additional sources of identity change, as does the need to relocate due to changes in health or financial circumstances. The challenges to adaptation faced by older adults should be contrasted with the extensive psychological coping resources that aging individuals develop over their lifetimes, which can mitigate against these potential threats to their well-being, a concept embodied in the notion of "successful aging." Many older adults are able to maintain continuity of their identities across these areas of change by drawing upon their lifetime of psychological coping resources and patterns of resilience (Fankhauser et al., 2010).

Cultural competence for working with older adults is a foundational component of the American Psychological Association's Guidelines for Psychological Practice with Older Adults (2014). Guideline 14 specifically states that "Psychologists strive to be familiar with and develop skill in applying culturally sensitive, specific psychotherapeutic interventions and environmental modifications with older adults and their families, including adapting interventions for use with this age group" (p. 50). Additionally, the Geropsychology Guidelines emphasize the need for mental health professionals to take into account the intersection of aging with gender, social class, sexual orientation, gender identity, and cultural background.

Specific applications of the concepts covered in Geropsychology Guidelines provide concrete ways that mental health professionals can adapt their work for the older adult population. Beginning with the appropriate use of assessment instruments developed for older adults and adapted as necessary to take into account their cultural background, language, and education, mental health professionals need to be aware of their own biases toward older adults and be able to address these through consultation and/or supervision. Apart from understanding how the aging process per se affects their patients, mental health professionals should also be aware of generational differences as applied to current cohorts of older adults. However, it is also necessary to take individual differences into account when applying culturally competent approaches to treatment.

For example, one older adult client may prefer not to be spoken to on a first-name basis, preferring instead more formal terms of salutation. Other older adults may instead prefer to be treated in a more egalitarian manner, particularly if they received a college education and feel more on a par with the mental health professional. Knowing the older individual's psychosocial history provides important clues to preferred modes of interaction, but even so, the mental health professional needs to be open to the possibility that assumptions based on this knowledge could be in error. Thus, learning about the sociohistorical influences on previous cohorts of adults can provide mental health professionals with valuable insights that can inform their approach to treatment.

Keeping in mind individual differences, mental health professionals should also take into account that cohort-based and cultural norms may dictate topics that the client prefers to share versus not discuss in a therapist's office. These norms may influence the patient's level of self-disclosure during an intake interview and/or on a self-report measure. For instance, in some cultures, discussions of death and dying are strongly stigmatized, and patients experiencing significant distress related to end-of-life issues may underreport these thoughts and worries. Another example is psychological versus physical help seeking and the stigma that a client's cultural background may impose on evaluating psychological well-being and/or seeking treatment for emotional concerns. Some older adult patients were raised with the belief that they need to solve problems on their own. They therefore enter the office worried that a mental health provider will "force" them to share personal details they prefer not to discuss, or that they will admit weakness by agreeing to fill out a self-report mood questionnaire.

Taking time to validate to the client that apprehension toward assessment is a common feeling for all clients and sharing the rationale for the assessment can become a conversation rather than a one-sided persuasion. Respecting their choice to not participate in an assessment can build rapport and validate that the mental health professional knows what is important to them.

Consider the example of an African American older adult client in his 70s who sought psychotherapy per his wife's request regarding his hypervigilance, increased irritability, and nightmares that started 30 years following combat-related trauma. During the intake session, the patient denied experiencing emotional distress, stated that he was only coming in to appease his wife, and refused to complete a PTSD screening form. Over time, the patient revealed that he was indeed experiencing distressing symptoms but saw this as a "curse" from a higher power for what had happened during combat, and not something psychological. His religious beliefs influenced his endorsement of symptoms, and prior to discussing themes of self-criticism, guilt, and religiously held belief in divine justice, it is quite unlikely that this patient would have endorsed symptoms when completing a PTSD screen initially. However, over time, with a deeper rapport and decreased guardedness, he eventually began completing the screening forms at each session's start.

Allowing older adult patients to share the concepts they learn in their own words is a useful approach for mental health professionals to take so that tools taught are understood and retained in a step-wise manner while not making assumptions about the specific client's capacities. In addition to pacing, older adults with memory difficulties may have difficulty holding on to information across sessions. For these patients, providing written materials and summaries may be a helpful way to boost retention and practice of tools learned across sessions. Especially for clients who have memory disorders and difficulty processing abstract information, it is necessary to use more concrete goals in treatment.

A major consideration in working with older adults is taking into account their biopsychosocial context and how that may interact with their presenting symptoms. Understanding the role of the current sociopolitical environment is also helpful in work with older adults. An older retired individual in therapy may be influenced by concerns about the current economic climate as it affects his or her pension, or an individual whose family is affected by changes in immigration policies may be impacted in important ways that affect his or her mental health. Specific influences on the older adult's social and economic well-being must also be recognized. For instance, if patients are struggling to pay their monthly rent and anxiety peaks at the end of the month, working with a case manager around these issues may be an important modification to traditional anxiety treatment.

Social and living contexts can impact mood and well-being in later life in many ways. An older adult who lives in a residential community may have access to activities that an older adult living at home in a rural area may not, and this can impact the feasibility of certain behavioral intervention possibilities. In addition, the culture of a senior living community, both in terms of staff and residents, may have a significant impact on the older adult's mood. For example, staff members who know residents on a first-name basis may be seen as social supports, whereas "cold-shoulder" providers may promote feelings of isolation and disconnectedness.

Finally, involving a client's social supports in psychotherapy is a unique and important component of family systems work in psychotherapy with older adults. Many older patients emotionally struggle alongside their caregivers, and family systems therapy can involve significant behavioral problem solving with families while in parallel promoting self-care strategies for caregivers. Integrating family members in the treatment process may be especially beneficial to patients with significant memory difficulties, both in helping to implement strategies at home and in reinforcing behaviors across the family as a whole.

Overall, the most important element of psychotherapy with older adults and their families is to tailor each treatment plan according to the client's needs, rather than making assumptions. It is crucial to dispel ageist heuristics and determine how to modify psychotherapy based on a client's stated requests.

Effective Strategies and Empirically-Supported Treatments

There is a growing body of work documenting the potential for effective and empirically supported treatments designed specifically for older adults. However, to be effective, these treatments must take into account the wide range of issues reflected in the biopsychosocial approach as applied to mental health and aging.

Empirically Validated Approaches to Specific Disorders in Older Adults

Depression

Cognitive behavioral therapy (CBT) has the greatest efficacy in improving symptoms in depressed older adults, as indicated in a large-scale meta-analysis (Pinquart & Sörensen, 2001) and more recent randomized control studies (Gould, Coulson, & Howard, 2012). CBT can also be modified in patients with memory difficulties and dementia, to involve caregivers in problem solving, with good effect (Teri, Logsdon, Uomoto, & McCurry, 1997).

As indicated earlier in the chapter, depression in later life is especially difficult to diagnose due to psychosocial factors that have similar outward presentations. Having a complete picture of factors likely contributing to changes in mood will help assess the root cause of the change. Using reliable and valid depression screening tools during office visits to track changes in emotional functioning can help detect changes in mood, even when the patient might not directly mention these concerns during the visit. Evidence suggests that depression screening and treatment significantly reduces risk of suicide in older adult populations (Lapierre et al., 2011).

Anxiety Disorders

A systematic review and meta-analysis of 27 randomized control trials demonstrated that older adults with generalized anxiety disorder (GAD) significantly benefited from both pharmacological and psychotherapeutic interventions (Pinquart & Duberstein, 2007), with active treatment more effective than control (Gonçalves & Byrne, 2012). The largest effect in symptom improvements for anxiety in older adults appears to be relaxation training rather than cognitive change (Thorp et al., 2009). Thus, an important adaptation for older adults in anxiety treatment may be to emphasize the use of relaxation techniques, such as progressive muscle relaxation, diaphragmatic breathing, and grounding strategies, and, depending on the cognitive level of the client, use of more concrete relaxation homework assignments.

Post-Traumatic Stress Disorder

Although most therapists feel comfortable engaging in psychoeducation about PTSD symptoms, enhancing social support, and teaching coping strategies to better manage symptoms in older adults with PTSD, many therapists avoid engaging in exposure-based interventions with older clients both due to fears and assumptions about poor outcomes, and lack of empirical data and randomized controlled trials to support efficacy in later life. However, a published case history using imaginal exposure for PTSD in a 57-year-old woman with childhood sexual trauma demonstrated effectiveness of the treatment (Russo, Hersen, & Van Hasselt, 2001). Other work has suggested that the use of life review therapy, in which clients overcome conflict by reflecting on the past in order to gain a sense of mastery and acceptance of their life accomplishments, is effective in treating trauma symptoms of PTSD (Maercker, 2002). An important challenge of older adults with lifetime PTSD is the presence of multiple comorbid chronic health conditions and poorer physical health (Pietrzak, Goldstein, Southwick, & Grant, 2012), which may lead to decreased activity and impact regular engagement in therapy.

Substance Use Disorders

Older adults demonstrate similar rates of abstinence to younger and middle-aged adults following group substance use treatments, regardless of whether the treatment is administered in similar-aged and mixed-age groups (Kuerbis

& Sacco, 2012). Very few randomized controlled trials have been conducted for substance use treatment in later-life cohorts, and most are limited by very small sample sizes. A recent literature review found that both clinic-based and mail-based CBT-focused interventions for alcohol use appear to be effective in reducing drinking among older adults (Quinn & Mowbray, 2018). A systematic review of the literature supported that older adults had self-reported improvements from psychological treatment for substance use problems either equal to or even greater than gains seen in younger adults (Moy, Crome, Crome, & Fisher, 2011). Unfortunately, the current treatment literature shows significant improvements from substance use treatment in older adults but focuses on interventions conducted in primary care and health clinics. Understanding whether specialized treatment of substance use disorders is more or less effective in the aging population would clarify an important gap in evidence-based treatment and how best to tailor it to the aging population.

Recommendations for Mental Health Professionals

As we have discussed, older adults have significant mental health needs that are vastly underserved by current mental health providers. Ageist assumptions regarding normative experiences of depression, dementia, asexuality, and lack of effectiveness of interventions in later life significantly contribute to the disparities in mental health care for elders. We suggest the following considerations for professionals working with older adults in mental health settings:

1. **Be aware of your biases.** Consider and question how some of your cultural stereotypes may influence your expectations of older clients and willingness to engage in specific treatments. Be critical of what motivates your clinical decision making and always take your cultural lens into account.
2. **Prioritize client preferences.** Ask clients to clarify their preferences and goals in your work together. How would they like to be addressed? What does therapy mean to them, and what are they expecting to gain? Discussing your own expectations relative to the client's expectations of treatment and establishing collaborative goals up front promotes a healthy therapeutic alliance. Formulating a treatment plan that addresses the client's priorities while dovetailing with your recommendations will strengthen client buy-in and adherence to treatment.
3. **Consider the whole individual.** Rather than making assumptions about a client's biopsychosocial world, assess the individual as a whole. Consider the environmental social support, economic resources, access to care and other factors that may factor into the client's overall well-being. Consider

medical comorbidities and cardiovascular risk factors that may impact the client's behavior and emotional well-being, such as chronic obstructive pulmonary disease, diabetes, and insomnia, among others.

4. **Consider many perspectives in assessment.** Working with older adults often means working with a client's family and other care providers to assess a client's daily activity level, social engagement, cognitive functioning, and overall health. Gathering information from multiple sources can provide collateral accounts of current symptoms, as well as help formulate a conceptualization of root mechanisms underlying current complaints.
5. **Stay informed.** Be cognizant of the prevalence of mental health disorders among older adults to promote accurate diagnosis and be informed of age-validated treatments as research progresses. Useful resources include the section on aging on the APA website, and the National Institute on Aging information page (https://order.nia.nih.gov/view-all-publications).
6. **If in doubt, consult or refer to a specialist.** When unsure whether your client is retaining information across sessions due to a memory disorder, or whether difficulty breathing at night may be influencing mood during the day, consult with a specialist. Referring your client to a geriatrics clinic for an evaluation, or to a specialist such as a neuropsychologist or sleep clinic, may provide both you and the client with information crucial to care.

Future Steps

Increasing education is a first step in helping close the geropsychology workforce gap. Incorporating the psychology of aging into curricula at the undergraduate level could help correct misconceptions about aging early in the training of future mental health professionals. Indeed, research suggests that intergenerational service learning programs, in which college students participate in small-group discussions together, lead to improvements after participation in attitudes toward older adults (Penick, Fallshore, & Spencer, 2014). Similar programs with medical students also show an increase in positive views of aging, and enhanced empathy with older adults when students engage in visits to art museums and discussion with older adults in the community (Gonzales, Morrow-Howell, & Gilbert, 2010).

Another manner of closing the geropsychology workforce gap is to boost education programs for primary care providers. Some policy reform suggestions have been made, but few programs have acted to correct this disparity (Boult, Counsell, Leipzig, & Berenson, 2010). For instance, Medicare could provide educational subsidies to strengthen geriatric graduate training in medical schools;

graduate clinical psychology and social work programs with geropsychology training could be provided with federal financial support; and health care professionals could be required to obtain continuing education credits to maintain licensure or be paneled. The recognition of geropsychology as a specialty in psychology prompted the development of board certification in geropsychology by the American Board of Professional Psychology (Molinari, 2011), which is beginning to produce highly trained providers of psychological services to older adults (Qualls, 2015).

In summary, clinicians working with older adults can benefit from advanced training as well as from taking advantage of the increasingly available resources on mental health and aging. With increasing recognition of both the strengths and mental health needs of older adults, psychotherapy for the aging population will become increasingly part of the mainstream training of all clinicians. We might hope that, as a result of greater attention being given to this underserved population, research on effective treatment approaches will be stimulated, both in graduate training departments and in the larger community and mental health settings that serve older adults.

References

Almeida, O. P., Calver, J., Jamrozik, K., Hankey, G. J., & Flicker, L. (2009). Obesity and metabolic syndrome increase the risk of incident depression in older men: The Health in Men study. *American Journal of Geriatric Psychiatry*, *17*(10), 889–898.

American Psychological Association. (2014). Guidelines for psychological practice with older adults. *American Psychologist*, *69*, 34–65.

Amore, M., Tagariello, P., Laterza, C., & Savoia, E. M. (2007). Beyond nosography of depression in elderly. *Archives of Gerontology and Geriatrics*, *44*(Suppl 1), 13–22.

Barnard, K., & Colon-Emeric, C. (2010). Extraskeletal effects of vitamin D in older adults: Cardiovascular disease, mortality, mood, and cognition. *American Journal of Geriatric Pharmacotherapy*, *8*(1), 4–33.

Bierman, A., & Lee, Y. (2018). Chronic pain and psychological distress among older adults: A national longitudinal study. *Research on Aging*, *40*(5), 432–455.

Boult, C., Counsell, S. R., Leipzig, R. M., & Berenson, R. A. (2010). The urgency of preparing primary care physicians to care for older people with chronic illnesses. *Health Affairs*, *29*(5), 811–818.

Brenes, G. A., Kritchevsky, S. B., Mehta, K. M., Yaffe, K., Simonsick, E. M., Ayonayon, H. N., . . . Penninx, B. W. (2007). Scared to death: Results from the Health, Aging, and Body Composition Study. *American Journal of Geriatric Psychiatry*, *15*(3), 262–265.

Brooks, J. M., Titus, A. J., Polenick, C. A., Orzechowski, N. M., Reid, M. C., MacKenzie, T. A., . . . Batsis, J. A. (2018). Prevalence rates of arthritis among us older adults with varying degrees of depression: Findings from the 2011 to 2014 National Health and Nutrition Examination Survey. *International Journal of Geriatric Psychiatry*, *33*(12), 1671–1679.

Butler, R. (1969). Ageism: Another form of bigotry. *The Gerontologist, 9*, 243–246.

Campayo, A., de Jonge, P., Roy, J. F., Saz, P., de la Camara, C., Quintanilla, M. A., . . . Lobo, A. (2010). Depressive disorder and incident diabetes mellitus: The effect of characteristics of depression. *American Journal of Psychiatry, 167*(5), 580–588.

Davison, E. H., Pless, A. P., Gugliucci, M. R., King, L. A., King, D. W., Salgado, D. M., . . . Bachrach, P. (2006). Late-life emergence of early-life trauma: The phenomenon of late-onset stress symptomatology among aging combat veterans. *Research on Aging, 28*(1), 84–114. doi:10.1177/0164027505281560

Depp, C. A., & Jeste, D. V. (2004). Bipolar disorder in older adults: A critical review. *Bipolar Disorders, 6*, 343–367.

DiGrande, L., Perrin, M. A., Thorpe, L. E., Thalji, L., Murphy, J., Wu, D., . . . Brackbill, R. M. (2008). Posttraumatic stress symptoms, PTSD, and risk factors among lower Manhattan residents 2–3 years after the September 11, 2001 terrorist attacks. *Journal of Traumatic Stress, 21*(3), 264–273.

Fankhauser, S., Wagner, B., Krammer, S., Aeschbach, M., Pepe, A., Maercker, A., & Forstmeier, S. (2010). The impact of social and interpersonal resources on adjustment disorder symptoms in older age: Motivational variables as mediators? *GeroPsych: The Journal of Gerontopsychology and Geriatric Psychiatry, 23*(4), 227–241.

Fowler, C., Gasiorek, J., & Giles, H. (2015). The role of communication in aging well: Introducing the communicative ecology model of successful aging. *Communication Monographs, 82*(4), 431–457.

Garcia-Fabela, L., Melano-Carranza, E., Aguilar-Navarro, S., Garcia-Lara, J. M., Gutierrez-Robledo, L. M., & Avila-Funes, J. A. (2009). Hypertension as a risk factor for developing depressive symptoms among community-dwelling elders. *Revista de Investigacion Clinica, 61*(4), 274–280.

Goldberg, J., Magruder, K. M., Forsberg, C. W., Friedman, M. J., Litz, B. T., Vaccarino, V., . . . Smith, N. L. (2016). Prevalence of post-traumatic stress disorder in aging Vietnam-era veterans: Veterans Administration Cooperative Study 569: Course and consequences of post-traumatic stress disorder in Vietnam-era veteran twins. *American Journal of Geriatric Psychiatry, 24*(3), 181–191.

Gonçalves, D. C., & Byrne, G. J. (2012). Interventions for generalized anxiety disorder in older adults: Systematic review and meta-analysis. *Journal of Anxiety Disorders, 26*(1), 1–11.

Gonzales, E., Morrow-Howell, N., & Gilbert, P. (2010). Changing medical students' attitudes toward older adults. *Gerontology & Geriatrics Education, 31*(3), 220–234.

Gould, R. L., Coulson, M. C., & Howard, R. J. (2012). Cognitive behavioral therapy for depression in older people: A meta-analysis and meta-regression of randomized controlled trials. *Journal of the American Geriatrics Society, 60*(10), 1817–1830.

Gum, A. M., King-Kallimanis, B., & Kohn, R. (2009). Prevalence of mood, anxiety, and substance-abuse disorders for older Americans in the National Comorbidity Survey-Replication. *American Journal of Geriatric Psychiatry, 17*, 782–792.

Haesler, E., Bauer, M., & Fetherstonhaugh, D. (2016). Sexuality, sexual health and older people: A systematic review of research on the knowledge and attitudes of health professionals. *Nurse Education Today, 40*, 57–71.

Hausdorff, J. M., Levy, B. R., & Wei, J. Y. (1999). The power of ageism on physical function of older persons: Reversibility of age-related gait changes. *Journal of the American Geriatrics Society, 47*(11), 1346–1349.

Heid, A. R., Pruchno, R., Cartwright, F. P., & Wilson-Genderson, M. (2017). Exposure to Hurricane Sandy, neighborhood collective efficacy, and post-traumatic stress symptoms in older adults. *Aging & Mental Health, 21*(7), 742–750.

Helmes, E., & Gee, S. (2003). Attitudes of Australian therapists toward older clients: Educational and training imperatives. *Educational Gerontology, 29*(8), 657–670.

Hess, T. M., Hinson, J. T., & Statham, J. A. (2004). Explicit and implicit stereotype activation effects on memory: Do age and awareness moderate the impact of priming? *Psychology and Aging, 19*(3), 495–505.

Hoge, M. A., Karel, M. J., Zeiss, A. M., Alegria, M., & Moye, J. (2015). Strengthening psychology's workforce for older adults: Implications of the Institute of Medicine's report to Congress. *American Psychologist, 70*(3), 265–278.

Hugo, F. N., Hilgert, J. B., de Sousa Mda, L., & Cury, J. A. (2009). Oral status and its association with general quality of life in older independent-living south-Brazilians. *Community Dentistry and Oral Epidemiology, 37*(3), 231–240.

Institute of Medicine. (2012). The mental health and substance use workforce for older adults: In whose hands? Retrieved from http://www.iom.edu/Reports/2008/Retooling-for-an-Aging-America-Building-the-Health-Care-Workforce.aspx

Jaremka, L. M., Andridge, R. R., Fagundes, C. P., Alfano, C. M., Povoski, S. P., Lipari, A. M., . . . Laderman, M. (2010). Prevalence of psychiatric illnesses in older ethnic minority adults. *Journal of the American Geriatrics Society, 58*(2), 256–264.

Kessler, R. C., Berglund, P., Demler, O., Jin, R., Merikangas, K. R., & Walters, E. E. (2005). Lifetime prevalence and age-of-onset distributions of DSM-IV disorders in the National Comorbidity Survey Replication. *Archives of General Psychiatry, 62*(6), 593–602.

Kuerbis, A., & Sacco, P. (2012). The impact of retirement on the drinking patterns of older adults: A review. *Addictive Behaviors, 37*(5), 587–595.

Lapierre, S., Erlangsen, A., Waern, M., De Leo, D., Oyama, H., Scocco, P., . . . Quinnett, P. (2011). A systematic review of elderly suicide prevention programs. *Crisis: The Journal of Crisis Intervention and Suicide Prevention, 32*(2), 88–98.

Lenze, E. J., Munin, M. C., Skidmore, E. R., Dew, M. A., Rogers, J. C., Whyte, E. M., . . . Reynolds, C. F., 3rd. (2007). Onset of depression in elderly persons after hip fracture: Implications for prevention and early intervention of late-life depression. *Journal of the American Geriatrics Society, 55*(1), 81–86.

Levy, B. R., Hausdorff, J. M., Hencke, R., & Wei, J. Y. (2000). Reducing cardiovascular stress with positive self-stereotypes of aging. *Journal of Gerontology Series B: Psychological Sciences and Social Sciences, 55*(4), P205–P213.

Levy, B. R., Slade, M. D., Kunkel, S. R., & Kasl, S. V. (2002). Longevity increased by positive self-perceptions of aging. *Journal of Personality and Social Psychology, 83*(2), 261–270.

Maercker, A. (2002). Life-review technique in the treatment of PTSD in elderly patients: Rationale and three single case studies. *Journal of Clinical Geropsychology, 8*(3), 239–249.

Mehta, K. M., Yaffe, K., Brenes, G. A., Newman, A. B., Shorr, R. I., Simonsick, E. M., . . . Covinsky, K. E. (2007). Anxiety symptoms and decline in physical function over 5 years in the health, aging and body composition study. *Journal of the American Geriatrics Society, 55*(2), 265–270.

Molinari, V. (2011). *Specialty competencies in geropsychology*. New York, NY: Oxford University Press.

Moy, I., Crome, P., Crome, I., & Fisher, M. (2011). Systematic and narrative review of treatment for older people with substance problems. *European Geriatric Medicine, 2*(4), 212–236.

Mroczek, D. K., & Kolarz, C. M. (1998). The effect of age on positive and negative affect: A developmental perspective on happiness. *Journal of Personality and Social Psychology, 75*, 1333–1349.

Paans, N. P. G., Dols, A., Comijs, H. C., Stek, M. L., & Schouws, S. N. T. M. (2018). Associations between cognitive functioning, mood symptoms and coping styles in older age bipolar disorder. *Journal of Affective Disorders, 235*, 357–361.

Peel, E. (2014). "The living death of Alzheimer's" versus "Take a walk to keep dementia at bay": Representations of dementia in print media and carer discourse. *Sociology of Health & Illness, 36*(6), 885–901.

Penick, J. M., Fallshore, M., & Spencer, A. M. (2014). Using intergenerational service learning to promote positive perceptions about older adults and community service in college students. *Journal of Intergenerational Relationships, 12*(1), 25–39.

Pietrzak, R. H., Goldstein, R. B., Southwick, S. M., & Grant, B. F. (2012). Physical health conditions associated with posttraumatic stress disorder in U S older adults: Results from wave 2 of the National Epidemiologic Survey on Alcohol and Related Conditions. *Journal of the American Geriatrics Society, 60*(2), 296–303.

Pinquart, M., & Duberstein, P. R. (2007). Treatment of anxiety disorders in older adults: A meta-analytic comparison behavioral and pharmacological interventions. *American Journal of Geriatric Psychiatry, 15*(8), 639–651.

Pinquart, M., & Sörensen, S. (2001). How effective are psychotherapeutic and other psychosocial interventions with older adults? A meta-analysis. *Journal of Mental Health and Aging, 7*(2), 207–243.

Potter, C. M., Kaiser, A. P., King, L. A., King, D. W., Davison, E. H., Seligowski, A. V., . . . Spiro, A., III. (2013). Distinguishing late-onset stress symptomatology from posttraumatic stress disorder in older combat veterans. *Aging & Mental Health, 17*(2), 173–179.

Qualls, S. H. (2015). Building competencies in professional geropsychology: Guidelines, training model, and strategies for professional development. In P. A. Areán (Ed.), *Treatment of late-life depression, anxiety, trauma, and substance abuse* (pp. 11–48). Washington, DC: American Psychological Association.

Quinn, A., & Mowbray, O. (2018). Effective treatments for older adult baby boomers with alcohol-use disorders: A literature review. *Journal of Social Work Practice in the Addictions, 18*(4), 389–410.

Robb, C., Chen, H., & Haley, W. E. (2002). Ageism in mental health and health care: A critical review. *Journal of Clinical Geropsychology, 8*(1), 1–12.

Royal College of Psychiatrists. (2009). Royal College of Psychiatrists' position statement PS2/2009. Age discrimination in mental health services: Making equality a reality. Retrieved from https://www.rcpsych.ac.uk/pdf/PS02_2009x.pdf

Russo, S. A., Hersen, M., & Van Hasselt, V. B. (2001). Treatment of reactivated posttraumatic stress disorder: Imaginal exposure in an older adult with multiple traumas. *Behavior Modification, 25*(1), 94–115.

Salari, S. M., & Rich, M. (2001). Social and environmental infantilization of aged persons: Observations in two adult day care centers. *International Journal of Aging and Human Development, 52*(2), 115–134.

Santos, M., Kovari, E., Hof, P. R., Gold, G., Bouras, C., & Giannakopoulos, P. (2009). The impact of vascular burden on late-life depression. *Brain and Research Reviews, 62*(1), 19–32.

Sareen, J., Cox, B. J., Clara, I., & Asmundson, G. J. (2005). The relationship between anxiety disorders and physical disorders in the U.S. National Comorbidity Survey. *Depression and Anxiety, 21*(4), 193–202.

Scogin, F., Floyd, M., & Forde, J. (2000). Anxiety in older adults. In S. K. Whitbourne (Ed.), *Psychopathology in later life* (pp. 117–140). New York: Wiley. 10.1080/13607860902774493

Substance Abuse and Mental Health Services Administration. (2017). Key substance abuse and mental health indicators in the United States: Results from the 2016 National Survey on Drug Use and Health. Publication No. SMA 17-5044, NSDUH Series H-52. Rockville, MD: Substance Abuse and Mental Health Services Administration.

Substance Abuse and Mental Health Services Administration. (2018). National Survey from the 2017 National Survey on Drug Use and Health: Detailed Tables. Rockville, MD: Center for Behavioral Health Statistics and Quality.

Teri, L., Logsdon, R. G., Uomoto, J., & McCurry, S. M. (1997). Behavioral treatment of depression in dementia patients: A controlled clinical trial. *Journals of Gerontology: Series B: Psychological Sciences and Social Sciences, 52*(4), P159–P166.

Thorp, S. R., Ayers, C. R., Nuevo, R., Stoddard, J. A., Sorrell, J. T., & Wetherell, J. L. (2009). Meta-analysis comparing different behavioral treatments for late-life anxiety. *American Journal of Geriatric Psychiatry, 17*(2), 105–115.

U.S. Department of Health and Human Services. (1999). *Mental health: A report of the Surgeon General*. Bethesda, MD: U.S. Public Health Service.

Whitbourne, S. K., & Collins, K. C. (1998). Identity and physical changes in later adulthood: Theoretical and clinical implications. *Psychotherapy, 35*, 519–530.

Whitbourne, S. K., & Meeks, S. (2010). Psychopathology, bereavement, and aging. In K. W. Schaie & S. L. Willis (Eds.), *Handbook of the psychology of aging* (pp. 311–323). New York, NY: Cambridge University Press.

World Health Organization. (2017). Mental health of older adults. Retrieved from http://www.who.int/news-room/fact-sheets/detail/mental-health-of-older-adults

Wuthrich, V. M., & Frei, J. (2015). Barriers to treatment for older adults seeking psychological therapy. *International Psychogeriatrics, 27*(7), 1227–1236.

14

Psychotherapy for Developmental Disabilities

Jonathan M. Campbell and Angela Scarpa

As defined in the Developmental Disabilities Assistance and Bill of Rights Act of 2000, a developmental disability is a severe, chronic disability that (a) is attributable to a mental or physical impairment or combination of mental and physical impairments; (b) is present prior to 22 years of age; (c) is likely to continue indefinitely; (d) results in substantial restrictions in several life activities, such as self-care, learning, daily living skills, and economic sufficiency; and (e) reflects the person's need for a combination and sequence of lifelong interdisciplinary care, treatment, or support services (Public Law 106-402, 2000). Many types of developmental disabilities fall within this large definition, such as cerebral palsy, Down syndrome, fragile X syndrome, intellectual disability (ID), and autism spectrum disorder (ASD). Although individuals with developmental disabilities share similarities due to delayed development, these individuals represent a highly heterogeneous group. The possibility for impairment across various domains of functioning, such as social, language, cognition, adaptive, and motor, necessitates tailored services that span various professions, such as medical, psychological, physical therapy, and speech-language therapy. Similarly, appropriate supports span multiple service delivery systems, such as medical, educational, vocational, and social services. Among the most common developmental disabilities are ID and ASD; therefore, these two groups of individuals are the focus of our chapter.

ID is defined as "a disorder with onset during the developmental period that includes both intellectual and adaptive functioning deficits in conceptual, social, and practical domains" (American Psychiatric Association, 2013, p. 33). "Adaptive functioning" refers to an individual's ability to manage everyday tasks within conceptual, social, and practical domains. Although intellectual functioning has traditionally been used to characterize level of severity for ID, contemporary practice relies on adaptive functioning to define levels of severity (e.g., mild, moderate, severe) based on the individual's ability to function within conceptual, social, and practical domains.

ASD is a specific and chronic neurodevelopmental disorder that begins early in life, affects approximately one in 59 children in the United States, and is characterized by deficits in social communication and interactions as well as the presence of restricted and repetitive behaviors and interests (Baio et al., 2018). ASD is considered a spectrum in that symptoms can vary widely from child to child in both form and severity, may or may not include cognitive or language impairments, and is often associated with additional psychiatric and medical comorbidities (Leyfer et al., 2006). Without intervention, ASD can lead to lifelong impairments in family and peer relationships, academic success, employment, and independent living.

The Scope and Description of the Problem

Elevated risk for psychological disorder is well established for individuals with developmental disabilities, with rates of comorbidity as high as 36% for children (Emerson & Hatton, 2007) and 74% for adults (Buckles, Luckasson, & Keefe, 2013) with ID. Similarly, up to 70% to 72% of individuals with ASD experience one or more comorbid psychological disorders (Rosen, Mazefsky, Vasa, & Lerner, 2018). Prevalence rates range widely due to various factors, such as the sampling procedures used, definitions of mental illness (e.g., whether or not disruptive behavior is considered a disorder), and assessment methods used to identify mental illness (Irvin & Beail, 2016). Across various studies, for both ID and ASD, three of the most common comorbid psychological conditions are anxiety, depression, and behavioral dysregulation disorders, such as attention-deficit/hyperactivity disorder and oppositional defiant disorder (Emerson & Hatton, 2007). Given the high rates of comorbidity of psychological disorders, initial diagnosis and assessment of behavioral and emotional concerns is crucial for appropriate treatment planning and improved prognosis for individuals with developmental disabilities.

Despite the heightened risk for co-occurring psychological disorders, individuals with developmental disabilities are underserved by psychosocial therapies. Epidemiological data document mental health utilization that falls well below prevalence estimates of psychological disorder. For example, Einfeld and Tonge (1996) reported that approximately half of caregivers did not seek out assistance for psychological disorders for their children with ID, and less than 10% of caregivers sought out assistance from professionals with appropriate training in both ID and mental health. Authors have identified potential barriers to help seeking related to caregivers' perceptions of mental health service delivery for their children; several of these barriers are discussed in the next section. Anecdotally, for example, Einfeld and Tonge (1996) report that caregivers often experience difficulty accessing specialized services for children with both ID and mental health concerns. The authors' suggestion is consistent with our clinical experiences. Unfortunately, limited access to and use of mental health services for individuals with developmental disabilities frequently leads to emergency department utilization to manage mental health crises (Spassiani, Chacra, & Lunsky, 2017).

Barriers to Service Delivery

As noted, individuals with developmental disabilities suffer from psychological disorders at rates greater than the general population; however, use of mental health services falls well below identified need. A host of variables have been identified in the literature attempting to account for the discrepancy between need and service use. Whittle, Fisher, Reppermund, Lenroot, and Troller (2018) define a useful organizational model to organize barriers and "enablers" to access and utilize mental health services for individuals with developmental disabilities. Adopting Gulliford et al.'s (2002) general model of access to health care, Whittle et al. (2018) identify barriers and enablers across four domains of access: (a) service availability, (b) utilization, (c) relevance/effectiveness, and (d) equity.

Service Availability

Both the supply of service and having access to service are major concerns (Gulliford et al., 2002). The limited number of mental health care providers constitutes a significant barrier to availability of mental health services. Rurality exacerbates this problem. Specialized services for individuals with developmental disabilities tend to aggregate in population centers; travel time, distance, and coordinating transportation create additional barriers for individuals and families living in rural areas. For ASD, availability of evidence-based ASD services is often lacking, and this situation is exacerbated in low-resource and rural communities (Antezana et al., 2017).

Utilization

Gaining access to service includes domains such as organizational, financial, and personal variables (Gulliford et al., 2002). For individuals with developmental disabilities, mental health services may be difficult to utilize due to separation (or "siloing") of such services within existing service structures, such as statewide divisions of intellectual disability and behavioral health. Individuals with co-occurring difficulties may find it difficult to access services within each office due to eligibility requirements. Fees for services are also barriers to utilization, including costs of transportation and caregiver loss of time at work to accompany an individual to therapy. In the specific case of ASD, many recommended interventions are prohibitively expensive for many families. Finally, for individuals with developmental disabilities, needs are often addressed by caregivers, who may or may not be aware of mental health concerns. Caregivers' limited awareness of mental health concerns may be due to various reasons, such as lack of knowledge about specific mental health issues, communication difficulties on behalf of the individual, beliefs that attribute psychological difficulties to developmental disability itself, and focus on other pressing needs of the individual, such as medical concerns.

Relevance and Effectiveness

The quality and the usefulness of the service provided are major concerns. Whittle et al. (2018) catalogue lack of professional training and diagnostic overshadowing as critical barriers within this domain. "Diagnostic overshadowing" is the tendency to attribute psychopathology to developmental disability or to view psychopathology as less significant than language and cognitive deficits (e.g., Rush, Bowman, Eidman, & Toole, 2004). Assessment instruments typically used in psychological evaluation, such as interviews and self-report scales, are often of limited use with individuals with developmental disabilities. Likewise, the most commonly used third-party behavior rating scales have not been validated for individuals with developmental disabilities.

With respect to ASD, challenges may occur with appropriately identifying ASD as well as identifying co-occurring mental health diagnoses. For example, reliable administration of current gold-standard instruments for diagnosing ASD (e.g., Autism Diagnostic Observation Schedule, 2nd edition; Lord, Rutter, DiLavore, Risi, Gotham, & Bishop, 2012) requires considerable training and experience. With the exception of specific measures used to diagnose ASD, most assessment instruments exclude children with ASD from their standardization samples and are inappropriate for self-report from children with ASD who have language or cognitive impairments (Mazefsky & White, 2013). Notwithstanding these challenges, co-occurring mental health conditions should be assessed upon ASD diagnosis in toddlers and children (Simonoff et al., 2008) for appropriate treatment. Recommended behavioral interventions for ASD, although they are effective and can lead to long-term societal cost savings, also require extensive professional training (Peters-Scheffer, Didden, Korzilius, & Matson,

2012). Many providers feel ill prepared to work with the ASD population due to inadequate training in evidence-based practices (Stahmer, Collings, & Palinkas, 2005).

Equity

Access in terms of equity refers to aspects of fairness and social justice, such as whether mental health services are equally accessible across race/ethnicity, socioeconomic status, and level of severity of disability. There are well-established delays in first identification of developmental disabilities across race. For example, ASD is identified earlier in White children than in non-Whites, and ASD is identified earlier in children from more affluent households than less affluent children (e.g., Mandell, Listerud, Levy, & Pinto-Martin, 2002). Individuals with more severe developmental disability also experience poorer access to service than individuals with milder symptoms (e.g., Whittle et al., 2018).

Creating Cultural Competency

Although there is no "culture" of developmental disability per se, it is important for mental health providers to understand stigmatizing attitudes, such as ableism, that accompany developmental disability. Ableism is a system of discrimination and exclusion that works against individuals with developmental disabilities as reflected in societal beliefs that "it's better not to have a disability than to have one, and it's better to do things the way nondisabled people do" (Storey, 2007, p. 56). Undergirding discrimination and exclusion are beliefs that individuals with developmental disabilities (a) are burdensome to society, (b) are to be pitied, (c) lack decision-making capacity, and (d) demonstrate defining character flaws. Individuals with developmental disability and mental illness may experience a "double stigma" (Spassiani et al., 2017, p. 85) during interactions with health care providers. A "double stigma" refers to the presence of two developmental and mental disabilities and is characterized by health care providers' lack of support, disregard, and dismissive responses to individuals' needs, as well as poor follow-up for mental health needs. Developmental disability and mental health concerns intersect with other social variables, such as geographic location, race, and socioeconomic status, to further produce disparities in mental health service delivery.

We recommend development and maintenance of competency through various strategies and approaches. Graduate training curricula should include specific content regarding mental health needs of individuals with developmental disabilities. Content may be infused across various courses, such as a multicultural course and introduction to psychotherapy. In our training programs, we have invited individuals and caregivers, as appropriate, to provide first-hand descriptions of stigmatizing attitudes and their impact on mental health services to share with graduate trainees. We have found such "guest lectures" to be powerful educational experiences for graduate students. Training programs should consider developing relationships with the local developmental disability community, both mental health agencies and support groups, to bring about better understanding of needs and provide initial training in provision of mental health services. Ideally, training programs would require supervised training with individuals with developmental disabilities. Ongoing professional training opportunities exist through the American Psychological Association's Division 33 (Intellectual and Developmental Disabilities/Autism Spectrum Disorder), an organization with the explicit mission to support professional education and clinical services that address the needs of individuals with developmental disabilities. The National Association for the Dually Diagnosed (NADD) is a not-for-profit association with the mission of advancing mental health care for individuals with developmental disabilities (www.thenadd.org). NADD hosts annual conferences and trainings to improve capacity to respond to mental health needs for individuals with developmental disabilities. NADD also publishes the *Journal of Mental Health Research in Intellectual Disabilities*, which focuses on mental health care for individuals with developmental disabilities.

In addition, mental health professionals should be reflective regarding their own stigmatizing beliefs about individuals with developmental disabilities. They should be aware of the importance of self-determination and self-advocacy for individuals with developmental disabilities (and families, as appropriate) and actively solicit opinions regarding treatment goals. Unfortunately, direct input from individuals with developmental disabilities is limited in the research literature; however, when asked, individuals provide a valuable description of what is helpful during psychotherapy. Like everyone else, individuals with developmental disabilities appreciate confidentiality, appreciate being heard, and value the therapeutic relationship (e.g., Jahoda, 2016).

Effective Strategies and Empirically-Supported Treatments

For individuals with developmental disabilities, psychosocial therapy has historically taken the form of behavioral modification grounded in operant conditioning and applied behavior analysis. The foci of behavioral modification are behavioral reduction of undesirable behavior, such as self-injury or aggression, and skill acquisition, such as communication and toileting. Behavioral modification techniques have proven to be efficacious in managing a host of behavioral challenges for those with developmental disabilities. For example, behavioral modification has been shown to decrease severe problem behavior for individuals across a wide range of ages, ability levels, and behavioral difficulties (e.g., Campbell, 2003). Likewise, behavioral modification has been shown to be effective in improving adaptive skills for individuals with developmental disabilities across a wide range of areas, such as communication, social, and adaptive living skills.

The contribution of psychotherapy in addressing mental health for individuals with developmental disabilities has a much more recent history. Greater advocacy for inclusion and access to institutions (e.g., public education) and the rise of empirically supported/evidence-based therapy movements within psychology have contributed to investigating the usefulness of traditional psychotherapeutic interventions with individuals with developmental disabilities, particularly ID and ASD. Given findings that mental illness affects individuals with developmental disabilities more often than the general population, this group of individuals should have access to psychotherapeutic interventions that have been shown to be efficacious for the general population.

Intellectual Disability

The overall evidence supporting the efficacy of psychotherapy for individuals with ID is mixed. For example, Vereenooghe and Langdon (2013) conducted a meta-analysis and concluded that psychotherapy was efficacious for reducing symptoms of anger, aggression, and depression; however, interpersonal functioning was not improved through psychotherapy. In contrast, Koslowski et al.'s (2016) meta-analysis concluded that psychotherapy was ineffective for individuals with mild to moderate ID for behavioral problems, depression, and anxiety. The authors reported that the effect size for depression fell in the moderate range but was not statistically significant (Koslowski et al., 2016). The reviews differed in inclusion criteria: The Koslowski et al. (2016) meta-analysis targeted mild to moderate ID while the Vereenooghe and Langdon (2013) meta-analysis included severe ID. Similar to Koslowski et al.'s (2016) findings, Osugo and Cooper (2016) concluded that the effectiveness of psychotherapy for individuals with mild ID is not well established.

Cognitive Behavioral Therapy

Cognitive behavioral therapy (CBT) is a psychotherapeutic approach that merges behavior and cognitive therapy, using short-term, problem-focused strategies based on empirical data and theory from learning and cognition. Within the larger psychotherapy outcome literature, CBT consistently emerges as a well-established treatment for various disorders, such as anxiety disorders and depression. For individuals with ID, psychotherapists may question the applicability of CBT as a psychotherapeutic approach due to individuals' limits with abstract reasoning, language understanding, and understanding connections between thoughts, emotions, and behavior. Nonetheless, CBT approaches have been evaluated with individuals with ID. Dagnan, Jackson, and Eastlake (2018) concluded that CBT for anxiety is promising but not yet well established for individuals with ID. In contrast, Hamers, Festen, and Hermans (2018) concluded that CBT is effective in treating depression for individuals with mild to moderate ID.

Cooney, Tunney, and O'Reilly (2018) reviewed evidence on whether individuals with ID demonstrate the cognitive skills needed to benefit from CBT, such as the ability to recognize emotions and link thoughts, feelings, and behaviors. They concluded that the research literature produced mixed findings. They found that emotion recognition is enhanced when photographs and visual depictions of emotions are used in CBT. Individuals with ID identify feeling and behaviors but often show difficulty with readily identifying thoughts. Individuals with ID also show the capacity to connect emotions with events; the ability to link these two together improves with greater verbal ability. Modifications to CBT are recommended to support individuals with ID (e.g., Jahoda, 2016). For example, visual aids should supplement verbal communication during therapy, and thought bubbles may be used to illustrate differing perspectives and interpretations of events. Role playing is also recommended to further highlight how different individuals may interpret the same event.

General Recommendations to Support Psychotherapy for Individuals with ID

Narrative reviews across disparate psychotherapeutic interventions (e.g., CBT, group, solution-focused) consistently recommend the following to support individuals with ID:

1. Include visual supports and aids during the psychotherapy process.
2. Use brief, clear language and reduce abstract language during psychotherapy.
3. Increase repetition of key therapeutic points.
4. Use a slower pace, incorporate breaks, and divide sessions.
5. Involve caregivers and direct care staff in intervention to consolidate gains in therapy and assist with therapeutic homework.

Autism Spectrum Disorder

Evidence-based practices for ASD vary widely depending upon the individual needs of the child but generally focus on language/communication for toddlers, emotional and behavioral problems for children, social skills for children and adolescents, and post-secondary needs as adolescents and young adults transition to life beyond school. A review published by the National Professional Development Center (Wong et al., 2015) identified 27 focused treatments that meet criteria for being evidence-based. We will focus on three of these practices that have been used by the second author to address different levels of functioning and targeted outcomes across ages: Pivotal Response Training (PRT), CBT approaches, and Social Skills Training (SST).

Pivotal Response Training

PRT is an approach based on applied behavior analysis in natural learning environments that targets pivotal skills (e.g., motivation, self-initiation, self-management, and focus on multiple cues) thought to have widespread influence on learning additional untargeted skills (Koegel, Ashbaugh, & Koegel, 2016). Social communication impairment is a core deficit in ASD that can include delayed acquisition and use of functional language, repetitive phrases, and restricted topics of interest (American Psychiatric Association, 2013). Our clinic has focused on using PRT within a parent or caregiver training/coaching model to target functional language for nonverbal or minimally verbal toddlers and preschoolers with ASD. (By "parent," we refer to anyone who is in the caregiving role for a child with ASD.)

PRT has been delivered effectively in both individual treatment with parent–child dyads and in a group model (Hardan et al., 2015, Minjarez, Mercier, Williams, & Hardan, 2013; Minjarez, Williams, Mercier, & Hardan, 2011). In PRT parent education, parents are taught antecedent–behavior–consequence principles of behavior analysis and motivational techniques, including:

1. Giving clear instructions and maintaining child attention
2. Interspersing maintenance tasks (already learned tasks) with acquisition tasks (new or difficult tasks)
3. Providing a choice between stimuli and/or tasks (e.g., a parent may prompt the child with "pretzels or cookies" to elicit a reply or may provide choices of toys a child could play with to assess and maintain the child's interest in the task)
4. Providing natural reinforcement contingent on a child's behavior, especially verbal behavior.

A systematic review concluded that PRT leads to increases in child self-initiations, functional language, and play skills, as well as decreases in problem behavior (Verschuur, Didden, Lang, Sigafoos, & Huskens, 2014).

Although parents can effectively learn PRT techniques to benefit their children, a consistent challenge to implementation is parental engagement, often as a result of parental stress and burnout. Parents may avoid or drop out of treatments that have a heavy parental component. Unfortunately, parents of children with ASD experience elevated stress levels compared to parents of children with other developmental disabilities and typical development (Hayes & Watson, 2013), and stress can be exacerbated in low-resource communities where other stressors exist, such as poverty and unemployment (Antezana, Scarpa, Valdespino, Albright, & Richey 2017). Elevated parenting stress can reduce parental efficacy (Rezendes & Scarpa, 2011) and is negatively associated with benefits obtained from services (Robbins, Dunlap, & Plienin, 1991). It is helpful to consider the family unit and sociodemographic circumstances, promote social support, and provide parents with coping skills during PRT.

Cognitive Behavioral Approaches for ASD

As with individuals with ID, CBT has been adapted for use with children and adolescents with ASD, particularly when there is little or no language and cognitive impairment (Attwood & Scarpa, 2013). The cognitive components of CBT primarily focus on helping clients identify and change maladaptive attitudes and beliefs that are maintaining negative emotions or behaviors; the behavioral components of CBT include techniques to change behavior through modifying antecedents and consequences in the situation.

Due to challenges inherent in ASD, children with ASD are at increased risk for emotion dysregulation and heightened negative affect, such as anger and anxiety (Mazefsky et al., 2013). Such difficulties can manifest in distressing disruptive outbursts (e.g., tantrums) and can potentially lead to later anxiety and depression (Mazefsky, Borue, Day, & Minshew, 2014). As such, targeting these problematic behaviors through CBT affective education and skill building can improve overall functioning. The CBT program Exploring Feelings teaches children how thoughts, feelings, and behaviors interact, with the goal of providing skills for monitoring and coping with anger and anxiety. This intervention program has been found to be an efficacious treatment for older children (age nine to 12) with high-functioning ASD and comorbid anger or anxiety problems (Sofronoff, Attwood, & Hinton, 2005; Sofronoff, Attwood, Hinton, & Levin, 2007). Pilot testing of the intervention, called the Stress and Anger Management Program (STAMP; Scarpa, Wells, & Attwood, 2013), which was developmentally adapted for young children (age five to seven) with ASD, also showed benefits through increased knowledge of emotion regulation skills and shorter and fewer emotional outbursts for children (Scarpa & Reyes, 2011).

STAMP is a manualized caregiver-assisted group CBT derivative of the Exploring Feelings program. It is unique in being the first CBT for children with ASD as young as five years, providing affective education, skill building, and cognitive restructuring components of traditional CBT in an engaging and developmentally appropriate group format (e.g., singing, stories), meeting once weekly for nine weeks. Details on STAMP components and implementation can be found in Scarpa, Reyes, and Attwood (2013) as well as in the manual (Scarpa, Wells, & Attwood, 2013). In essence, children are first provided with an affective education and vocabulary to understand and identify positive and negative emotions (e.g., happiness, anxiety), followed by weekly introduction of tools or coping strategies, which are added to their "emotional toolbox." The strategies consist of physical, relaxation, social, cognitive, and special interest tools aimed at helping the children to self-soothe physiological responses, redirect behavior, or reframe cognitions in the service of managing negative emotions.

Parents/caregivers are viewed as integral to the therapeutic process in assisting children with home practice and generalization of behavior (Hassenfeldt, Lorenzi, & Scarpa, 2015). Therefore, STAMP includes simultaneous parent and child groups, wherein parents receive psychoeducation about autism and emotion regulation while also observing (via live video) the tools being taught to the children in another room. Pilot results indicate parents' confidence in their ability to handle the child's angry or anxious behaviors (Scarpa & Reyes, 2011); anecdotally, parents have commented during these sessions that they are also learning and benefiting from tools to cope with their own negative emotions, thus having a side benefit of helping parents cope with the additional demands placed upon them.

Although STAMP has shown promising results for both young children with ASD and their parents, additional research is needed to replicate the findings, test generalization of behavior outside the home and clinic, and understand the mechanisms at work. Overall, this program supports the benefits of CBT when adapted appropriately for youth with ASD and is unique in being the first CBT to be used in children with ASD as young as five years old. Regarding implementation, we have found it helpful to modify traditional CBT for this population by including caregiver training, providing children with a schedule for each session, adding visual aids, and using stories and games to teach and illustrate techniques.

Social Skills Training

Regardless of cognitive or verbal ability, people who have ASD are, by definition, limited by their social impairments. They often become more aware of ASD-related social difficulties and experience associated problems with anxiety and depression during adolescence (Carter, Davis, Klin, & Volkmar, 2005; White, Oswald, Ollendick, & Scahill, 2009), making the teen years an important time to intervene on social skills. SST refers to programs that teach people with ASD ways to appropriately interact with others and have positive relationships. SST components often include instruction on basic concepts, modeling, role playing or practice, and feedback to teach both basic and advanced skills such as making appropriate eye contact, using gestures, exchanging information, starting and ending a conversation, and handling conflict. According to a systematic review, there is significant evidence for benefits of social skills group interventions for adolescents with autism (Miller, Vernon, Wu, & Russo, 2014).

The Program for the Education and Enrichment of Relationship Skills (PEERS; Laugeson & Frankel, 2010) is a manualized SST developed for adolescents with ASD, with the goal of helping these teens make and keep friends using techniques that are typical and expected for their age group. PEERS for adolescents is implemented over 14 weekly sessions, covering the following topics, each of which is broken down into micro-skills or steps:

1. Conversational skills, such as trading information, two-way conversations, entering and exiting a conversation
2. Use of electronic communication
3. Choosing appropriate friends
4. Appropriate use of humor
5. Planning and handling get-togethers
6. Good sportsmanship
7. Dealing with teasing, embarrassing feedback, bullying, a bad reputation, rumors, and gossip
8. Handling disagreements/arguments.

Two randomized controlled trials of PEERS ($n = 33$ and $n = 28$ adolescents) have yielded large between-group effects on parent-reported social skills as well as improvements on social skills knowledge, social responsiveness, and number of get-togethers (Laugeson, Frankel, Gantman, Dillon, & Mogil, 2012; Laugeson, Frankel, Mogil, & Dillon, 2009). Results have also been replicated in young adults with ASD and in other countries (e.g., Laugeson, Gantman, Kapp, Orenski, & Ellingson, 2015).

Although results consistently indicate that PEERS is an effective social skills intervention for teens with ASD, some important caveats are noted. PEERS is intended for adolescents with ASD who are not cognitively impaired (i.e., IQ > 70), express clear motivation to make and keep friends and willingness to engage in the treatment, and do not have excessive anxiety. The effectiveness of the intervention is limited if any of these criteria are not met. As such, teens with ASD and low motivation or high social anxiety, for example, may not engage in the behavioral rehearsals and social exposures needed in this program. Treatment that targets their anxiety may be called for before returning to PEERS. Those with cognitive impairment may not fully comprehend the terminology used in PEERS, but benefits might be maximized to the extent that extra time and effort is made to ensure their understanding of the material.

Future Steps

Various recommendations are presented in the literature regarding improving access to and utilization of psychological services, and three consistent themes emerge. First, there is a consistent call for building capacity of service providers to identify and respond to mental health concerns for those with developmental disabilities. Interdisciplinary training is consistently recommended due to the various needs of individuals with developmental disabilities. Federally funded training programs, such as University Centers of Excellence in Developmental Disabilities (https://www.aucd.org/template/page.cfm?id=667) and Leadership in Neurodevelopmental Disorders (https://www.aucd.org/template/page.cfm?id=473), and interdisciplinary personnel preparation programs for special educators and related service providers are examples of mechanisms to accomplish interdisciplinary training. As noted earlier in the chapter, we recommend didactic content and supervised experiences within graduate training that focus on the mental health needs of individuals with developmental disabilities. Due to the known risk for psychological disorders, clinicians working with individuals with developmental disabilities should inquire about changes in functioning (e.g., loss of interest, changes in appetite) to screen for comorbid behavioral and psychological conditions.

Innovative Service Delivery

Public schools serve as the de facto service delivery provider for most individuals with developmental disabilities. Within the United States, the Individuals with Disabilities Education Act (IDEA), along with its reauthorizations, protects the right of students with developmental disabilities between the ages of three and 22 years to a free and appropriate public education (FAPE) in the least restrictive environment possible (Public Law 108-446, 2004). A key component of FAPE is development and implementation of an individualized education program (IEP), which details the educational, communicative, social, and behavioral needs of students with developmental disabilities. The IEP includes provision of additional services and supports needed for students with developmental disabilities, such as speech therapy, occupational therapy, behavioral interventions, and psychological services. Given these circumstances, public schools represent a service delivery setting for implementation of the evidence-based interventions described in the chapter. Clinical interventions traditionally developed and evaluated in clinic settings have begun to be implemented and evaluated in school settings. Implementation science models may prove helpful in the delivery of evidence-based interventions within schools, including use of response-to-intervention and stepped-care models (e.g., Hume & Campbell, 2019; Wood, McLeod, Klebanoff, & Brookman-Frazee, 2015). In each case, service delivery is initiated with minimal intensity, with increases in intensity if individuals do not respond to intervention.

Outside of schools, mental health services may be delivered within other community setting and primary care settings. Medical home models have been proposed to offer continuity of care over the lifespan as well as a single entry point to access medical and mental health services for individuals with developmental disabilities (Carbone, Behl, Azor, & Murphy, 2010). Telehealth has been utilized to counter distance and logistical barriers and has proven helpful for early identification and behavioral consultation for individuals with developmental disabilities.

Collaboration Across Service Providers and Agencies

Fractured service delivery also creates barriers to mental health services. Interagency collaboration reduces redundancy of service and increases the likelihood of care coordination. Collaboration also increases access to expertise across disciplines, which may address knowledge deficits, such as diagnostic overshadowing, within a service team. Such collaboration may need to occur across disparate systems of care and support, such as state agencies focused on public health, behavioral health, education, vocational-rehabilitation services, and Medicaid funding (National Association of State Mental Health Program Directors, 2004). Several states have launched interagency collaboration efforts to improve outcomes for individuals with ASD, such as the Office of Autism in Kentucky and the Virginia Autism Council. Within each council, institutes of higher education partner with the state agencies to provide consultation but also keep abreast of community needs for families and individuals.

Within schools, various service providers, such as school psychologists, school counselors, speech therapists, and physical therapists, respond to the educational and social-emotional needs of students with developmental disabilities. Some school districts feature school-based mental health centers within their structures, such as the Shelby County Schools Mental Health Center in Tennessee (http://www.scsk12.org/exceptional/mental.php?PID=1027). Mental health providers operating outside of school systems need to understand the scope of mental health services provided within schools to understand how they may best serve individuals with developmental disabilities. Such understanding may be achieved through contacting directors of special education services to inquire about the services provided and opportunities for collaboration. Using a systems framework, Laundy (2015) advocates for building successful collaborative teams within schools. Teams could include the appropriate general and special education teachers, psychotherapist, speech therapist, occupational therapist, psychiatrist, social worker, paraprofessionals, family members, and others who work with the student who wish to be involved. One model for collaborative consultation in the IEP process, for example, is the Collaborative Model for Promoting Competence and Success for Students with ASD (COMPASS), an evidence-based school consultation model (Ruble, Dalrymple, & McGrew, 2012). The goal of COMPASS is to use information gathered from caregivers, teachers, and other professionals to achieve mutually discussed and identified IEP goals. A randomized controlled trial found that children enrolled in COMPASS were able to reach educational goals at a significantly higher level than children enrolled in treatment as usual (Ruble, Dalrymple, & McGrew, 2010).

Concluding Comments

Psychological disorders commonly co-occur with developmental disabilities, yet mental health services are underdeveloped for this group. Evidence-based interventions exist to address mental health concerns for individuals with developmental disabilities, such as cognitive behavioral and behavioral approaches. Barriers to access and utilization of services include low numbers of appropriately trained providers, costs of services, and fragmented service delivery; barriers are exacerbated by minority race status, low socioeconomic status, and rurality. Stigmatizing attitudes toward individuals with developmental disabilities also contribute to poor experiences with mental health providers. Interdisciplinary training, adoption of innovative service delivery models, and care coordination are identified as potential solutions to these barriers.

References

American Psychiatric Association. (2013). *Diagnostic and statistical manual of mental disorders* (5th ed.). Washington, DC: Author.

Antezana, L., Scarpa, A., Valdespino, A., Albright, J., & Richey, J. A. (2017). Rural trends in diagnosis and services for autism spectrum disorder. *Frontiers in Psychology, 8*, 590.

Attwood, T., & Scarpa, A. S. (2013). Modifications of cognitive-behavioral therapy for children and adolescents with high-functioning ASD and their common difficulties. In A. Scarpa, S. W. White, & T. Attwood (Eds.), *CBT for children and adolescents with high functioning autism spectrum disorders* (pp. 27–44). New York, NY: Guilford.

Baio, J., Wiggins, L., Christensen, D. L., Maenner, M. J., Daniels, J., Warren, Z., . . . Dowling, N. F. (2018). Prevalence of autism spectrum disorder among children aged 8 years—Autism and Developmental Disabilities Monitoring Network, 11 wites, United States, 2014. *MMWR Surveillance Summaries, 67*(No. SS-6):1–23.

Buckles, J., Luckasson, R., & Keefe, E. (2013). A systematic review of the prevalence of psychiatric disorders in adults with intellectual disability, 2003-2010. *Journal of Mental Health Research in Developmental Disabilities, 6*, 181–207.

Campbell, J. M. (2003). Efficacy of behavioral interventions for reducing problem behavior in persons with autism: A quantitative synthesis of single-subject research. *Research in Developmental Disabilities, 24*, 120–138.

Carbone, P. S., Behl, D. D., Azor, V., & Murphy, N. A. (2010). The medical home with children with autism spectrum disorders: Parent and pediatrician perspectives. *Journal of Autism and Developmental Disorders, 40*, 317–324.

Carter, A., Davis, N., Klin, A., & Volkmar, F. (2005). Social development in autism. In F. R. Volkmar, R. Paul, A. Klin, & D. Cohen (Eds.), *Handbook of autism and pervasive developmental disorders* (3rd ed., pp. 312–334). Hoboken, NJ: Wiley.

Cooney, P., Tunney, C., & O'Reilly, G. (2018). A systematic review of the evidence regarding cognitive therapy skills that assist cognitive behavioural therapy in adults who have intellectual disability. *Journal of Applied Research in Intellectual Disabilities, 31*, 23–42.

Dagnan, D., Jackson, I., & Eastlake, L. (2018). A systematic review of cognitive behavioural therapy for anxiety in adults with intellectual disabilities. *Journal of Intellectual Disability Research, 62*, 974–991.

Developmental Disabilities Assistance and Bill of Rights Act of 2000, Pub. L. No. 106-402, 114 Stat. 1677 (2000).

Einfeld, S. L., & Tonge, B. J. (1996). Population prevalence of psychopathology in children and adolescents with intellectual disability: II. Epidemiological findings. *Journal of Intellectual Disability Research, 40*, 99–109.

Emerson, E., & Hatton, C. (2007). Mental health of children and adolescents with intellectual disabilities in Britain. *British Journal of Psychiatry, 191*, 493–499.

Gulliford, M., Figueroa-Munoz, J., Morgan, M., Hughes, D., Gibson, B., Beech, R., & Hudson, M. (2002). What does "access to health care" mean? *Journal of Health Services Research and Policy, 7*, 186–188.

Hamers, P. C. M., Festen, D. A. M., & Hermans, H. (2018). Non-pharmacological interventions for adults with intellectual disabilities and depression: A systematic review. *Journal of Intellectual Disability Research, 62*, 684–700.

Hardan, A. Y., Gengoux, G. W., Berquist, K. L., Libove, R. A., Ardel, C. M., Phillips, J., . . . Minjarez, M. B. (2015). A randomized controlled trial of Pivotal Response Treatment Group for parents of children with autism. *Journal of Child Psychology and Psychiatry, 56*, 884–892.

Hassenfeldt, T. A., Lorenzi, J., & Scarpa, A. (2015). A review of parent training in child interventions: Applications to cognitive-behavioral therapy for children with high-functioning autism. *Review Journal of Autism and Developmental Disorders, 2*, 79–90.

Hayes, S. A., & Watson, S. L. (2013). The impact of parenting stress: A meta-analysis of studies comparing the experience of parenting stress in parents of children with and without autism spectrum disorder. *Journal of Autism and Developmental Disorders, 43*, 629–642.

Hume, K. A., & Campbell, J. M. (2019). Introduction to special section on peer interventions for autism spectrum disorder in school settings. *School Psychology Review, 48*(2), 115–122.

Individuals with Disabilities Education Improvement Act of 2004. Pub. L. No. 108-446, 118 Stat. 2647. (2004).

Irvine, M., & Beail, N. (2016). Identifying and meeting the emotional and mental health needs of people who have intellectual disabilities through psychological therapies. In N. Beail (Ed.), *Psychological therapies and people who have intellectual disabilities* (pp. 11–18). Leicester, UK: British Psychological Society.

Jahoda, A. (2016). Cognitive behavioural therapy. In N. Beail (Ed.), *Psychological therapies and people who have intellectual disabilities* (pp. 29–33). Leicester, UK: British Psychological Society.

Koegel, L. K., Ashbaugh, K., & Koegel, R. L. (2016). Pivotal response treatment. In R. Lang, T. B. Hancock, & N. N. Singh (Eds.), *Early intervention for young children with autism spectrum disorder* (pp. 85–112). Switzerland: Springer International Publishing.

Koslowski, N., Klein, K., Arnold, K., Kosters, M., Schutzwohl, M., Salize, H. J., & Puschner, B. (2016). Effectiveness of interventions for adults with mild to moderate intellectual disabilities and mental health problems: Systematic review and meta-analysis. *British Journal of Psychiatry, 209*, 469–474.

Laugeson, E. A., & Frankel, F. (2010). *Social skills for teenagers with developmental and autism spectrum disorders: The PEERS treatment manual.* New York, NY: Routledge.

Laugeson, E. A., Frankel, F., Gantman, A., Dillon, A. R., & Mogil, C. (2012). Evidence-based social skills training for adolescents with autism spectrum disorders: The UCLA PEERS program. *Journal of Autism and Developmental Disorders, 42*, 1025–1036.

Laugeson, E. A., Frankel, F., Mogil, C., & Dillon, A. R. (2009). Parent-assisted social skills training to improve friendships in teens with autism spectrum disorders. *Journal of Autism and Developmental Disorders, 39*, 596–606.

Laugeson, E. A., Gantman, A., Kapp, S. K., Orenski, K., & Ellingsen, R. (2015). A randomized controlled trial to improve social skills in young adults with autism spectrum disorder: The UCLA PEERS® program. *Journal of Autism and Developmental Disorders, 45*, 3978–3989.

Laundy, K. C. (2015). *Building school-based collaborative mental health teams: A systems approach to student achievement.* Camp Hill, PA: TPI Press/The Practice Institute.

Leyfer, O. T., Folstein, S. E., Bacalman, S., Davis, N.O., Dinh, E., Morgan, J., . . . Lainhart, J. (2006). Comorbid psychiatric disorders in children with autism: Interview development and rates of disorders. *Journal for Autism and Developmental Disorders, 36*, 849–861.

Lord, C., Rutter, M., DiLavore, P., Risi, S., Gotham, K., & Bishop, S. (2012). *Autism Diagnostic Observation Schedule, Second Edition (ADOS-2) manual.* Torrance, CA: Western Psychological Services.

Mandell, D. S., Listerud, J., Levy, S. E., & Pinto-Martin, J. A. (2002). Race differences in the age at diagnosis among Medicaid-eligible children with autism. *Journal of the American Academy of Child & Adolescent Psychiatry, 41*, 1447–1453.

Mazefsky, C. A., Borue, X., Day, T. N., & Minshew, N. J. (2014). Emotion regulation patterns in adolescents with high-functioning autism spectrum disorder: Comparison to typically developing adolescents and association with psychiatric symptoms. *Autism Research, 7*, 344–354.

Mazefsky, C. A., Herrington, J., Siegel, M., Scarpa, A., Maddox, B. B., Scahill, L., & White, S. W. (2013). The role of emotion regulation in autism spectrum disorder. *Journal of the American Academy of Child & Adolescent Psychiatry, 52*, 679–688.

Mazefsky, C. A., & White, S. W. (2013). The role of assessment in guiding treatment planning for youth with ASD. In A. Scarpa, S. W. White, & T. Attwood (Eds.), *CBT for children and adolescents with high-functioning autism spectrum disorders* (pp. 45–72). New York, NY: Guilford.

Miller, A., Vernon, T., Wu, V., & Russo, K. (2014). Social skill group interventions for adolescents with autism spectrum disorders: A systematic review. *Review Journal of Autism and Developmental Disorders, 1*, 254–265.

Minjarez, M. B., Mercier, E. M., Williams, S. E., & Hardan, A. Y. (2013). Impact of Pivotal Response Training group therapy on stress and empowerment in parents of children with autism. *Journal of Positive Behavior Interventions, 15*, 71–78.

Minjarez, M. B., Williams, S. E., Mercier, E. M., & Hardan, A. Y. (2011). Pivotal Response group treatment program for parents of children with autism. *Journal of Autism and Developmental Disorders, 41*, 92–101.

National Association of State Mental Health Program Directors. (2004). *Serving individuals with co-occurring developmental disabilities and mental illnesses: Systems barriers and strategies for reform.* Retrieved from https://www.nasmhpd.org/sites/default/files/ServingIndividualswithCoOccurring.pdf

Osugo, M., & Cooper S. A. (2016). Interventions for adults with mild intellectual disabilities and mental ill-health: A systematic review. *Journal of Intellectual Disability Research, 60*, 615–622.

Peters-Scheffer, N., Didden, R., Korzilius, H., & Matson, J. (2012). Cost comparison of early intensive behavioral intervention and treatment as usual for children with autism spectrum disorder in the Netherlands. *Research in Developmental Disabilities, 33*, 1763–1772.

Rezendes, D. L., & Scarpa, A. (2011). Associations between parental anxiety/depression and child behavior problems related to autism spectrum disorders: The roles of parenting stress and parenting self-efficacy. *Autism Research and Treatment, 2011*, 395190.

Robbins, F. R., Dunlap, G., & Plienis, A. J. (1991). Family characteristics, family training, and the progress of young children with autism. *Journal of Early Intervention, 15*, 173–184.

Rosen, T. E., Mazefsky, C. A., Vasa, R. A., & Lerner, M. D. (2018). Co-occuring psychiatric conditions in autism spectrum disorder. *International Review of Psychiatry, 30*, 40–61.

Ruble, L. A., Dalrymple, N. J., & McGrew, J. H. (2010). The effects of consultation on individualized education program outcomes for young children with autism: The collaborative model for promoting competence and success. *Journal of Early Intervention, 32*, 286–301.

Ruble, L. A., Dalrymple, N. J., & McGrew, J. H. (2012). *Collaborative model for promoting competence and success for students with ASD.* New York, NY: Springer.

Rush, K. S., Bowman, L. G., Eidman, S. L., Toole, L. M., & Mortenson, B. P. (2004). Assessing psychopathology in individuals with developmental disabilities. *Behavior Modification, 28*, 621–637.

Scarpa, A., & Reyes, N. M. (2011). Improving emotion regulation with CBT in young children with high functioning autism spectrum disorders: A pilot study. *Behavioural and Cognitive Psychotherapy, 39*, 495–500.

Scarpa, A., Reyes, N., & Attwood, T. (2013). Cognitive behavioral treatment for stress and anger management in young children with ASD: The Exploring Feelings program. In A. Scarpa, S. W. White, & T. Attwood (Eds.), *CBT for children and adolescents with high functioning autism spectrum disorders* (pp. 147–172). New York, NY: Guilford.

Scarpa, A., Wells, A., & Attwood, T. (2013). *Exploring feelings for young children with high-functioning autism or Asperger's disorder: The STAMP treatment manual*. Philadelphia, PA: Jessica Kingsley Publishers.

Simonoff, E., Pickles, A., Charman, T., Chandler, S., Loucas, T., & Baird, G. (2008). Psychiatric disorders in children with autism spectrum disorders: Prevalence, comorbidity, and associated factors in a population-derived sample. *Journal of the American Academy of Child & Adolescent Psychiatry, 47*, 921–929.

Sofronoff, K., Attwood, T., & Hinton, S. (2005). A randomised controlled trial of a CBT intervention for anxiety in children with Asperger syndrome. *Journal of Child Psychology and Psychiatry, 46*, 1152–1160.

Sofronoff, K., Attwood, T., Hinton, S., & Levin, I. (2007). A randomized controlled trial of a cognitive behavioural intervention for anger management in children diagnosed with Asperger syndrome. *Journal of Autism and Developmental Disorders, 37*, 1203–1214.

Spassiani, N., Chacra, M. S. A., & Lunsky, Y. (2017). "Why are you here? Can't you cope at home?" The psychiatric crisis of people with intellectual disabilities and the community's response. *Journal of Mental Health Research in Intellectual Disabilities, 10*, 74–92. https://doi.org/10.1080/19315864.2016.1278290

Stahmer, A. C., Collings, N. M., & Palinkas, L. A. (2005). Early intervention practices for children with autism: Descriptions from community providers. *Focus on Autism and Other Developmental Disabilities, 20*, 66–79.

Storey, K. (2007). Combating ableism in schools. *Preventing School Failure, 52*, 56–58.

Vereenooghe, L., & Langdon, P. E. (2013). Psychological therapies for people with intellectual disabilities: A systematic review and meta-analysis. *Research in Developmental Disabilities, 34*, 4085–4102.

Verschuur, R., Didden, R., Lang, R., Sigafoos, J., & Huskens, B. (2014). Pivotal response treatment for children with autism spectrum disorders: A systematic review. *Review Journal of Autism and Developmental Disorders, 1*, 34–61.

White, S. W., Oswald, D., Ollendick, T., & Scahill, L. (2009). Anxiety in children and adolescents with autism spectrum disorders. *Clinical Psychology Review, 29*, 216–229.

Whittle, E. L., Fisher, K. R., Reppermund, S., Lenroot, R., & Troller, J. (2018). Barriers and enablers to accessing mental health services for people with intellectual disability: A scoping review. *Journal of Mental Health Research in Intellectual Disabilities, 11*, 69–102.

Wong, C., Odom, S. L., Hume, K. A., Cox, A. W., Fettig, A., Kucharczyk, S., . . . Schultz, T. R. (2015). Evidence-based practices for children, youth, and young adults with autism spectrum disorder: A comprehensive review. *Journal of Autism and Developmental Disorders, 45*, 1951–1966.

Wood, J. J., McLeod, B. D., Kelbanoff, S., & Brookman-Frazee, L. (2015). Toward the implementation of evidence-based interventions for youth with autism spectrum disorders in schools and community agencies. *Behavior Therapy, 46*, 83–95.

SECTION 5
OTHER CHALLENGES

15

Ethics Issues and Challenges When Bringing Psychotherapy to the Underserved

Jeffrey E. Barnett

As noted throughout this book, there are many areas across the globe with unmet mental health treatment needs, and in many geographic areas where mental health services are plentiful, there are groups of individuals who nevertheless remain underserved. These underserved communities could benefit from the talents and skills possessed by mental health professionals who wish to offer their services in these settings. Doing so is consistent with the values of the mental health professions as articulated in their codes of ethics, which focus on social justice activities and offering one's services for a reduced fee or free of charge (pro bono). While it is laudable that mental health professionals with altruistic tendencies will seek to offer such much-needed assistance, this must be done with significant advance planning and forethought, to include attention to a number of ethics, legal, and clinical issues, to ensure that these services are provided in a helpful, clinically relevant, and appropriate manner. This chapter addresses the ethics, legal, and clinical issues every mental health professional should consider prior to and while offering mental health treatment services to members of underserved communities.

Assessing the Community's Needs and Advance Planning

An important first step is to consider the needs of the community in question, prior to making a decision about attempting to address these needs. Failure to understand the community's needs may result in efforts to assist those in need that prove to be ineffective at best, and actually harmful at worst. While we may have highly praiseworthy intentions, our assistance is not always welcomed or desired. It is important to first ensure that assistance is desired. Then, it is important to find out what the specific needs of this particular community are. This may involve research to educate oneself about the community and communication with community leaders or other representatives of the community. It is the members of the community in question who know best about the needs of their community. After obtaining information about the community's mental health needs and why local resources are not sufficient to meet them, it is then important to engage in a process of self-assessment, reflection, and consultation to ensure that we possess the necessary clinical *and* multicultural competence to be effective in providing the needed mental health treatment services.

For mental health professionals who will be traveling out of their local area to provide needed mental health treatment services, knowledge of the new area, its climate, how to dress, if there is electricity, if there is potable water, where one will stay, what expenses one should anticipate, and where one will provide treatment services are all important pieces of information to obtain as part of the process of planning to travel to a new area to provide these services. When traveling abroad, issues such as a passport that will not expire within 30 days of initiating the travel, needed visas, required immunizations, State Department advisories about unsafe areas, and related issues are all important to address before accepting the assignment and leaving the country.

Clinical Competence

To ensure that we provide mental health treatment services effectively, we must possess the appropriate level and range of clinical competence. Each mental health profession has a code of ethics that requires professionals to possess the competence to provide effective clinical services. For example, the Ethical Principles of Psychologists and Code of Conduct (Ethics Code, APA, 2017a) requires in Standard 2.01, Boundaries of Competence, that psychologists provide clinical services "with populations and in areas only within the boundaries of their competence, based on their education, training, supervised experience, consultation, study, or professional experience" (p. 4). Further, in Standard 2.04, Bases for Scientific and Professional Judgments, the Ethics Code requires that "psychologists' work is based upon established scientific and professional knowledge of the discipline" (p. 5). This necessitates that psychologists take active steps to remain current with developments in their discipline as they are relevant to the populations they will be treating, and is consistent with Standard 3.04, Avoiding Harm.

Clinical competence is defined by Epstein and Hundert (2002) as "the habitual and judicious use of communication, knowledge, technical skills, clinical reasoning, emotions, values, and reflection in daily practice for the benefit of the individual and the community served" (p. 226). At the most basic level, clinical competence requires us to possess sufficient knowledge, skills, attitudes, and values and to be able to apply them in a thoughtful and effective manner (Haas & Malouf, 2005). While ethics codes and licensing laws can only set minimal standards that must be achieved, it is widely accepted that a positive or aspirational approach to ethics is more desirable (Handelsman, Knapp, & Gottlieb, 2009). This approach is consistent with the underlying values of the mental health professions as articulated by Beauchamp and Childress (2013): beneficence, nonmaleficence, fidelity, autonomy, justice, and self-care. In each of these areas we are guided to strive to do our best at all times, never being satisfied with meeting minimal expectations and standards.

When considering providing professional services to members of underserved communities, we should not automatically assume that we possess the competencies needed to be of assistance to these potential clients. In addition to the research and advance preparation that has been described, we must thoughtfully assess our own competence. While this is a necessary step, it is not sufficient for determining if we possess the needed level of clinical competence. Health professionals are notoriously poor at self-assessment of competence (Dunning, Johnson, Ehrlinge, & Kruger, 2003), and we must seek input from colleagues who are recognized experts in those areas of practice. These expert colleagues can provide us with feedback on our current level of competence, any areas of noted deficiency or weakness, and recommendations for education and training opportunities to bring us up to the desired level of competence.

Of particular relevance to providing clinical services to underserved communities, the APA Ethics Code (APA, 2017a) requires in Standard 2.01(d):

> When psychologists are asked to provide services to individuals for whom appropriate mental health services are not available and for which psychologists have not obtained the competence necessary, psychologists with closely related prior training or experience may provide such services in order to ensure that services are not denied if they make a reasonable effort to obtain the competence required by using relevant research, training, consultation, or study. (p. 5)

Similarly, the American Counseling Association (ACA)'s Code of Ethics (2014) states that "[c]ounselors practice in specialty areas new to them only after appropriate education, training and supervised experience. When developing skills in new specialty areas, counselors take steps to ensure the competence of their work and protect others from harm" (p. 8).

Thus, in addition to self-assessment and consultation with expert colleagues to determine our level of clinical competence, even in situations where we are motivated to ensure that individuals receive much-needed services, we must take reasonable steps to ensure we possess the competence necessary to make certain we can assist these individuals and not harm them. Consistent with this expectation, Standard 2.01(c) requires that "[p]sychologists planning to provide services . . . involving populations, areas, techniques, or technologies new to them undertake relevant education, training, supervised experience, consultation, or study" (APA, 2017a, p. 5).

Multicultural Competence

Awareness of, and attention to, individual differences and how they impact mental health issues are inextricably intertwined with clinical competence. One cannot be clinically competent if one is not multiculturally competent. The ACA Code of Ethics (ACA, 2014) includes in its standard on professional competence that "multicultural counseling competency is required across all counseling specialties" and that "counselors gain knowledge, personal awareness, sensitivity, dispositions, and skills pertinent to being a culturally competent counselor in working with a diverse client population" (p. 8). Similarly, the Code of Ethics of the National Association of Social Workers (NASW, 2008) states that "[s]ocial workers should have a knowledge base of their clients' cultures and be able to demonstrate competence in the provision of services that are sensitive to clients' cultures and to differences among people and cultural groups" (para. 35). Representative of the other mental health professions' codes of ethics, the American Association for Marriage and Family Therapy's Code of Ethics (2015) requires marriage and family therapists to provide assessment and treatment services "without discrimination on the basis of race, age, ethnicity, socioeconomic status, disability, gender, health status, religion, national origin, sexual orientation, gender identity or relationship status" (p. 1). The codes of ethics of each of the mental health professions require that mental health professionals possess an understanding of individual differences and how they may impact the professional services we provide, emphasizing that to be able to competently provide clinical services to individuals of diverse backgrounds we must possess a sufficient understanding of all potential individual differences and how they may be relevant to understanding the individuals to be treated, their worldview, and their views of mental health issues and treatment.

Further guidance is provided in relevant APA guidelines for practitioners that are online at http://www.apa.org/practice/guidelines/. Guidelines differ from ethics code standards in that standards are enforceable and guidelines are aspirational. Further, guidelines are consensus statements from experts in each area addressed that are endorsed by the APA. These guidelines for practitioners include:

- Guidelines for Psychological Practice with Transgender and Gender Nonconforming People
- Guidelines for Psychological Practice with Girls and Women
- Guidelines for Psychological Practice with Older Adults
- Guidelines for the Practice of Telepsychology
- Practice Parameters: Screening and Diagnosis of Autism
- Guidelines for Psychological Practice with Lesbian, Gay & Bisexual Clients
- Guidelines for Assessment of and Intervention with Persons with Disabilities
- Guidelines for the Evaluation of Dementia and Age-Related Cognitive Change.

Additionally, the APA has promulgated clinical practice guidelines to include the Clinical Practice Guideline for the Treatment of Posttraumatic Stress Disorder, which may be of particular relevance for psychologists who provide clinical services to survivors of abuse, torture, war, and natural disasters.

The Multicultural Guidelines: An Ecological Approach to Context, Identity, and Intersectionality (APA, 2017b) include a number of guidelines that are of particular relevance for psychologists considering providing mental health treatment services to members of underserved communities. These include:

- Psychologists are encouraged to recognize that, as cultural beings, they may hold attitudes and beliefs that can detrimentally influence their perceptions of and interactions with individuals who are ethnically and racially different from themselves.
- Psychologists are encouraged to recognize the importance of multicultural sensitivity/responsiveness, knowledge, and understanding about ethnically and racially different individuals.
- Psychologists strive to apply culturally appropriate skills and culturally adaptive interventions in clinical and other applied psychological practices.

All mental health professionals considering providing mental health services to members of underserved communities should consider their own attitudes, values, and beliefs, to include biases and prejudices we may hold. Additionally, we must understand and value individual differences, taking an approach of understanding and treating the whole person. For example, a lack of understanding of a collectivistic culture and how this may impact the informed consent process and decision making in treatment might result in alienating potential clients. This could then result in the community not being willing to participate in the treatment services being offered. Similarly, mental health professionals should understand how mental health issues are expressed and treated in that community.

In some settings, it is not appropriate to apply Western conceptualizations of mental health issues or to apply Western treatment techniques without first adapting them to be consistent with the values and beliefs of the community.

Not all commonly used treatment techniques can easily be adapted for use with all populations. Mental health professionals will need to do research and seek education, training, and supervised experience before adapting treatment techniques for use with other groups. It also will be helpful to spend time immersed in the underserved community to better understand community members' needs, customs, values, and beliefs, as well as to develop credibility as one who understands, who is not a threat, and who truly wants to be of assistance to them. For communities that have been marginalized or oppressed, either in the recent past or historically, it will be important to ensure that, even inadvertently, we are not repeating these patterns by acting as oppressors have in the past. We must be able to convey our valuing of, and respect for, the community's culture, values, beliefs, and practices. In some communities, this may involve participating in traditional ceremonies, eating traditional foods, wearing traditional clothing, and integrating traditional healers from the community into the treatments we provide.

It is also important not to offend or alienate members of the community by violating their norms or mores. Views on boundaries such as the use of touch, interpersonal space, self-disclosure, and acceptance of gifts may vary in different communities. For example, in some communities it is inappropriate for a man to be in a room alone with a woman or to touch her (even to shake her hand); in some communities, it is considered inappropriate for a woman to dress "immodestly" so that her hair, arms, and legs are exposed. Some cultural groups expect a significant amount of self-disclosure by mental health professionals as a means of developing comfort in sharing about themselves. Other groups give gifts or food they have made as an expression of appreciation, and declining to accept them may be considered a significant insult (Vasquez, 2007). Some groups may expect gifts as a sign of friendship and respect, as mental health professionals enter their community. A rigid adherence to strict boundaries may prove to be alienating and offensive, rendering one's clinical competence ineffective, again illustrating the importance of integrating multicultural competence into one's general clinical competence.

Thus, knowledge of all relevant information about the community one is planning to serve is essential. This is an ongoing process that one never completes. At a minimum, it is important to do one's homework before leaving home to travel to the underserved community, learning all one can about that community and its members. One must keep in mind that communities are diverse and not homogenous or monolithic, so there will be individual differences among community members. For example, some cultures may be in transition between traditional and more modern practices. Additionally, community members will each have multiple types of diversity and individual differences that make up each individual's experiences and worldview (Rosenthal, 2016). An openness to learning about individuals different from ourselves and a respect for their values, beliefs, and practices are essential so we can assist them in a competent and effective manner. Similarly, we need to learn about how we (based on our personal demographics) are likely to be viewed by the community we want to serve. These issues are of vital importance for mental health professionals to consider before attempting to provide treatment services to underserved communities.

As Turner et al. (2016) highlight, many members of underserved communities do not seek out mental health treatment services because they perceive professionals as lacking cultural competence and not integrating the community's cultural values into the treatments they offer. Cultural adaptations of treatments that psychotherapists regularly use with members of majority groups should be evidence-based. Evidence-based practice for mental health clinicians is defined as "the integration of the best available research with clinical expertise in the context of patient characteristic, culture, and preferences" (APA, 2006, p. 273). Further, as La Roche, Matista, and D'Angelo (2011) explain, culturally adapted treatments should be based on each group's unique cultural characteristics, preferences, and needs.

Language Differences and the Use of Interpreters

One important individual difference that may be present in a wide range of underserved communities is language. In addition to cultural differences, language differences are likely to be present and can be a barrier to individuals seeking and receiving needed mental health treatment (Mercado & Hinojosa, 2017). This may be especially relevant when offering mental health services in other countries and to immigrant and refugee communities (Miller, Martell, Pazdirek, Caruth, & Lopez, 2005). The NASW Code of Ethics (NASW, 2008) states that "[i]n instances when clients are not literate or have difficulty understanding the primary language used in the practice setting, social workers should take steps to ensure clients' comprehension. This may include providing clients with . . . a qualified interpreter or translator whenever possible" (para. 26). Unless the mental health clinician possesses sufficient facility with the other language, the use of interpreters may be the only way to provide needed assistance to members of that community.

There are a number of clinical, ethical, and practical matters and issues to consider when attempting to provide mental health services when one is not fluent in the client's language. As Sluzki (1984) describes, the use of an interpreter injects a third party into the treatment, when usually mental health treatment involves just the clinician and the client(s). Several important adjustments may need to be made so that treatment may be provided effectively. First, it is important to ensure the interpreter's fluency with both languages and familiarity with mental health terminology that likely will be used. The interpreter should also be familiar with cultural nuances and local language usage, such as sayings and expressions used in that community. Assessing each of these is important to do prior to utilizing a particular interpreter with a client.

Next, it is important to establish ground rules with the interpreter to include translating verbatim what is said by each party. It is important that interpreters not provide commentary, make recommendations to the client, or interpret what they think either party means or intends to say; they should not omit anything that is said from the translation. Working with an interpreter can be challenging, and it may take some practice to develop comfort with it. At times, it may be necessary to have two interpreters, one interpreting to the professional and one interpreting to the client(s). Many interpreters become fatigued interpreting in both directions, especially if there is strong emotional content that they also have to contend with that may be outside their usual experience, given that they typically are not mental health professionals.

While the use of a trained interpreter is optimal, as Villalobos et al. (2016) report, at present there are no credentialing agencies for interpreters and no uniform standards for evaluating interpreter effectiveness. While these authors recommend bilingual psychotherapists as the ideal situation, a next-best scenario is the use of a trained interpreter (Karliner, Jacobs, Chen, & Mutha, 2007). This interpreter should have no close relationship with the client. For example, it would be inappropriate to use the client's child as the interpreter due to the dynamics of the relationship between them, the intimate content that is likely to be discussed in the treatment sessions, and the inappropriateness of the child being exposed to this information. While it is likely that the interpreter will be a member of the client's community, if possible, utilizing someone without a close personal relationship with the client is preferable.

It is then important to conduct a comprehensive informed consent process with both the client and the interpreter. Each party needs to understand confidentiality expectations and how the client's private information will be protected. While we cannot guarantee that the interpreter will never violate confidentiality, conducting an orientation to mental health services and training on relevant ethics issues and expectations will be important. Intermittent reminders and review of ethics obligations over time will likely prove helpful as well.

The National Council on Interpreting in Health Care Working Paper Series offers a number of working papers prepared by experts on the use of interpreters in health care settings. Topics addressed include translation guidelines, terminology frequently used by health care interpreters, standards of practice for interpreters, a guide to interpreter positioning in the health care setting, and models for the provision of health care interpreter training. These useful guides are available at http://www.ncihc.org/publications.

Knowledge of Local Laws and Regulations

When providing mental health treatment to underserved groups, it is likely that one may be asked to provide these services outside the jurisdiction where one is licensed. This raises a number of issues that must be considered and addressed to ensure that we do not violate the law, place ourselves at legal risk, or place our clients at risk of harm. An important first step is to research the licensure laws in other jurisdictions. Psychology licensure laws in the United States may be accessed at http://www.asppb.net/?page=BdContactNewPG. Members of other mental health professions should investigate licensing board websites for their profession. When planning to practice in a jurisdiction where one is not licensed, one should become familiar with the other jurisdiction's licensing requirements. Many jurisdictions have temporary licensure allowances so that mental health professionals licensed elsewhere may practice on a time-limited basis in their jurisdiction, something particularly helpful when offering time-limited disaster response services. When planning to provide professional services in another country, one should find out if licensure is required in that country and, if so, how to obtain it. Licensing requirements vary by country, with some countries not having any licensing of mental health professionals. In such situations, it is recommended that mental health clinicians still practice ethically by following the dictates of their profession's code of ethics and their relevant licensure law and accompanying regulations.

In addition to licensing requirements, other laws to be aware of in the jurisdiction where the services are to be provided include mandatory reporting of suspected abuse or neglect of minors; mandatory reporting requirements for suspected elder abuse or neglect, or for vulnerable adult abuse, neglect, self-neglect, and exploitation requirements; and laws concerning the duty to warn, protect, and treat (dangerousness reporting requirements). Since laws and requirements vary by jurisdiction, this may be a complex situation that necessitates consultation with ethics and legal experts, especially those in the jurisdiction(s) where the services are rendered. Should one follow the laws in the jurisdiction where one are licensed or the laws where one is providing treatment services? What if these laws are inconsistent, conflict with each other, or are contradictory? It is possible that following the laws of one jurisdiction may place the psychologist at legal risk in the other jurisdiction. Thus, ethics and legal consultation prior to providing mental health treatment services in underserved areas outside of one's licensing jurisdiction is important for obtaining guidance on how to address such situations.

One should also become aware of other local laws, beyond those required for practice. For example, there may be laws around eating in public, customs around head coverings, and even curfews that one needs to follow. In some areas, even free speech may not be a right.

The Practice of Tele-Mental Health

Tele-mental health is the use of different technologies such as telephone, email, and video conferencing to provide clinical services across distances. This may be quite useful for providing mental health treatment to prospective clients in underserved communities, especially when it is not feasible for the mental health clinician to travel to these areas. It may also be helpful when clients are homebound, lack transportation, or are in remote locales. While tele-mental health can be very effective in providing underserved communities with access to needed mental health treatment services, it also brings with it a number of ethics, legal, and clinical challenges that should be addressed to ensure that it is being applied appropriately and effectively.

Consistent with discussions earlier in the chapter, when using tele-mental health to bring mental health treatment to underserved areas, one must consider licensure issues, other relevant laws, clinical competence, multicultural competence, technological competence, informed consent, confidentiality, decisions about when tele-mental health may or may not be the most appropriate treatment delivery method, and responding to emergencies.

As with in-person inter-jurisdictional practice, when practicing tele-mental health, one must consider licensure requirements in the jurisdiction where one is providing the clinical service as well as in the jurisdiction where the client is receiving the service. Thus, this may require that the mental health clinician be licensed in multiple jurisdictions or risk being in violation of licensure laws. Additionally, clinicians should be familiar with relevant laws in all jurisdictions in which they practice. The practice of tele-mental health can create many more challenges in this regard than will arise through in-person treatment since one may provide treatment to individuals in separate jurisdictions, nationally and internationally, each hour of the day.

The practice of tele-mental health also enables clinicians to easily have contact with clients from around the world. While this can be an amazing opportunity for those who would not otherwise be able to receive needed mental health treatment, it also can put the clinician in contact with clients from a wide range of diverse backgrounds, to include different cultures and languages. This may create significant challenges with regard to multicultural competence. Just because one has the technological capability to access and communicate with clients does not mean that it is appropriate to do so. Those who are enamored with the use of technology and the amazing reach of tele-mental health may be at risk of providing clinical services outside the scope of their multicultural and clinical competencies.

A similar situation exists with regard to clinical competence in general. It may be tempting to utilize this technology to provide mental health services that are desperately needed, but if one does not possess the necessary clinical competence, clients are put at risk of harm and the mental health professional risks ethics, regulatory, and legal consequences. As a general rule, one should not provide clinical services through tele-mental health that one is not competent to provide in person. The use of tele-mental health should not lower our ethical obligation to provide only services for which we are clinically competent.

Additionally, clinicians should be familiar with the literature on tele-mental health and understand that not all forms of tele-mental health are equivalent and not all are equally appropriate for the provision of mental health treatment. There is a broad literature on the use of various forms of tele-mental health in the treatment of a wide range of mental health issues. But, as an example, the use of email has not found to be supported for ongoing psychotherapy or counseling (Mallen, Vogel, & Rochlen, 2005). Yet, video conferencing has been found to be effective in the treatment of a wide range of disorders; in fact, it has been found that the therapeutic alliance in video conferencing treatment can be comparable to the therapeutic alliance developed in in-person treatment (Barnett & Kolmes, 2016).

Mental health professionals should first screen all potential clients for the appropriateness of tele-mental health treatment. Some individuals would be better served by in-person treatment; examples include clients who are actively suicidal and those with serious mental illnesses such as schizophrenia. But, for many clients, tele-mental health may provide a means for receiving needed treatment. Yet, all clients may at times experience crises or emergencies. It is important that mental health clinicians become familiar with resources in the client's local area before such situations arise. Then, when needed, referrals may be made for emergency services or even for hospitalization if it is needed.

In addition to clinical and multicultural competence, the mental health professional must possess technological competence to provide tele-mental health services effectively. One must be familiar with the hardware and software being used to be able to troubleshoot problems that may arise and interfere with the ability of clinician and client to communicate effectively with each other. Additionally, the mental health professional should assess each client's familiarity with the systems involved and provide any training needed so that each client may participate fully. It also is important to ensure a secure internet connection to protect clients' privacy. Encryption software should be utilized when communicating by email to further protect confidential information from unauthorized access. Clinicians will want to use only software programs that comply with the Health Insurance Portability and Accountability Act (HIPAA). Not all tele-mental health platforms are HIPAA compliant; thus, using them may place confidential communications at risk. Certainly, if appropriate software and communication platforms are not available, informed consent should be obtained (see the next paragraph) such that the client acknowledges and agrees to the risk that the communication might not be confidential. Mental health professionals should keep all security software up to date, to include virus, malware, and firewall protections. Failure to do so can place clients' confidential materials at risk of unauthorized disclosures.

As with all forms of treatment, the provision of mental health treatment via tele-mental health requires a comprehensive informed consent agreement at the outset of the treatment relationship. One's standard informed consent agreement used in in-person treatment will need to be modified to include several additional issues that are associated with tele-mental health in particular (Joint Task Force for the Development of Telepsychology Guidelines for Psychologists, 2013). This informed consent agreement should include important factors such as fees and financial arrangements, confidentiality and its limits, the likely course of treatment, technology and internet requirements for participation in treatment, procedures to follow if the internet or telephone connection is lost during a treatment session, emergency procedures, and how to contact the clinician between regularly scheduled treatment sessions. It also is important to ensure that clients have realistic expectations about the clinician's availability and responsiveness to communications between sessions. For example, will you respond to emails within 24 hours of receiving them, or should the client expect you to respond immediately to text messages, regardless of the time of day they are received or their length and complexity? All fees should be clarified in advance, to include if the clinician will charge for responding to emails and text messages. For many clinicians, there is a big difference between responding to an occasional brief email and receiving multi-page emails from clients who expect a detailed response to each issue.

Fee Issues

When planning to provide mental health services in underserved communities, one should keep fee and payment issues in mind. Many communities are underserved because residents lack the financial resources to afford needed mental health treatment. This may be due to not being able to afford insurance premiums, not being able to afford co-pays and deductibles, and not being able to afford fee-for-service treatment. Thus, when offering mental health treatment services in these communities one must exercise sensitivity to such issues.

Options that exist for bringing affordable mental health treatment to underserved communities include offering these services on a sliding fee scale, for a significantly reduced fee, or free of charge (pro bono). The APA Ethics Code (APA, 2017a) states in Principle B: Fidelity and Responsibility, "Psychologists strive to contribute a portion of their professional time for little or no compensation or personal advantage" (p. 3). In some settings, community members may not be accustomed to paying for mental health services; this may, in fact, be a new concept to them. In many communities, barter is an established method of enabling community members to obtain needed goods and services. Barter is allowed by the codes of ethics of each of the mental health professions as long as it is requested by the client and is not exploitative of the client. Additionally, as is highlighted in the ACA Code of Ethics (ACA, 2014) "Counselors consider the cultural implications of bartering and discuss relevant concerns with clients and document such agreements in a clear written contract" (p. 6).

Mental health professionals should not assume that members of underserved communities will be familiar with the professional's standard practices. Some information sharing with clients may be necessary, and, of course, all fee and payment issues should be addressed up front as part of the informed consent agreement. As is stated in Standard 10.01, Informed Consent to Therapy, of the APA Ethics Code, "psychologists inform clients/patients as early as is feasible in the therapeutic relationship about the nature and anticipated course of therapy, fees, . . ." (APA, 2017a, p. 13).

When one is offering professional services as a volunteer, such as when doing disaster relief work or when volunteering one's services through a nonprofit agency or nongovernmental organization, it is still best to ensure that prospective clients are informed of all relevant informed consent issues so that they have realistic expectations for the professional experience. This should include discussion of any reasonably anticipated limits to the professional services being offered, to include those caused by finances. This might include if only a specific limited number of treatment sessions will be offered to each client free of charge or if the mental health professional will be in that community for a limited time period. How the client's treatment needs will be addressed after the free sessions are exhausted or when the mental health professional leaves the community should be addressed at the outset, especially if fees will be charged for subsequently available services.

Atypical Situations

In many situations, such as in disaster relief work, mental health clinicians may need to provide treatment services outside of the typical office setting. At times, mental health clinicians will be faced with the choice of modifying their usual clinical and ethics practices so that clients may receive much-needed treatment. A rigid adherence to usual practices may not be feasible in some settings and situations. With disasters, some treatment services may need to be provided on site. Additionally, in some locations, there may not be facilities that enable clinicians to have an office, or even a private space, in which to treat clients. Mental health professionals may need to be flexible and adaptive with regard to where clinical services are offered. At the same time, great sensitivity to confidentiality and privacy concerns is needed. Yet, in some cultures, privacy may be viewed very differently than in the clinician's culture, and we must be respectful of our clients' needs and wishes even if they may make us uncomfortable and go against our views of best practices.

Such issues should be addressed through the informed consent process so that clients understand possible implications of participating in mental health treatment in nontraditional settings. At the same time, we must not impose our beliefs on clients; as the NASW Code of Ethics (NASW, 2008) articulates, "Social workers respect and promote the right of clients to self-determination" (para. 24). This is an area where mental health clinicians will need to be alert to their countertransference reactions and seek consultation when they experience negative reactions to clients that may adversely impact the treatment relationship and process.

Vicarious Traumatization and Self-Care

Work as a mental health clinician can be very rewarding, but it also can be emotionally challenging and exhausting at times. Mental health clinicians must monitor their own functioning and attend to how the practice of psychology is impacting their functioning. The ACA Code of Ethics (ACA, 2014) includes in Ethics Standard C.2, Professional Competence, that "[c]ounselors continually monitor their effectiveness as professionals and take steps to improve when necessary. Counselors take reasonable steps to seek peer supervision to evaluate their efficacy as counselors" (p. 8). Additionally, the APA Ethics Code (APA, 2017a) requires that "[w]hen psychologists become aware of personal problems that may interfere with their performing work-related duties adequately, they take appropriate measures, such as obtaining professional consultation or assistance, and determine whether they should limit, suspend, or terminate their work-related duties" (p. 5).

When providing mental health treatment services to underserved groups, mental health professionals will experience all the usual challenges and stressors of being a clinician, such as working with challenging clients, working long hours, dealing with client crises, documentation requirements, and the like. Additionally, if they are leaving home to provide these services, additional stressors experienced may include being away from loved ones, living in challenging circumstances and being without the comforts of home, adjusting to a new culture and setting, facing clinical situations for which one is not prepared, perhaps working very long hours trying to meet vast needs with very limited resources, and facing traumatic and disturbing circumstances.

Mental health clinicians who provide treatment to clients who are the victims of trauma, to include physical and sexual abuse, torture, and other degradations, may find themselves traumatized by this clinical work. Being exposed to the violence and trauma experienced in some settings and listening to the intimate details of the traumatic experiences some clients have been through can be very traumatizing to clinicians themselves, resulting in the clinician experiencing symptoms of post-traumatic stress disorder. This phenomenon has been referred to as vicarious traumatization or secondary traumatic stress (Figley & Ludick, 2017). Clinicians treating these clients are susceptible to what Wise and Barnett (2016) describe as "the emotional toll of working with traumatized patients" (p. 210). This type of clinical work, and work with clients in general, necessitates the promotion of wellness and the ongoing practice of self-care.

Self-care refers to the intentional practice of positive actions that promote the mental health professional's emotional, physical, relational, and spiritual wellness. As Coster and Schwebel (1997) state, its goal is "the enduring quality in one's professional functioning over time and in the face of professional and personal stressors" (p. 5). Mental health clinicians all experience distress in response to the many challenges and stressors in our professional and personal lives. Failure to adequately attend to these stressors may result in distress developing into burnout over time. In illustrating this point, Baker (2003) has described burnout as "the terminal phase of therapist distress" (p. 21). Burnout is described as including feelings of emotional exhaustion, depersonalization (loss of compassion and caring toward clients), and loss of feelings of professional accomplishment and satisfaction. A primary goal of self-care is to reduce the risk of developing burnout, to prevent compassion fatigue from developing, and to prevent the development of problems with professional competence that may result from the experience of these difficulties.

Self-care is especially important for mental health clinicians providing treatment services to underserved communities. Failure to adequately manage the many stresses involved and their impact on our wellness and functioning can easily lead to a decrease in effective functioning, both professionally and personally. Positive self-care behaviors may include getting adequate sleep, eating a healthy diet, and exercising regularly. It may also include taking regularly scheduled breaks from work, managing one's schedule to include a mix of clients and professional activities, and engaging in enjoyable and relaxing activities such as meditation, yoga, and mindfulness activities (Barnett & Cooper, 2009). As the codes of ethics of each of the mental health professions require, it is also important to seek peer support, to utilize colleagues for consultation, and when indicated to seek personal psychotherapy.

Mental health professionals at times may engage in maladaptive coping strategies, instead of or in addition to positive self-care activities. Examples include self-medication with food, alcohol, and other substances; working more hours in response to ongoing stressors and demands; ignoring or minimizing the emerging signs of burnout or compassion fatigue; and isolating oneself personally and professionally. It is easy to convince oneself that all is fine and or that all will be fine if we just work harder to get through a particularly stressful time. As caregivers, it is easy for us to overlook our own needs, reactions, and vulnerabilities, erroneously thinking that our near-total focus on our clients is an indication of our commitment to them and to helping them. Unfortunately, as has been highlighted, if we do not take adequate care of ourselves, over time, our ability to effectively care for others will deteriorate.

Professional isolation is an especially pernicious influence in regard to self-care and the promotion of effective functioning. As has been emphasized, we tend to be very poor at accurately self-assessing our competence and our ability to function effectively. The more distress we are experiencing, the more traumatizing the situation we are immersed in, and the more challenging the clients we work with, the more we need the support of colleagues. Johnson, Barnett, Elman, Forrest, and Kaslow (2013) recommend that each mental health professional participate in a "competence constellation," a community of colleagues who look out for each other. Participation in such a network of colleagues is essential for managing the stresses and challenges of clinical work in underserved communities. To achieve maximum benefit from participation in these networks of colleagues, we must be open and honest about the stresses we face and the distress we experience, we must be open to support from our colleagues and accept their recommendations, and we must accept how stressful and traumatizing this clinical work can be. The best way to manage this is by actively utilizing the support, caring, feedback, and assistance from our close colleagues. As members of these competence constellations, we must each also actively support our colleagues, working to monitor their functioning, listening to their descriptions of the distress they are experiencing, and offering them needed support and assistance. For without the active caring and support of each other, our ability to meet our clients' needs in these challenging situations will be quite limited over time.

Summary and Recommendations

Providing mental health treatment services to underserved communities is a very commendable activity. It is consistent with the highest ethical ideals of the mental health professions. Yet, it brings with it a number of challenges, and it requires that we possess the necessary clinical and multicultural competence to be of assistance to those who are in such great need of our help. Advance preparation and planning, targeted education and clinical training, and a respect for the diverse groups we hope to serve are all important to ensure that we are able to be of actual assistance to these communities.

It is important that we attend to clinical, ethical, and legal issues, such as not practicing outside our areas of clinical competence, providing clinical services in culturally adaptive ways, following all applicable laws, and possessing the necessary technological competence to practice tele-mental health safely and effectively. Key issues to consider, questions to ask, and steps to take when considering providing mental health treatment services to underserved populations include:

- Ensure you possess the required competence to provide the services needed. For natural disasters and mass casualty situations, do you possess disaster relief training?
- Know the community. Learn about its culture, customs, norms, and mores.
- Participate in immersion experiences if possible to learn about the communities you will be serving.
- Find out about language issues. Will interpreters be needed? If so, ensure they are competent in the role to include language and cultural nuances, will follow confidentiality requirements, don't have a disqualifying preexisting multiple relationship with clients, and will translate verbatim without adding or deleting communications.
- Find out about practical matters such as supplies to bring, how to dress, what the climate is like, vaccinations needed, visas needed, and where you will stay.
- Learn local laws and regulations in advance of your trip. Do you need to be licensed or need to obtain formal approval in advance of providing professional services there?

- Always follow your profession's ethics code and be guided by the aspirational values of your profession in all that you do.
- When faced with dilemmas or challenging situations and unsure how to proceed, actively consult with experienced and trusted colleagues.
- Monitor countertransference reactions to clients in the communities being served and seek consultation, and personal psychotherapy if needed, to ensure that clients receive the best treatment possible.
- Will you have a local contact person or organization? If so, make contact with them in advance to learn all you can to prepare you for your work in this community.
- When considering the use of technology to access and provide services to underserved populations, ensure that the mode of treatment is appropriate for each client's clinical needs, know local resources for addressing crises and emergencies, and take appropriate precautions to protect each client's confidentiality.
- Keep in mind that without multicultural competence, there can be no clinical competence. Seek to continually learn about the cultures and individual differences of those you serve.
- When adapting treatments for use with underserved populations, ensure that standards of evidence-based practice are met and that the treatments are culturally responsive to the needs of the clients.
- Mental health clinicians planning to offer assistance in the wake of a natural or manmade disaster should ensure they possess the requisite competence, to include completing Red Cross Mental Health Volunteer disaster relief training (American Red Cross, 2017).
- Clinicians seeking to provide disaster relief assistance should do so under the auspices of a recognized group such as the American Red Cross and not attempt to do so independently.
- Stay focused on practicing ethically, but remain flexible in your approach so that individuals may receive much-needed treatment in a timely manner. Take advantage of available options and alternatives rather than focusing on a standard of perfection.
- Understand the factors that can adversely impact your competence and take active steps to promote your ongoing competence.
- Actively practice self-care and the promotion of wellness.

Remember that it takes a village; do not isolate yourself from your network of colleagues, but actively engage with them to seek from them, and provide to them, ongoing support and assistance as you do this very important work.

References

American Association for Marriage and Family Therapy. (2015). AAMFT Code of Ethics. Retrieved from http://www.aamft.org/iMIS15/AAMFT/Content/Legal_Ethics/Code_of_Ethics.aspx

American Counseling Association. (2014). ACA Code of Ethics. Retrieved from https://www.counseling.org/resources/aca-code-of-ethics.pdf

American Psychological Association. (2017a). Ethical principles of psychologists and code of conduct. Retrieved from http://www.apa.org/ethics

American Psychological Association. (2017b). *Multicultural guidelines: An ecological approach to context, identity, and intersectionality.* Retrieved from http://www.apa.org/about/policy/multicultural-guidelines.pdf

American Psychological Association Presidential Task Force on Evidence-Based Practice. (2006). Evidence-based practice in psychology. *American Psychologist, 61*(4), 271–285.

American Red Cross. (2017). Become a disaster mental health volunteer. Retrieved from http://www.redcross.org/become-a-disaster-mental-health-volunteer

Baker, E. K. (2003). *Caring for ourselves: A therapist's guide to personal and professional well-being.* Washington, DC: American Psychological Association.

Barnett, J. E., & Cooper, N. (2009). Creating a culture of self-care. *Clinical Psychology: Science and Practice, 16*(1), 16–20.

Barnett, J. E., & Kolmes, K. (2016). The practice of tele-mental health: Ethical, legal, and clinical issues for practitioners. *Practice Innovations, 1*(1), 53–66.

Beauchamp, T. L., & Childress, J. F. (2013). *Principles of biomedical ethics* (7th ed.). New York, NY: Oxford University Press.

Coster, J. S., & Schwebel, M. (1997). Well-functioning in professional psychologists. *Professional Psychology: Research and Practice, 28*, 5–13.

Dunning, D., Johnson, K., Ehrlinger, J., & Kruger, J. (2003). Why people fail to recognize their own incompetence. *Current Directions in Psychological Science, 12*, 83–87.

Epstein, R. M., & Hundert, E. M. (2002). Defining and assessing professional competence. *Journal of the American Medical Association, 287*, 226–235.

Figley, C. R., & Ludick, M. (2017). Secondary traumatization and compassion fatigue. In S. N. Gold (Ed.), *APA handbook of trauma psychology: Foundations in knowledge* (pp. 573–593). Washington, DC: American Psychological Association.

Haas, L. J., & Malouf, J. L. (2005). *Keeping up the good work: A practitioner's guide to mental health ethics* (4th ed.). Sarasota, FL: Professional Resource Press.

Handelsman, M. M., Knapp, S., & Gottlieb, M. C. (2009). Positive ethics: Themes and variations. In S. J. Lopez & C. R. Snyder (Eds.), *Oxford handbook of positive psychology* (2nd ed., pp. 105–113). New York, NY: Oxford University Press.

Health Insurance Portability and Accountability Act of 1996 (HIPAA), Public Law 104-191. Retrieved from https://www.hhs.gov/hipaa/for-professionals/index.html

Johnson, W. B., Barnett, J. E., Elman, N., Forrest, L., & Kaslow, N. J. (2013). The competence constellation model: A communitarian approach to support professional competence. *Professional Psychology: Research and Practice, 44*(5), 343–354.

Joint Task Force for the Development of Telepsychology Guidelines for Psychologists. (2013). Guidelines for the practice of telepsychology. *American Psychologist, 68*, 791–800.

Karliner, L. S., Jacobs, E. A., Chen, A. H., & Mutha, S. (2007). Do professional interpreters improve clinical care for patients with limited English proficiency? A systematic review of the literature. *Health Services Research*, *42*(2), 727–754.

La Roche, M. J., Batista, C., & D'Angelo, E. (2011). A content analysis of guided imagery scripts: A strategy for the development of cultural adaptations. *Journal of Clinical Psychology*, *67*(1), 45–57.

Mallen, M. J., Vogel, D. L., & Rochlen, A. B. (2005). The practical aspects of online counseling: Ethics, training, technology, and competency. *The Counseling Psychologist*, *33*(6), 776–818.

Mercado, A., & Hinojosa, Y. (2017). Culturally adapted dialectical behavior therapy in an underserved community mental health setting: A Latina adult case example. *Practice Innovations*, *2*(2), 80–93.

Miller, K. E., Martell, Z. L., Pazdirek, L., Caruth, M., & Lopez, D. (2005). The role of interpreters in psychotherapy with refugees: An exploratory study. *American Journal of Orthopsychiatry*, *75*, 27–39.

National Association of Social Workers. (2008). Code of Ethics of the National Association of Social Workers. Retrieved from https://www.socialworkers.org/pubs/code/code.asp

Rosenthal, L. (2016). Incorporating intersectionality into psychology: An opportunity to promote social justice and equity. *American Psychologist*, *71*(6), 474–485.

Sluzki, C. E. (1984). The patient–provider–translator triad: A note for providers. *Family Systems Medicine*, *2*(4), 397–400.

Turner, E. A., Cheng, H., Llamas, J. D., Tran, A. G. T. T., Hill, K. X., Fretts, J. M., & Mercado, A. (2016). Factors impacting the current trends in the use of outpatient psychiatric treatment among diverse ethnic groups. *Current Psychiatry Reviews*, *12*(2), 199–220.

Vasquez, M. J. T. (2007). Sometimes a taco is just a taco! *Professional Psychology: Research and Practice*, *38*(4), 406–408.

Villalobos, B. T., Bridges, A. J., Anastasia, E. A., Ojeda, C. A., Hernandez Rodrigues, J., & Gomez, D. (2016). Effects of language concordance and interpreter use on therapeutic alliance in Spanish-speaking integrated behavioral health care patients. *Psychological Services*, *13*(1), 49–59.

Wise, E. H., & Barnett, J. E. (2016). Self-care for psychologists. In J. C. Norcross, G. R. VandenBos, & D. K. Freedheim (Eds.), *APA handbook of clinical psychology: Vol. 5. Education and profession* (pp. 209–222). Washington, DC: American Psychological Association.

16

From Exploratory to Experimental

Matching Method to Need in Research with Underserved Populations

Elizabeth Nutt Williams

As the chapters in this book have highlighted, there are numerous populations considered underserved in mental health treatment, including racial minorities, members of the LGBTQ community, military service members and veterans, and individuals with low socioeconomic status, among others. Clearly there is need for mental health services (Vigo, Thornicroft, & Atun, 2016), and clearly there is underutilization of existing resources (Cook et al., 2014). Ideally, we would find ways to match the needs to the resources. We also need research that matches the needs of the underserved to the most useful methodologies for identifying barriers and treatment solutions. The purpose of this chapter is to explore current research strategies and to consider additional, less often employed methodologies in this area of research.

There is quite a bit of research on health disparities in general (Cook, McGuire, & Miranda, 2007). Some researchers have focused on studying issues of access (Williams & Jackson, 2005), while others have studied quality of care (Kilbourne et al., 2018). Both are important. We want to ensure that individuals who need mental health care have access and choose to seek help, but we also want to ensure that treatment is helpful and has been tailored to the needs of the varying populations (Kawaii-Bogue, Williams, & MacNear, 2017).

Most of the research in this area, it appears, has been primarily done within medical and psychiatric research centers. Yet psychologists and other mental health professionals also have much to offer this area of research. Those trained as scientists have expertise in a wide range of research methodologies; for example, both clinical and counseling psychologists are typically trained as scientist-practitioners (Belar, 2000). Psychologists and other mental health professionals are also experts on behavioral health (American Psychological Association, 2003) and, as such, can assist in understanding the behaviors of help seeking and help avoidance. Many mental health professionals are also experts on psychotherapy research, focusing on both the processes and outcomes of psychotherapy (Gelso, Williams, & Fretz, 2014). We can help identify not only whether clinical outcomes were met but how best to individualize treatment for clients (Fuertes & Williams, 2017), considering multicultural elements within the process (Comas-Diaz, 2014). So why are we not seeing more research on underserved populations?

One reason might be that doing research on underserved populations is difficult in three primary ways. First, it is often difficult to access the appropriate population. While large-scale medical studies can access hospital records around the United States, much research in psychology and other mental health professions is housed in academic institutions. As such, the population of choice is often college students (see discussion later in the chapter). College students, however, represent a unique segment of the population—with generally more young adult, educated, middle-class, and White individuals (National Center for Education Statistics, 2018) than other sectors of the population. For example, much of the help-seeking literature designed to examine the stigma of seeking help for mental health concerns has been validated on college student samples (Vogel, Wade, & Ascheman, 2009). While it is certainly important to ensure that young adults are seeking and receiving treatment when they need it, there are other populations that might have very different experiences. We know much less about why adults in rural areas, those with less formal education, and those without economic means seek or choose not to seek treatment. Even within populations that do seek treatment, such as veterans, there is uneven access (Hester, 2017).

When research is designed specifically to address populations outside of the college student population, it can be difficult to accurately measure meaningful social identity variables (Cook, McGuire, & Zaslavsky, 2012). For example, it is difficult to find a common strategy for assessing socioeconomic status (Liu et al., 2004); some studies have measured income reported, while others ask for self-identification of status. Without a common approach to the measurement, it is difficult to meaningfully compare samples and findings. Researchers must also make difficult choices about how to collect data. Many studies of health disparities have used large-scale surveys (e.g., Lo, Cheng, & Howell, 2014), many of which rely on the population's participation in community programs (e.g., Fripp & Carlson, 2017), while others have used internet surveys (e.g., Steele et al., 2017). Yet not all populations in need are already involved in community projects, nor do all have access to the Internet (though that may be changing, with the increasing percentage of usage of smartphones) (Pew Research Center, 2018).

Finally, there are discrete areas of research exploring ways to identify need (e.g., Shah, Luo, Winterbauer, & Madamala, 2016), measure help-seeking attitudes and behaviors (e.g., Vogel, Wade, & Haake, 2006), and examine clinical outcomes in underserved populations (e.g., Kilbourne et al., 2018). Yet, those areas of research do not always connect. Thus, we need more research that provides integration (such as meta-analyses) and that uses a wider variety of methodologies to address the critical research questions. In this chapter we will review the strategies most often reported in the literature and recommend alternative strategies to enhance the science as well as clinical care of underserved populations.

Overview of Methods

When reviewing the literature, it becomes apparent that most of the research on underserved populations is correlational in nature. Most research studies have distributed measures to different populations looking for relationships or have done research using a variety of national surveys and datasets. The research on help-seeking stigma and racial bias has most often been done with college student populations, though there has been research with a variety of adult and adolescent populations of need as well. Most non–college-based research has been part of larger data-collection projects on national or statewide programs and utilization rates. These general strategies are reviewed in the following section.

Research with College Students

It has been a popular approach in the literature on help-seeking attitudes and behaviors to study college student participants. Many studies use Vogel and Wade's work (Vogel et al., 2006, 2009) on self-stigma and public stigma of help-seeking attitudes as a basis for their work on college students' utilization of counseling services. There have been some very useful studies regarding racism and ethnic minority identities in this population, which may well be translatable to other (non-college) populations. For example, Cheng, Kwan, and Sevig (2013) used structural equation modeling to test the relationships among psychological distress, psychocultural variables (e.g., ethnic identity, other-group orientation, and perceived discrimination), and perceived stigma regarding seeking psychological help. Among a sample of African American, Asian American, and Latinx students, they found that higher levels of distress and perceived discrimination predicted higher levels of perceived stigma surrounding help seeking for all three ethnic groups. In particular, they also found for African American students that higher levels of ethnic identity predicted lower levels of self-stigma of help seeking. They noted that all students tend to underutilize mental health services on college campuses (Zivin, Eisenberg, Golllust, & Golberstein, 2009) and that underutilization is even more pronounced among ethnic minority students. To address these concerns regarding stigma and under-utilization of counseling services, they suggested employing programs that are designed to normalize help seeking, provide psychoeducation, promote positive relations across ethnic groups, and support the identity development of individuals.

Similarly, Tummala-Narra et al. (2018), in a study with Asian American college students, found connections among ethnic identity, perceived racism, and help-seeking attitudes. Using multiple online measures, the researchers found that perceived racism (both subtle and blatant) was associated with greater mental health concerns but not help-seeking attitudes. However, unlike Cheng et al.'s (2013) study, help-seeking attitudes were negatively associated with ethnic identity commitment and exploration (which were also negatively associated with mental health outcomes). Clearly the relationship between ethnic identity and help-seeking attitudes is a complex one that needs further research. One approach has been to identify the barriers to seeking help. Miranda, Soffer, Polanco-Roman, Wheeler, and Moore (2015) found, for example, that racial minority college students report financial concerns, lack of time, and stigma as barriers to treatment. Kearney, Draper, and Baron (2005) found that disparities in attendance of counseling sessions were related to stigma as well as to perceptions of mental health professionals lacking cultural competence. So, even for students who do seek help, utilization rates are lower among ethnic minorities and may negatively impact how much they benefit from treatment over time.

Another subpopulation in college students that has been examined using correlational designs is men, as men are less likely than women to seek psychological help (Goodwin, Hoven, Lyons, & Stein, 2002). Wasylkiw and Clairo (2018) examined help-seeking stigma in men by studying the relationships between conformity to masculine norms and self-compassion. They found that male athletes in particular were more likely to endorse masculine stereotypes than non-athletes, but they were also more likely to have higher scores on self-compassion (confirming prior meta-analytic work by Yarnell et al., 2015). To further complicate their findings, higher endorsement of masculine norms was negatively associated with help-seeking attitudes, whereas higher levels of self-compassion were predictive of more positive help-seeking attitudes. They suggested that self-compassion may have a moderating effect on the relationship between group membership (e.g., male athletes) and help-seeking attitudes, though additional work using different methodologies will be needed to more clearly understand the causal links involved.

While research with college student populations may limit the generalizability of findings to other populations, some of the findings may in fact be translatable. More research is needed to examine whether these same variables (gender, ethnic identity, racism, and stigma) have the same effect across populations and what types of approaches mitigate these barriers.

Research with Other Populations

A number of studies have attempted to study these variables outside of the college population. Researchers have made similar links between ethnic identity and help seeking in adult samples. For example, Fripp and Carlson (2017) studied the relationship between attitude (or core beliefs) toward help seeking, concerns about stigma, and the decision to seek counseling in African Americans and Latinos in the community. Using linear regression analysis, they found that attitudes were a unique (though weak) predictor of the decision to seek help but that attitudes were influenced by perceived stigma of being treated unfairly by professionals based on their ethnic identity. These findings are quite similar to the barriers to treatment found in college student populations.

In the LGBTQ community, similar health disparities exist, and cross-sectional correlational data have been the primary approach to gathering information about LGBTQ adults. For example, Steele et al. (2017) used a cross-sectional survey design to compare experiences of untreated depression among heterosexual cisgender women, cisgender lesbians, cisgender bisexual women, and transgender persons. Using a mixed-methods, community-based approach, the researchers surveyed participants via a measure posted to a website. Fliers were distributed in the area to recruit participants, who were given a $10 gift card as an incentive to complete the online survey. They found that transgender and bisexual participants were the most likely to report unmet needs. They cited discrimination, lower levels of social support, and exclusion from traditional health care systems as factors in explaining the underutilization of treatment.

Even for populations that do have access to traditional health care resources, such as active-duty members of the military and veterans, research suggests underutilization of mental health care. For example, using a survey design, Brunner et al. (2018) studied female veterans' perceptions of timely access to care. Overall, the veterans were happy with their ability to get an appointment in a timely manner at the Veterans Affairs clinics however, two specific problems were identified: the specific available hours of the clinics and accessing information between visits. The researchers suggested, based on their survey work, that alternative approaches to care (e.g., ways to contact providers outside of traditional clinic visits) might be very helpful, allowing traditional clinic hours to be accessed by more people who may have more acute needs.

Burton et al. (2018) studied the needs of those with more serious mental health needs and found far fewer veterans were being seen by providers. Even when veterans were seen at the Veterans Affairs clinics, many would discontinue treatment (more so by those who were homeless, younger, or unmarried, or had a diagnosis of bipolar disorder) and were not contacted for re-engagement. The researchers argue that this lack of follow-up is a "compounded risk" to treatment disruption, potentially leading to persistent disengagement. They emphasized the importance of tracking patients during treatment transitions and looking for creative approaches to care (such as home-based care or telehealth options).

These various survey-based studies help us understand the experiences of the underserved in a variety of populations, suggesting new ways to consider the barriers to treatment they experience in the community as well as potential new solutions for matching needs to care. These smaller survey studies help us understand the needs of particular communities, though they may not address more widespread concerns about access to care. The following section outlines the most common approach to research in this area: the use of large-scale, multisite datasets that allow for very broad social analysis.

Use of Large-Scale Census and Survey Work

Most of the research on underserved populations appears to make use of large-scale, multisite data-collection approaches. For example, Wang, Demler, and Kessler (2002) established, using the National Comorbidity Survey (www.hcp.med.harvard.edu/ncs/), that only 15% of respondents with serious mental illnesses in this cross-sectional study of households across the nation received what they identified as minimally adequate treatment. One of the predictors of receiving inadequate treatment was being African American. Similarly, Lo et al. (2014), using the National Health Interview Survey (www.cdc.gov/nchs/nhis/index.htm), examined race differences in prevalence of serious mental illness, finding lower utilization-of-treatment rates among African Americans and higher levels of chronic mental illness. Similarly, Wells et al. (2001) used a national survey of adults to assess unmet needs related to alcohol and drug abuse and other mental health treatment. They found that among those with perceived need, African Americans were likely to report less access to or delay of care. Whites were more likely than other ethnic groups to receive treatment. The researchers emphasized the importance of both access to care and the need to improve quality of care for diverse ethnic groups.

Census data have also been used to help examine issues of access to treatment. For example, Sharma et al. (2017) used U.S. Census (http://quickfacts.census.gov/qfd/) data and data from the California Board of Psychology to assess if geographic access to licensed mental health providers was a barrier to underserved populations. They found higher concentrations of licensed mental health providers (particularly licensed clinical social workers and psychologists) in areas that were wealthier, Whiter, older, and more educated. Interestingly, the distribution of marriage and family therapists was more even across geographic areas.

An area of rapidly growing research is on Latinx individuals. Ault-Brutus and Alegría (2018) used the National Comorbidity Survey (www.hcp.med.harvard.edu/ncs/) to measure perceived need and utilization of treatment among Blacks and Latinos across a decade. They found that perceived need did not differ over time or across groups, but disparities in accessing mental health care significantly worsened over time. Similarly, Cancel-Tirado et al. (2018), using the Rural Families Speak About Health Project (www.ruralfamiliesspeak.org), a multistate cross-sectional dataset, compared health, well-being, and health care in rural communities among Latinx and non-Latinx low-income families. Consistent with other studies, they found that Latinx families were significantly disadvantaged. Likewise, Snowden et al. (2017) examined MediCal paid claims for per-user expenditures on mental health treatment for Latinx and White children. They found more spending on White than Latinx children. However, they also found that having culture- and language-sensitive programs available helped prevent the disparity from growing (though it did not reduce overall disparity).

In an attempt to examine programs similar to those suggested by Snowden et al. (2017), Parra-Cardona and DeAndrea (2016) studied help seeking and online options. They pulled data on nearly 40,000 Latinx adults from the National Survey on Drug Use and Health (NSDUH; www.samhsa.gov/data/data-we-collect/nsduh-national-survey-drug-use-and-health) and found that most Latinx adults with identified mental health needs identified cost of treatment as a major barrier to seeking in-person treatment. They also found that fewer than 0.25% of Latino adults (compared with 3% of adults in general) sought online mental health support. They suggested that online treatment may be a reasonable response to more costly in-person treatments, but also noted concerns with the low comparative usage of technology, suggesting that this "digital divide" may represent another barrier to those seeking mental health treatment.

Many studies have attempted to uncover the barriers to seeking treatment across the country. For example, Alang (2015) also used the NSDUH to examine sociodemographic disparities and unmet need. Alang found that predominant barriers were cost, stigma, perception of effectiveness of providers, and structural barriers (lack of time, transportation, and information), which were particularly problematic for African American and rural individuals, particularly for those without insurance. Similarly, Alegría et al. (2012) found a negative impact of insurance coverage in explaining disparities among diverse populations. Dickey, Budge, Katz-Wise, and Garza (2016) also identified lack of insurance as a deterrent to seeking help within the transgender community.

Some of the large-scale studies have been longitudinal in nature. For example, Fuller-Rowell, Curtis, Chae, and Ryff (2018) studied the consequences of socioeconomic disadvantage, perceived discrimination, and health over nearly 20 years. They found perceived discrimination (using measures of inequality at work and everyday perceived discrimination) to be a significant explanatory variable in the relationship between socioeconomic disadvantage and health, suggesting that experiences with discrimination, rather than simply being poor, represent an important factor in health and access to care. Similarly, Fuller-Rowell, Evans, and Ong (2012), in an earlier wave of the study, found that the effect of poverty on health was mostly explained by discrimination as a mediating variable.

All of these large, multisite, multiyear studies have given us a clear picture of the disparities in mental health care—access and quality. They have been invaluable in helping us gain a nationwide understanding of the issues at hand. They are also an excellent contrast to smaller-scale community studies and studies on college campuses. Yet, despite the quality of these studies, it is notable that they have tended to stick with just two methodological approaches—the use of correlational and descriptive survey data. Through correlational studies, we can understand the ways important variables are related and see possible causal connections suggested (for example, through studies using structural equation modeling). Large-scale descriptive studies allow us a peek into the lived experiences of people all over the country (and, potentially, the globe). However, they also limit us in depth of understanding and in terms of being able to assess causal connections. The following section suggests the use of less frequently used methodologies in the area of understanding the needs and treatment experiences of the underserved.

Recommended Methodologies

As there is now a growing volume of research on underserved populations, and as much of that research has found consistent results over time and across populations, it may be time for the application of a greater variety of methodologies, which will allow for more in-depth exploration as well as the testing of causal models. In fact, as Snowden and Yamada called for more theoretically grounded research in this area in 2005, we are beginning to see more meta-analytic work and the development of theory-based models in the literature. For example, as a follow-up to decades of research examining the effect of matching client and psychotherapist race/ethnicity on the process and outcome of psychotherapy, Cabral and Smith (2011) conducted a meta-analysis of race matching between clients and psychotherapists to examine issues of client preference and psychotherapy outcome. They found that while clients overall do show some preference for psychotherapists of their own race/ethnicity, they found also no benefit to treatment outcomes of this kind of matching. Cabral and Smith suggest that because there was also substantial variability across studies, their findings do "not suggest that race/ethnicity does not matter for a client, but rather that racial/ethnic dynamics are so complex that prediction is problematic. Individuals' experiences with race/ethnicity must be acknowledged more than aggregate trends" (p. 546). Thus, a logical follow-up to this meta-analysis would be exploratory, qualitative studies of individual client experiences.

Similarly, Griner and Smith (2006) conducted a meta-analysis on culturally adapted treatments, given the increasing cultural diversity around the globe as well as the need to improve the access and quality of treatment for underserved individuals with mental health needs. They studied 76 prior studies (which were predominantly experimental) and found a moderately strong effectiveness of culturally adapted interventions, including interventions delivered in a client's native language and interventions designed specifically for particular cultural groups. They urged future researchers to increase the "rigor of experimentation" used (p. 543) to more clearly test specific contexts and adaptations that would be most beneficial to clients. The two meta-analyses provided as examples here show how the cumulative research can help suggest both more exploratory, individualized examination of client experiences as well as more experimental work on testing new models. We need to be able to test models that suggest new ways to both prevent and remediate problems with access and quality of treatment, and we need to better understand the unique experiences of underserved populations in much greater depth. Approaching the research from these two ends of the methodological spectrum (exploratory to experimental) will allow for both causal testing and attention to psychotherapy processes and outcomes, ideally encouraging greater tailoring of treatments to individual needs.

Exploratory Studies

Qualitative and exploratory studies allow researchers to delve deeply into the lived experiences of key informants. While we understand quite a bit about broad-level experiences (e.g., of Latinx adults, of African Americans, of those living in poverty), we do not have a true understanding of what those individuals experience vis-à-vis help seeking, access to care, and quality of treatment. Qualitative research is a critical next step in our methodological approaches so that we may better understand the experiences of the underserved from a client-focused perspective (Fuertes & Williams, 2017).

Some excellent qualitative studies have already been conducted in this area with a few specific underserved populations (e.g., the homeless, men, veterans). For example, Liu, Stinson, Hernandez, Sheppard, and Haag (2009) conducted a Consensual Qualitative Research (CQR; Hill, Thompson, & Williams, 1997) study exploring masculinity, homelessness, and social class and their implications for mental health treatment. Their key informants (homeless men) reported increases in anxiety, depression, and substance abuse related to being homeless and expressed the desire for greater mental health services, especially longer-term, one-on-one counseling. As one of the interviewees said, "Thirty days ain't going to do it" (p. 139). While their findings provide added depth to understanding the complex personal experiences of homelessness and mental health, the authors clearly articulated the need for mental health professionals to provide services that recognize the resilience and dignity of the men within a supportive and empathic environment.

In another CQR (Hill et al., 1997) study of men, Wolf, Williams, Darby, Herald, and Schultz (2018) explored the implications of feminist multicultural (FMC) therapeutic approaches to treating male clients. While there has been theoretical work suggesting that FMC counseling would be beneficial for male clients, there was little empirical evidence exploring this concept. As men are less likely than women to seek mental health treatment (Goodwin et al., 2002), Wolf et al. invited psychotherapists to discuss the ways in which they have used the FMC model with men. They found that psychotherapists reported that the FMC model not only works well for male clients but that it uniquely allows them to explore issues of masculinity in relation to their mental health experiences. They suggested that FMC psychotherapy might provide a new model for men to explore the impact of privilege and oppression with a safe therapeutic environment, which might be uniquely important in some male-dominated populations such as the military. The hope would be that, in doing so, men might be more willing to seek help for mental health concerns.

A recent interview study (Bovin et al., 2018) has also explored the experiences of veterans (predominantly men) who have sought mental health treatment. Their content analysis provided a model of both facilitating factors and barriers to seeking help. The authors noted that using a qualitative approach allowed them to "uncover unexpected findings by capturing veterans' lived experiences of accessing care" (p. 6). For example, while their purpose was to study factors that influence the initiation of care, they found that veterans discussed their "pathways" to accessing care; rather than direct access of care, they reported more often connecting with mental health care through other services (primary care, disability services, non–Veterans Affairs services, and mandated care). Having a deeper understanding of how veterans with need make decisions about accessing treatment will be beneficial for creating more relevant pathways and treatment approaches for them. The qualitative studies presented here have allowed for a deeper understanding of individuals' experiences with mental health, treatment, and barriers to access. With a more nuanced understanding of the unique lived experiences of individuals in underserved populations, we will be able to design more effective strategies for reducing disparities in both mental health care access and quality of care.

Experimental Designs

Moving beyond more exploratory and descriptive studies of direct experiences, we also are well poised to use experimental methodology to test causal variables related to health disparities and underserved populations. At this point, there is very little experimental research in this area, as some studies have needed to rely on quasi-experimental designs. As one example, Guo, Kim, Bear, and Lau (2017), in a quasi-experimental design, studied the impact of access to universal mental health screening in schools. Using a large sample (2,494 Asian and Latinx middle school students), Guo et al. found that those students with access to universal screening did have a higher likelihood of receiving a referral for treatment; however, the universal screening did not significantly predict treatment initiation (therefore not reducing disparities as expected).

Using a quasi-experimental approach with adult samples, Lanoye et al. (2017) found a decrease in inpatient utilization rates among patients who were treated in integrated care settings (where psychological health care and behavioral health care were integrated into a primary care clinic in the United States) compared to the control group. Tepper et al. (2017) found, using a quasi-experimental approach in the United Kingdom, that patients (with psychotic and bipolar disorders) who participated in an integrated behavioral health program had significantly fewer emergency visits and hospitalizations. While lacking in internal validity, these quasi-experimental designs do suggest possible causal connections among treatment options for further analysis.

To address the need for higher internal validity by using a true experimental approach, several experiments have been conducted to test issues related to race/ethnicity in health care. For example, Wells et al. (2013) conducted a community-partnered cluster-randomized comparative effectiveness trial of "community engagement" compared to "resources for services." They defined "resources for services" as toolkits received by community organizations for their use (including webinars), whereas "community engagement" was defined as organizations whose agency administrators were invited to co-produce toolkits with academic experts. They randomized the intervention received by participants in Los Angeles with participating partner institutions and found that community engagement was more effective than resources for services in improving health outcomes for community members. As they were able to randomly assign participants to varying conditions (while controlling for additional variables was challenging in this field experiment), they could establish with greater confidence the causal link between community engagement and health outcomes, suggesting the importance of establishing collaborative networks to help provide the highest quality of care. More of this type of field experiment is critical to help us understand how to better serve populations that have consistently been underserved.

As an example of another field experiment, Alcantara, Li, Wang, Canino, and Alegría (2016) conducted a randomized controlled trial in Boston and San Juan, randomly assigning participants to (a) usual care, (b) face-to-face Engagement and Counseling for Latinos (ECLA) intervention, or (c) telephone ECLA. Overall, the ECLA intervention produced significant reduction in worry, with the greatest worry reduction in the telephone condition. New service delivery ideas (such as telephone-delivered counseling) may need to be considered with underserved populations. This study provides an excellent example of how experimental design can be used to test new treatment delivery systems.

In a lab-based experiment, Abdou and Fingerhut (2014) studied the impact of stereotype threat (or being made aware of one's social identities in a way the makes an individual aware of negative stereotypes about groups to which they belong) on health care. They recruited Black and White women for an online "virtual" health care situation and randomly assigned them to an experimental (stereotype threat) or control condition. They found that Black women exposed to stereotype threat reported significantly higher anxiety than in the control condition while in the virtual "waiting room." The researchers suggest that stereotype threat may be an overlooked social barrier in understanding racial/ethnic health disparities. These various quasi-experimental and experimental designs allow for a more rigorous testing of potentially useful models of treatment and prevention, as well as the unveiling of additional variables (such as stereotype threat) that have received limited attention within the health care arena.

Conclusions and Recommendations

This chapter has reviewed the most common types of studies in the area of disparities in mental health treatment (access and quality) with underserved populations. As the predominant methodologies have been descriptive and correlational in nature (with both smaller community samples and larger national surveys), additional methodologies would now be helpful to extend our knowledge base. In particular, both exploratory (qualitative) and experimental (including quasi-experimental) studies will help us deepen our understanding of individual client experiences and allow for a more causally based approach to understanding and testing both preventive and remediative models of mental health treatment. Additional meta-analyses will also prove useful as tools to integrate information. In particular, the use of meta-analysis may help us identify and agree upon specific definitions and measures of a variety of social identity variables (e.g., socioeconomic status) as well as examine ways in which findings translate across populations (e.g., college students to community samples).

The research findings to date are clear: Health disparities exist and are persistent. We know that social identity issues (e.g., gender, race/ethnicity, sexual orientation, socioeconomic status) play a role in access, as does perceived discrimination. In addition to understanding barriers to treatment, we need to focus on what works for underserved populations. Based on the previous research, more experimental studies of different treatment modalities (e.g., telehealth), the impact of integrated care and geographic access, and the use of culture- and language-sensitive programs as starting points for good treatment seem timely. Additional qualitative studies of individual experiences within various underserved populations will also help us devise innovative treatment approaches as yet undiscovered. By matching the method to the need, we will be able to find new ways to help underserved populations decide to seek help, access the care they need, and receive the best psychotherapeutic treatments available.

Acknowledgment

I would like to thank Kierston Hill, my research assistant, for her help gathering relevant research for the chapter.

References

Abdou, C. M., & Fingerhut, A. W. (2014). Stereotype threat among Black and White women in health care settings. *Cultural Diversity and Ethnic Minority Psychology, 20,* 316–323.

Alang, S. M. (2015). Sociodemographic disparities associated with perceived causes of unmet need for mental health care. *Psychiatric Rehabilitation Journal, 38,* 293–299.

Alcantara, C., Li, X., Wang, Y., Canino, G., & Alegría, M. (2016). Treatment moderators and effectiveness of engagement and counseling for Latinos intervention on worry reduction in a low-income primary care sample. *Journal of Consulting and Clinical Psychology, 84,* 1016–1022.

Alegría, M., Lin, J., Chen, C. N., Duan, N., Cook, B., & Meng, X. L. (2012). The impact of insurance coverage in diminishing racial and ethnic disparities in behavioral health services. *Health Services Research, 47,* 1322–1344.

American Psychological Association. (2003). Health service psychologists as primary health care providers. Retrieved from http://www.apa.org/about/ policy/chapter-10b.aspx#psychologists-healthcare

Ault-Brutus, A., & Alegría, M. (2018). Racial/ethnic differences in perceived need for mental health care and disparities in use of care among those with perceived need in 1990–1992 and 2001–2003. *Ethnicity & Health, 23,* 142–157.

Belar, C. D. (2000). Scientist-practitioner ≠ science + practice: Boulder is bolder. *American Psychologist*, *55*, 249–250.

Bovin, M. J., Miller, C. J., Koenig, C. J., Lipschitz, J. M., Zamora, K. A., Wright, P. B., . . . Burgess, J. J. (2018). Veterans' experiences initiating VA-based mental health care. *Psychological Services*, Advance online publication. doi:10.1037/ser0000233.

Brunner, J., Schweizer, C. A., Canelo, I. A., Leung, L. B., Strauss, J. L., & Yano, E. M. (2018). Timely access to mental health care among women veterans. *Psychological Services* [Epub ahead of print], doi:10.1037/ser0000226

Burton, C. Z., Abraham, K. M., Grindle, C. M., Visnic, S., Hack, S. M., McCarthy, J. F., & Bowersox, N. W. (2018). Outreach to veterans with serious mental illness who are lost to care: Predictors of outreach contact. *Psychological Services*, *15*, 40–44.

Cabral, R. R., & Smith, T. B., (2011). Racial/ethnic matching of clients and therapists in mental health services: A meta-analytic review of preferences, perceptions, and outcomes. *Journal of Counseling Psychology*, *58*, 537–554.

Cancel-Tirado, D. I., Feeney, S. L., Washburn, I. J., Greder, K. A., & Sano, Y. (2018). Health, well-being, and health care access in rural communities: Comparing Latino and non-Latino White low-income families. *Family & Community Health: The Journal of Health Promotion & Maintenance*, *41*, 73–82.

Cheng, H., Kwan, K. K., & Sevig, T. (2013). Racial and ethnic minority college students' stigma associated with seeking psychological help: Examining psychocultural correlates. *Journal of Counseling Psychology*, *60*, 98–111.

Comas-Díaz, L. (2014). Multicultural psychotherapy. In F. T. L. Leong, L. Comas-Díaz, G. C. Nagayama Hall, V. C. McLoyd, & J. E. Trimble (Eds.), *APA handbook of multicultural psychology, Vol. 2. Applications and training* (pp. 419–441). Washington, DC: American Psychological Association.

Cook, B., McGuire, T., & Miranda, J. (2007). Measuring trends in mental health care disparities, 2000–2004. *Psychiatric Services*, *58*, 1533–1539.

Cook, B. L., McGuire, T. G., & Zaslavsky, A. M. (2012). Measuring racial/ethnic disparities in health care: Methods and practical issues. *Health Services Research*, *47*, 1232–1254.

Cook, B. L., Zuvekas, S. H., Carson, N., Wayne, G. F., Vesper, A., & McGuire, T. G. (2014). Assessing racial/ethnic disparities in treatment across episodes of mental health care. *Health Services Research*, *49*, 206–229.

Dickey, L. M., Budge, S. L., Katz-Wise, S. L., & Garza, M. V. (2016). Health disparities in the transgender community: Exploring differences in insurance coverage. *Psychology of Sexual Orientation and Gender Diversity*, *3*, 275–282.

Fripp, J. A., & Carlson, R. G. (2017). Exploring the influence of attitude and stigma on participation of African American and Latino populations in mental health services. *Journal of Multicultural Counseling and Development*, *45*, 80–94.

Fuertes, J. N., & Williams, E. N. (2017). Client-focused psychotherapy research. *Journal of Counseling Psychology*, *64*, 369–375.

Fuller-Rowell, T. E., Curtis, D. S., Chae, D. H., & Ryff, C. D. (2018). Longitudinal health consequences of socioeconomic disadvantage: Examining perceived discrimination as a mediator. *Health Psychology*, *37*, 491–500.

Fuller-Rowell, T. E., Evans, G. W., & Ong, A. D. (2012). Poverty and health: The mediating role of perceived discrimination. *Psychological Science*, *23*, 734–739.

Gelso, C. J., Williams, E. N., & Fretz, B. R. (2014). *Counseling psychology* (3rd ed.). Washington, DC: American Psychological Association.

Goodwin, R. D., Hoven, C. W., Lyons, J. S., & Stein, M. B. (2002). Mental health service utilization in the United States: The role of personality factors. *Social Psychiatry and Psychiatric Epidemiology, 37*, 561–566.

Griner, D., & Smith, T. B. (2006). Culturally adapted mental health intervention: A meta-analytic review. *Psychotherapy, 43*, 531–548.

Guo, S., Kim, J. J., Bear, L., & Lau, A. S. (2017). Does depression screening in schools reduce adolescent racial/ethnic disparities in accessing treatment? *Journal of Clinical Child & Adolescent Psychology, 46*, 523–536.

Hester, R. D. (2017). Lack of access to mental health services contributing to the high suicide rates among veterans. *International Journal of Mental Health Systems, 11*, 47–50.

Hill, C. E., Thompson, B., & Williams, E. N. (1997). A guide to conducting consensual qualitative research. *The Counseling Psychologist, 25*, 517–572.

Kawaii-Bogue, B., Williams, N. J., & MacNear, K. (2017). Mental health care access and treatment utilization in African American communities: An integrative care framework. *Best Practices in Mental Health, 13*, 11–29.

Kearney, L. K., Draper, M., & Barón, A. (2005). Counseling utilization by ethnic minority college students. *Cultural Diversity and Ethnic Minority Psychology, 11*, 272–285.

Kilbourne, A. M., Beck, K., Spaeth, R. B., Ramanuj, P., O'Brien, R. W., Tomoyasu, N., & Pincus, H. A. (2018). Measuring and improving the quality of mental health care: A global perspective. *World Psychiatry, 17*, 30–38.

Lanoye, A., Stewart, K. E., Rybarczyk, B. D., Auerbach, S. M., Sadock, E., Aggarwal, A., . . . Austin, K. (2017). The impact of integrated psychological services in a safety net primary care clinic on medical utilization. *Journal of Clinical Psychology, 73*, 681–692.

Liu, W. M., Ali, S. R., Soleck, G., Hopps, J., Dunston, K., & Pickett, T. (2004). Using social class in counseling psychology research. *Journal of Counseling Psychology, 51*, 3–18.

Liu, W. M., Stinson, R., Hernandez, J., Shepard, S., & Haag, S. (2009). A qualitative examination of masculinity, homelessness, and social class among men in a transitional shelter. *Psychology of Men & Masculinity, 10*, 131–148.

Lo, C. C., Cheng, T. C., & Howell, R. J. (2014). Access to and utilization of health services as pathway to racial disparities in serious mental illness. *Community Mental Health Journal, 50*, 251–257.

Miranda, R., Soffer, A., Polanco-Roman, L., Wheeler, A., & Moore, A. (2015). Mental health treatment barriers among racial/ethnic minority versus white young adults 6 months after intake at a college counseling center. *Journal of American College Health, 63*, 291–298.

National Center for Education Statistics. (2018). *Digest of education statistics, 2016* (NCES 2017-094), Chapter 3. Washington, DC: U.S. Department of Education. Retrieved from https://nces.ed.gov/pubs2017/2017094.pdf

Parra-Cardona, J. R., & DeAndrea, D. C. (2016). Latinos' access to online and formal mental health support. *Journal of Behavioral Health Services & Research, 43*, 281–292.

Pew Research Center. (2018, February). Mobile fact sheet. Retrieved from www.pewinternet.org/fact-sheet/mobile/

Shah, G. H., Luo, H., Winterbauer, N., & Madamala, K. (2016). Addressing psychological, mental health and other behavioural healthcare needs of the underserved populations in the United States: The role of local health departments. *Perspectives in Public Health, 136*, 86–92.

Sharma, R. N., Casas, R. N., Crawford, N. M., & Mills, L. N. (2017). Geographic distribution of California mental health professionals in relation to sociodemographic characteristics. *Cultural Diversity and Ethnic Minority Psychology*, *23*, 595–600.

Snowden, L. R., Wallace, N., Cordell, K., & Graaf, G. (2017). Increased mental health treatment financing, community-based organization's treatment programs, and Latino-White children's financing disparities. *Journal of Mental Health Policy and Economics*, *20*, 137–145.

Snowden, L. R., & Yamada, A. M. (2005). Cultural differences in access to care. *Annual Review of Clinical Psychology*, *1*, 43–166.

Steele, L. S., Daley, A., Curling, D., Gibson, M. F., Green, D. C., Williams, C. C., & Ross, L. E. (2017). LGBT identity, untreated depression, and unmet need for mental health services by sexual minority women and trans-identified people. *Journal of Women's Health*, *26*, 116–127.

Tepper, M. C., Cohen, A. M., Progovac, A. M., Ault-Brutus, A., Leff, H. S., Mullin, B., . . . Cook, B. (2017). Mind the gap: Developing an integrated behavioral health home to address health disparities in serious mental illness. *Psychiatric Services*, *68*, 1217–1224.

Tummala-Narra, P., Li, Z., Chang, J., Yang, E. J., Jiang, J., Sagherian, M., . . . Alfonso, A. (2018). Developmental and contextual correlates of mental health and help-seeking among Asian American college students. *American Journal of Orthopsychiatry*, *88*(6), 636–649.

Vigo, D., Thornicroft, G., & Atun, R. (2016). Estimating the true global burden of mental illness. *Lancet Psychiatry*, *3*, 171–178.

Vogel, D. L., Wade, N. G., & Ascheman, P. L. (2009). Measuring perceptions of stigmatization by others for seeking psychological help: Reliability and validity of a new stigma scale with college students. *Journal of Counseling Psychology*, *56*, 301–308.

Vogel, D. L., Wade, N. G., & Haake, S. (2006). Measuring the self-stigma associated with seeking psychological help. *Journal of Counseling Psychology*, *53*, 325–337.

Wang, P. S., Demler, O., & Kessler, R. C. (2002). Adequacy of treatment for serious mental illness in the United States. *American Journal of Public Health*, *92*, 92–98.

Wasylkiw, L., & Clairo, J. (2018). Help seeking in men: When masculinity and self-compassion collide. *Psychology of Men & Masculinity*, *19*, 234–242.

Wells, K. B., Jones, L., Chung, B., Dixon, E. L., Tang, L., Gilmore, J., . . . Miranda, J. (2013). Community-partnered cluster-randomized comparative effectiveness trial of community engagement and planning or resources for services to address depression disparities. *Journal of General Internal Medicine*, *28*, 1268–1278.

Wells, K., Klap, R., Koike, A., & Sherbourne, C. (2001). Ethnic disparities in unmet need for alcoholism, drug abuse, and mental health care. *American Journal of Psychiatry*, *158*, 2027–2032.

Williams, D. R., & Jackson, P. B. (2005). Social sources of racial disparities in health. *Health Affairs*, *24*, 325–334.

Wolf, J., Williams, E. N., Darby, M., Herald, J., & Schultz, C. (2018). Just for women? Feminist multicultural therapy with male clients. *Sex Roles*, *78*, 439–450.

Yarnell, L. M., Stafford, R. E., Neff, K. D., Reilly, E. D., Knox, M. C., & Mullarkey, M. (2015). Meta-analysis of gender differences in self compassion. *Self and Identity*, *14*, 499–520.

Zivin, K., Eisenberg, D., Golllust, S. E., & Golberstein, E. (2009). Persistence of mental health problems and needs in a college student population. *Journal of Affective Disorders*, *117*, 180–185.

Index

Tables are indicated by *t* following the page number

For the benefit of digital users, indexed terms that span two pages (e.g., 52–53) may, on occasion, appear on only one of those pages.